MARILYN MELTZER, M.A. •

SUSAN [illegible] A. •

LEARNING STRATEGIES IN NURSING

READING STUDYING & TEST-TAKING

EDITION

2

W.B. SAUNDERS COMPANY

A Division of Harcourt Brace & Company

Philadelphia London Toronto Montreal Sydney Tokyo

W.B. SAUNDERS COMPANY
A Division of Harcourt Brace & Company

The Curtis Center
Independence Square West
Philadelphia, Pennsylvania 19106

Library of Congress Cataloging-in-Publication Data

Meltzer, Marilyn.
Learning strategies in nursing: reading, studying, and test-taking / Marilyn Meltzer, Susan Marcus Palau.—2nd ed.

p. cm.

Rev. ed. of: Reading and study strategies for nursing students. © 1993.

Includes bibliographical references and index.

ISBN 0–7216–6342–7

1. Nursing—Study and teaching. 2. Study skills. I. Palau, Susan Marcus. II. Meltzer, Marilyn. Reading and study strategies for nursing students. III. Title. [DNLM: 1. Education, Nursing. 2. Learning—nurses' instruction. 3. Reading—nurses' instruction. 4. Vocabulary—nurses' instruction. WY 18 M528r 1997]

RT73.M396 1997 610.73'071—dc20

DNLM/DLC 96–20650

LEARNING STRATEGIES IN NURSING:
Reading, Studying, and Test-Taking, Second Edition ISBN 0–7216–6342–7

Printed in the United States of America.

Last digit is the print number: 9 8 7 6 5 4 3 2 1

LEARNING STRATEGIES IN NURSING

READING STUDYING & TEST-TAKING

To Sheldon, Michael, Sara, and Simon
M.M.

To Joe, Serena, Pepy, and Telly, and to Clowe's memory
S.M.P.

Preface

Learning Strategies in Nursing: Reading, Studying, and Test-Taking is intended for those nursing students who need to improve their reading and study skills. The purpose of this text is to teach students the strategies necessary for reading the assigned texts in their courses. This book is designed to have nursing students practice basic concentration, vocabulary, and reading and study skills on materials in their own area of study. The exercise materials are taken exclusively from nursing texts so that the skills are not presented in isolation but are practically applied within the nursing field.

In this second edition, we have included critical thinking practice. This will help students analyze and evaluate information that they have read in their textbooks. It also allows them to perform better in the workplace. We have also expanded the test-taking strategies to ensure greater success in school.

• ORGANIZATION

Unit 1, Improving Concentration, helps students to become organized and focused. The techniques transform students from passive to active readers and provide a foundation for improving comprehension.

Unit 2, Vocabulary Development, gives nursing students specific ways for learning the specialized vocabulary in nursing texts, which is often a hurdle for students. They can learn and retain new words through a variety of approaches including word structure, context clues, and using inferences and index cards.

Unit 3, Reading Comprehension, shows students how to recognize the main ideas, details, and organizational plans of textbook materials. The strategies help students better comprehend and retain what they are reading.

Unit 4, Study Skills, provides nursing students with the necessary tools for better understanding of their textbooks and classroom lectures.

Unit 5, Test-Taking Strategies, helps students learn how to prepare for and get better results on examinations.

Each chapter in Units 1 through 5 includes the following:

- objectives
- key words
- skills presentations
- examples
- practice exercises
- vocabulary check
- critical thinking log
- chapter summary.

Unit 6, Reading Selections, gives students the opportunity to apply the following skills to 15 selections from nursing textbooks:

- prereading
- identifying key vocabulary
- summarizing
- answering multiple choice questions
- critical thinking/evaluation.

• USING THE TEXTBOOK

Learning Strategies in Nursing: Reading, Studying, and Test-Taking is designed to be used in one semester; the 15 chapters can be completed weekly. The Reading Selections in Unit 6 can be used in conjunction with Chapters 1 through 15 or done after the student has completed Chapter 15.

This text can be used in a traditional classroom setting or can be used by the nursing student for self-study on an individual basis or in consultation with an instructor. The answer key at the back can be used by the instructor for graded assignments or used by the student for self-evaluation.

• SETTING UP THE COURSE

Participants in the reading and study strategies course can be any student who scores below the 12th grade level on the nursing school entrance examination or on standardized adult reading tests. Nursing programs may want to consider making this course a requirement for prefreshman or freshman students. In any case, the course would be especially helpful for returning adult students who need special learning strategies to get back to academic work. Instructors who teach bridge courses for licensed practical/vocational nurses who are entering registered nursing courses will find the book useful to introduce students to the expected higher level of academic work.

If this textbook is to be used in a classroom setting, the instructor should provide guided practice: working closely with the students at the beginning of the exercises in each chapter, then allowing the students to practice the exercises independently toward the end of the chapter. If the students are studying independently with the text, they are encouraged to work through the chapters sequentially. Because the text is divided into four independent units, they can be done in any order. The instructor can assess the students' work in class, or students can evaluate their own work using the Answer Key individually or in small groups. The classroom can also be structured so that the students are working together in small groups (collaborative learning), or the students can work individually at their own pace.

• MOTIVATING THE STUDENTS

When doing the lessons in this textbook, students will have strategies to help them concentrate. They will comprehend and retain textbook information that will help them do well in nursing school. These strategies are concrete, providing plans for organizing study time. The information is provided that the nursing students need to learn to feel more in control of the time and academic pressures that they face. Once the students see the positive results gained from using this text, motivation problems will be solved.

• ACKNOWLEDGMENTS

We would like to thank our word processors, Michael Meltzer, Mary Espencheid, and Sara Meltzer-Shemia. We would also like to thank the following people at W.B. Saunders Company who helped in the preparation of the book: Thomas Eoyang, Mary Anne Folcher, David Prout, Rita Martello, Christine Cantera, Dave Ward, Marjory Fraser, Frank Polizzano, I. Stacey Polk, and Melanie Nordlinger.

MARILYN MELTZER
SUSAN MARCUS PALAU

Contents

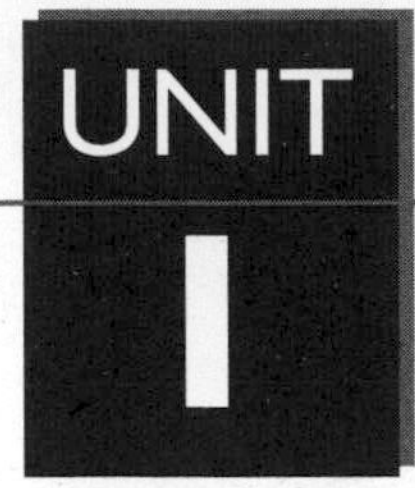

IMPROVING CONCENTRATION

As a nursing student, you are probably finding yourself in a bewildering new world of facts, theories, and words. Every day the classroom and clinic offer new challenges to your intellect.

Your nursing textbooks present a vast array of facts in intimidating volumes. This may be the first time in your academic career that you are expected to read so much material in so little time. Therefore you need to read your nursing textbooks as efficiently as possible. To be an efficient reader you must concentrate.

Many nursing students find it difficult to concentrate on their textbook assignments. Their minds wander, they do not connect ideas, and when they are finished, they do not retain the information.

Tested strategies can increase your reading concentration. Concentration is the first step to improving reading comprehension and retention.

Unit 1 introduces the technique of improving concentration. Chapter One, "Time Management," helps you to set priorities, schedule your study time, and work in a focused, purposeful style. Chapter Two, "Prereading Strategies," introduces techniques for becoming actively involved with the author's ideas. Chapter Three, "Monitoring Your Comprehension," helps you keep track of your comprehension as you read and introduces five strategies for getting back on track when your concentration falters.

A vocabulary check is included at the end of each chapter in Units 1 through 4. This vocabulary exercise reinforces the words that are essential to understanding the information in each chapter.

Reading textbooks with concentration requires your active participation. Unit 1 gives you the strategies needed to learn how to concentrate on your nursing studies.

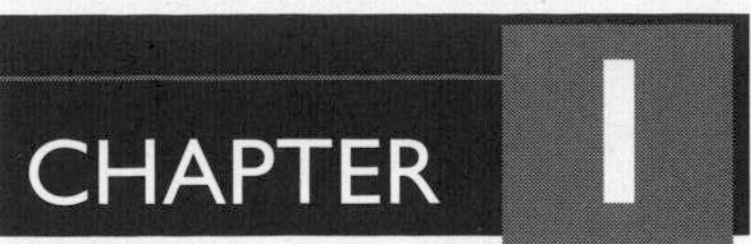

Time Management

• OBJECTIVE

To organize your time so that you will improve your study habits.

• KEY WORDS

Pay attention to the key words, which are listed below. They are underscored the first time they appear in this chapter. Try to determine the meanings of these words from the surrounding words in the passage. If you need further help, use your dictionary or the glossary in the back of this book.

As you read the exercises in this chapter, write additional words you need to learn in the spaces provided.

GENERAL VOCABULARY

anxiety	internal
avoidance	priority
concrete	procrastination
consistency	____________
excessive	____________
external	____________
extracurricular	____________

• QUESTIONS TO THINK ABOUT BEFORE READING

When you are doing assignments, do you:

1. Fall behind? Yes ________ No ________

2. Procrastinate? Yes ________ No ________

3. Save difficult assignments for last? Yes ________ No ________

4. Waste time? Yes ________ No ________

5. Find it difficult to get started? Yes ________ No ________

• USING TIME MANAGEMENT

If you've answered yes to these questions, you have to learn about time management. Time management helps you to get organized and focused. You will learn to control your time rather than letting time control you. The most successful students have learned time management.

Getting Organized

There are different ways to manage your study time more efficiently. Following a few simple steps will enable you to set goals so that you can successfully complete your assignments.

The most anxiety-producing situation for any student is to fall behind in completing assignments. Establishing goals will help you to solve this problem. You will learn how to set goals so that you can keep up with all your nursing studies and eliminate the anxiety that comes with procrastination.

Setting and Prioritizing Goals

To manage your time most efficiently during the course of the semester, you should think about the goals you want to achieve by the end of the semester and place these goals in the order of importance to you (prioritizing). When setting semester goals, you must think about how you need to have your life structured. Are you required to take three or four courses? Do you want a part-time job? Are there home and family responsibilities that you must meet? Are you allowing time for hobbies and other recreational interests? List on notebook paper everything you want to accomplish for the semester. Make sure that your goals are balanced. You will not be happy with just studying and working; give yourself the opportunity to relax.

When you prioritize these goals, you will notice that some activities have greater urgency than others. In nursing school, studying for your major, or your nursing course, should have priority over some lesser activity. When you order your goals, some priorities will limit other goals. For example, studying for a nursing exam may not allow you to go to the gym that week. However, keep in mind that in prioritizing, the most important goals should be met first. Be realistic about what you expect to accomplish in a semester. If you overextend yourself, you may have difficulty meeting any of your goals. Determine what is most important to you and focus on achieving these chosen goals. Table 1–1 is an example of how one student set and prioritized semester goals.

TABLE 1–1 One Student's Semester Goals

Setting Semester Goals	*Prioritizing Goals*
• Taking full-time schedule at nursing school	**1** Taking full-time schedule at nursing school
• Working part-time 10 hours a week	**2** Preparing family meals
• Practicing in choir	**3** Working part-time 10 hours a week
• Exercising in gym	**4** Practicing in choir
• Preparing family meals	**5** Exercising in gym

Using Calendars

Once you have set and prioritized your goals, calendars can help you organize your time efficiently. By using monthly, weekly, and daily calendars, you will be able to follow any schedule you establish to meet your goals.

Each of these calendars has its own function:

- Monthly calendar—to plan long-range assignments
- Weekly calendar—to learn consistency
- Daily calendar—to help you set priorities

MONTHLY CALENDAR

Some helpful information to place on your monthly calendar (Fig. 1–1):

- Exam dates
- Due dates of papers
- Special projects

EXERCISE 1–1

Directions. Fill in the monthly calendar (see Fig. 1–1). What other information might you add to the monthly calendar?

____

____

____

____

WEEKLY CALENDAR

The weekly calendar (Fig. 1–2) helps you to organize your time and think about consistency. Consistency is staying with a regular schedule. Successful students do assignments at scheduled times. They are not haphazard. They establish a study time and place.

JANUARY

SUN	MON	TUE	WED	THURS	FRI	SAT
	1	2	3	4	5	6
7	8	9	10	11 med-surg exam	12	13
14	15	16	17	18	19	20
21	22	23	24	25	26	27
28	29	30	31			

Figure 1–1 Monthly calendar.

How to Use the Weekly Calendar

Fill in the hours you sleep, have meals, work at part-time employment, and attend classes. Look at the hours left. Circle the hours each day that are free for study. Be realistic. Allow time for extracurricular activities and recreation. Circle the hours you intend to use for study each day with a red pen. Now decide where you will study. Many students find that they are less distracted when they study in a school or neighborhood library than when they work at home. It doesn't matter where you choose to study, but your study area should be quiet, well lit, and free from distractions.

Once you have decided when and where you will study each day, you are beginning to get organized. The next step is sticking to the schedule you planned on your weekly calendar. Learning consistency will help you to manage time.

EXERCISE 1–2

Directions. Fill in the weekly calendar. As you go through the week, make a checkmark (√) next to each task you complete. You'll see at a glance whether you're accomplishing your goals.

Write out a weekly calendar each Sunday. You may have to make changes, but at least you will have a concrete plan for scheduling your time.

TIME	SUN	MON	TUES	WED	THURS	FRI	SAT
7-8 AM							
8-9							
9-10							
10-11							
11-12							
12-1 PM							
1-2							
2-3							
3-4							
4-5							
5-6							
6-7							
7-8							
8-9							

Figure 1–2 Weekly calendar.

Self-Monitoring

At this point in your time management, you must evaluate whether your schedule is allowing you to meet your established goals. One good way of doing this is to monitor your activities as they relate to your weekly schedule. Ask yourself the following questions:

- Are my nonscheduled activities interfering with my school activities?
- Does my study schedule accurately reflect my prioritized goals?
- Am I allowing myself enough time to study?
- Is my weekly schedule flexible enough to allow for the unexpected?
- Does my weekly schedule show that I am wasting time?
- Did I establish a good balance between work and recreation in my schedule?

When you have answered these questions, you may need to rethink your weekly schedule. Keep monitoring and evaluating your weekly calendar to determine whether it is helping you to organize your time efficiently.

DAILY CALENDAR

The daily calendar helps you learn to set priorities. Each evening, think about what you want to accomplish the next day. Start by writing a "to-do" list.

To-Do List

A to-do list is an informal listing of all the activities you need to do for the following day. This to-do list encompasses both academic and nonacademic tasks. Each night as you think about the next day's activities, write down everything you need to do on a piece of paper. Then number these activities in the order you want to accomplish them. Make sure that you write down specific activities and assignments. Do not be vague. Then transfer this information to the time slots in your daily calendar.

Table 1–2 is an example of a nursing student's to-do list. In step 1 the student wrote down all necessary activities. In step 2 he prioritized the activities according to when he wanted to do them. Note how specific the student was when listing school assignments.

EXERCISE 1–3

Directions. Fill in the daily calendar (Fig. 1–3). Again, be realistic when you set your goals. Make a checkmark (√) next to each assignment that you complete. You will then monitor what you are accomplishing each day. Set your priorities. Decide which tasks are the most important to complete.

Identifying Time Wasters

Using calendars helps you to avoid wasting time. Some common time wasters are:

Procrastination: "I'll do it later." Procrastination, or delaying what needs to be done, is the greatest source of anxiety for students. Do it now—not later. Your grades will improve and you'll be more relaxed. Do not save difficult assignments for last. Do them first, when concentration is best. Avoidance only increases anxiety.

Excessive socializing: Students can allow socializing to get in the way of completing assignments if they don't stick to a schedule. In your weekly and daily calendars leave some realistic time for socializing. Staying on schedule eliminates the tendency to allow socializing to take up too much of your time.

Distractions: Students are often distracted. Both external and internal distractions get in the way of efficient studying.

EXTERNAL DISTRACTIONS

External distractions are elements in your surroundings that prevent you from paying attention to your studies.

TABLE 1–2 To-Do List

Step 1	*Step 2*
• Do grocery shopping	**2** Do grocery shopping
• Read Chapter 5 in *Anatomy and Physiology*	**1** Read Chapter 5 in *Anatomy and Physiology*
• Pick up shirts at cleaner's	**3** Pick up shirts at cleaner's
• Pay phone bill	**7** Pay phone bill
• Review clinical notes	**4** Review clinical notes
• Write first draft of English essay	**5** Write first draft of English essay
• Make dental appointment	**6** Make dental appointment

(✓) When Completed

9:00 - 9:30	
9:30 - 10:00	
10:00 - 10:30	
10:30 - 11:00	
11:00 - 11:30	
11:30 - 12:00	
12:00 - 12:30	
12:30 - 1:00	
1:00 - 1:30	
1:30 - 2:00	
2:00 - 2:30	
2:30 - 3:00	
3:00 - 3:30	
3:30 - 4:00	
4:00 - 4:30	
4:30 - 5:00	
5:00 - 5:30	
5:30 - 6:00	
6:00 - 6:30	
6:30 - 7:00	
7:00 - 7:30	
7:30 - 8:00	
8:00 - 8:30	
8:30 - 9:00	

Figure 1–3 Daily calendar.

Learning consistency, by establishing a study place and time, helps to eliminate external distractions. You should plan to study away from the telephone, television, and other distractions.

INTERNAL DISTRACTIONS

Internal distractions are your thoughts and feelings that prevent you from concentrating on your schoolwork.

Using the daily calendar to establish priorities helps to eliminate internal distractions. Instead of worrying about the things you can't control, you can focus on managing your time and completing the tasks on your daily calendar. Sticking to a schedule keeps you organized and improves your concentration.

Remember, if you set and prioritize goals and use monthly, weekly, and daily calendars, you will learn to manage time. Time management is an essential skill for nursing school students.

• VOCABULARY CHECK

Directions. Below are 10 words taken from the key words section of this chapter. Circle the letter of the best definition from the four choices.

1. Consistency
- **a** instability
- **b** contentment
- **c** disorder
- **d** regularity

2. Priority
- **a** goal placed in order of importance
- **b** activity done beforehand
- **c** task left uncompleted
- **d** action done previously

3. Extracurricular
- **a** an assignment for extra credit
- **b** additional course information
- **c** outside the regular course of work
- **d** illogical circular reasoning

4. Concrete
- **a** abstract
- **b** hard
- **c** false
- **d** definite

5. Procrastination
- **a** delaying what needs to be done
- **b** rearranging events
- **c** failing to establish goals
- **d** forgetting crucial assignments

6. Anxiety
- **a** bodily pain
- **b** chronic pain
- **c** emotional pain
- **d** pain reduction

7. Avoidance
- **a** reaching out to something
- **b** withdrawing from something
- **c** rejecting the truth
- **d** answering a complaint

8. Internal
- **a** outside the body
- **b** inside the body
- **c** away from the body
- **d** damaging to the body

9. External
- **a** outside the body
- **b** inside the body
- **c** away from the body
- **d** damaging to the body

10. Excessive
- **a** too regular
- **b** too few
- **c** too much
- **d** too little

• CRITICAL THINKING LOG

List the strategies you learned in this chapter.	Select the strategy that is most useful for your school success.	How can you apply this strategy to your nursing studies?

• SUMMARY

Time management helps you to become a successful nursing student. The first step in time management is setting and prioritizing goals. The use of calendars will help to manage your time most efficiently. Monthly calendars are useful for long-range planning. Weekly calendars help you to learn to be consistent and to follow a regular study routine. Daily calendars allow you to set priorities and focus on completing everyday activities in order of importance. You will eliminate the time wasters of procrastination, excessive socializing, and distractions. Time management will help you to become an accomplished nursing student.

CHAPTER 2

Prereading Strategies

• OBJECTIVE

To learn to use prereading strategies to improve reading concentration and comprehension.

• KEY WORDS

Pay attention to the key words, which are listed on the following pages. They are underscored the first time they appear in this chapter. Try to determine the meanings of these words from the surrounding words in the passage. If you need further help, use your dictionary or the glossary in the back of this book.

Look up the medical terminology in your medical dictionary or the glossary. As you read the exercises in this chapter, write additional words you need to learn in the spaces provided.

MEDICAL TERMINOLOGY	GENERAL VOCABULARY
analgesia	credence
dressing	delegate
gastrointestinal	document
inflammatory	extraneous
interventions	impending

irrigate	inherent
ostomy	lifestyle
regimen	locus
sterile	motivated
trauma	multidisciplinary
______________	______________
______________	______________
______________	______________
______________	______________

• QUESTIONS TO THINK ABOUT BEFORE READING

When you are assigned chapters in your nursing textbook, do you:

1. Find it hard to get started? Yes ______ No ______
2. Find it difficult to identify the main idea? Yes ______ No ______
3. Have trouble concentrating? Yes ______ No ______
4. Have difficulty understanding what you are reading? Yes ______ No ______
5. Have trouble connecting ideas in the chapter? Yes ______ No ______

• USING PREREADING STRATEGIES

If you've answered yes to these questions, you will find that prereading strategies will help you to tackle assignments in your nursing textbooks.

Many students open a text and just begin reading. They then find it difficult to get involved with the chapter information and complain that the assignment is boring. Instead of giving up before you begin, use prereading strategies as a way to become actively involved with the reading material.

Prereading strategies enable you to concentrate and comprehend textbook assignments by helping you to:

- Get started.
- See how the parts fit into the whole.
- Organize information into main ideas and supporting details.
- Become familiar with the subject matter.
- Read your assignments more efficiently.

• FIVE PREREADING STRATEGIES

The following five prereading strategies will help you to stay involved with the material and actively read with a purpose.

Read the Chapter Title

The title gives you the topic of the chapter. It tells you who or what the chapter is about. Write the title of this chapter.

___

Read the Introduction and Summary

The beginning paragraph or paragraphs will usually indicate the contents of the chapter. Carefully reading the introduction gives you a focus. You will know what to concentrate on as you read the rest of the chapter. In a phrase write what the introduction is about.

___

The summary is usually found in the last paragraph or paragraphs. The summary concisely restates the main ideas of the chapter. Read the summary of this chapter. List the important ideas.

___

___

___

___

Read All Headings

Headings are the titles that are in larger or darker print for emphasis. These are the main topics of the chapter. When done properly, these headings are the outline of the chapter. The largest headings should indicate the most important divisions of the chapter. List all the boldface headings in this chapter.

___

___

___

___

___

___

___

Look at Key Words

Pay attention to all words in *italics* (the slanted, thinner type) or **boldface** (the heavier, darker type) and <u>underscored</u> words. These words have been selected because their meanings are important to your understanding the ideas in the chapter. Key words are essential to your comprehending the information in your nursing textbooks.

Read the list of key words in this chapter.

Write any of the key words you need to learn.

______________ ______________ ______________

______________ ______________ ______________

______________ ______________ ______________

______________ ______________ ______________

Examine All Graphic Aids

Graphic aids are the illustrations, tables, graphs, and charts found in the chapter. Don't skip over graphic aids. Authors often use graphic aids to explain important ideas in the chapter.

Are there any graphic aids in this chapter?

____

____

EXAMPLE 2–1

Below is an example of how you can use the five prereading strategies to preview an excerpt from a nursing textbook (Iyer et al., *Nursing Process and Nursing Diagnosis,* 3rd ed., pp. 240–241; underscores added). Following this excerpt is an example of questions with answers that demonstrate how prereading strategies can help your reading concentration and comprehension.

Identify Factors Influencing Ability to Learn

There are a number of factors that affect the client's ability to learn, including preexisting knowledge, level of education, age, perceived locus of control, state of health, and lifestyle.

Clients' current *level of knowledge,* including their misconceptions and misinformation, frequently affects their ability to learn. Some knowledge is prerequisite for additional learning. For example, clients who need to change a sterile dressing may encounter great difficulty if they do not know the basics of good hand-washing.

Level of education frequently defines clients' knowledge of health and disease. If the information presented is above that level, the client may be unable to learn. The reverse may also be true. If information is presented at a level significantly below the client's level of education, the client might feel insulted and therefore fail to learn the material.

Age also affects ability to learn. The very young child may have difficulty in grasping concepts unless they are presented in very concrete terms. Some elderly clients may have ingrained ideas of "myths" that affect their ability to accept new changes. Additionally, they may have physiological deficits that interfere with their ability to learn (e.g., vision or hearing problems).

Not all clients desire information. Some prefer to delegate the responsibility for promoting, maintaining, or restoring their health to family members or health care personnel. Others in a state of denial may refuse to acknowledge the need to learn about their illness. Therefore, it is very difficult for these clients to learn effectively.

The client's perceptions about *locus of control* will also affect readiness to learn. Locus of control is defined as the belief in one's ability to control reinforcements or results. If an individual perceives that results come from outside forces, such as luck, fate, or powerful others, this person is said to have an *external* control orientation. An individual with an *internal* control orientation perceives that the outcomes of one's own behavior are contingent upon one's own behavior and abilities (Bigbee, 1983). A client who has an internal control orientation will be more likely to be motivated to learn than individuals who believe that fate is in charge of their health status.

The client must be *physically and emotionally prepared* for the teaching-learning experience. Plan to use interventions directed toward relief of pain, fear, anxiety, or fatigue before attempting to involve the client in learning activities. The state of health of the client may affect ability to learn. The client with a critical illness, severe debilitation, or sensory-perception deficits may be unable to process or absorb information. This may also be the case for clients with terminal disease, since they may lack motivation or ability.

The client's lifestyle may affect ability to learn. This is particularly pertinent when considering low socioeconomic groups and people of certain cultures. The client's learning problem may be associated with deficits in the types of experiences that make learning a desirable outcome. The client may not be stimulated in his or her culture to learn content perceived to be unnecessary or unimportant. Certain personality types—e.g., dependent or irresponsible persons—may also have inherent motivational problems.

Develop Realistic and Attainable Outcomes

The learning outcomes for each client involve knowledge, attitudes, and skills. For example, you may be required to teach the client who needs an ostomy so that the client will be able to

- describe how the surgery has altered the gastrointestinal tract (knowledge).
- explain how the ostomy will affect the client's relationship with spouse (attitude).
- list types of equipment necessary to manage the ostomy (knowledge).
- cleanse the stomal area and apply a pouch (skill).
- irrigate the ostomy (skill).
- express confidence in the ability to manage the ostomy (attitude).

1. What are the headings? ("Identify Factors Influencing Ability to Learn" and "Develop Realistic and Attainable Outcomes")
2. What is the introductory paragraph about? (It highlights the factors that affect a client's ability to learn. These factors are preexisting knowledge, level of education, age, motivation, perceived locus of control, state of health, and lifestyle.)
3. Is there a summary paragraph? (No)
4. List the key words in this selection. Use the glossary if you need help finding the meanings of these words.

interventions ____________

locus ____________

sterile ____________

dressing ____________

motivated ____________

delegate ____________

lifestyle ____________

inherent ____________

gastrointestinal ___________

ostomy ___________

irrigate ___________

5. What is this reading selection about? (A nurse must recognize the factors that affect a client's ability to learn and develop realistic outcomes.)

EXERCISE 2–1

Directions. Use the five prereading strategies to get actively involved with the following chapter from a nursing textbook (Iyer et al., *Nursing Process and Nursing Diagnosis,* 3rd ed., pp. 205, 206, 208, 210, 211, 213, 217–219; underscores added). Answer the questions at the end of the chapter.

TYPES OF CARE PLANS

There are several different types of care plans in use. Those that are most common include individually constructed, standardized, computerized, and multidisciplinary plans.

Individually Constructed

Plans written from scratch are documented on forms that are divided into columns with the usual headings of Nursing Diagnoses, Outcomes, and Interventions.

Advantages. The individually written plan enables the documentation of the nursing diagnoses, outcomes, and interventions that are most pertinent to a particular client. No extraneous or inapplicable information is included in the care plan.

Disadvantages. Development and documentation of this type of care plan are time-consuming.

Standardized

Standardized care plans have been introduced into several types of agencies to facilitate the preparation and use of care plans. Standardized care plans consist of actual, high-risk, or wellness nursing diagnoses, outcomes, and interventions that are printed in a care plan format. The plans of care may be organized according to the client's medical diagnosis or nursing diagnosis (see Fig. 6–5). Individualization is possible through the use of blank spaces, as illustrated in Figure 6–5. The nurse may cross off items that do not apply to the client or add additional nursing diagnoses, outcomes, and interventions. The care plans may be developed by the nursing staff of a particular agency or may be derived from the literature. Standardized care plans have been published in articles or books. Figure 6–5 is a standardized plan for the client with pain.

Standardized care plans may be used in one of two ways: (1) they may be placed in a centrally located area and referred to by nurses when developing handwritten individually constructed care plans, or (2) they may be placed directly on the Kardex or chart, dated, and signed.

Advantages. The advantages of standardized care plans include the following:

1. They are usually developed by clinical experts who have researched the literature carefully. They are useful in educating nurses who are not familiar with a certain medical or nursing diagnosis.
2. They reduce the amount of time spent in writing plans. This increases the efficiency of nursing care planning.
3. They provide information specific to a particular client and require less time to complete. Additionally, because they outline the expected nursing care, they enhance the quality of the delivery and documentation of care.

ACUTE PAIN

Pain related to effects of surgery, effects of ischemia, inflammatory process, effects of trauma, effects of invasive procedures, and prolonged immobility

Outcomes
Reports pain promptly when experiencing it
Verbalizes decreased pain within 30 minutes following initiation of comfort measures

Interventions

1. Help client identify pain relief measures that have been helpful in the past.
2. Explore with client feelings and attitudes related to use of pain medication and fear of addiction.
3. Instruct client/family:
   - ☐ to report pain promptly
   - ☐ to describe using 0–10 scale
   - ☐ regarding prescribed regimen for pain relief
   - ☐ to evaluate and report effectiveness of interventions
4. Assess for pain using verbal and nonverbal messages ________ including location, quality, intensity, duration, precipitating/aggravating/relieving factors, and associated symptoms.
5. Explain source of pain/discomfort if known.
6. Collaborate with physician to establish a pain control regimen:
   - ☐ Medications
   - ☐ Use of hot/cold application
   - ☐ Patient controlled analgesia
   - ☐ TENS
7. Provide therapeutic comfort measures based on appropriateness and client willingness/desire.
   - ☐ Position change (specify position of comfort) ______________________________

     ____
   - ☐ Back rub/massage
   - ☐ Relaxation techniques and guided imagery
   - ☐ Diversional activities (specify) __________
   - ☐ Alteration in environment (specify) ____________
8. Reassure and support client/family during episodes of pain.
9. Provide quiet environment and organize care to promote periods of uninterrupted rest.
10. Medicate prior to activities to promote participation.
11. Assess and document findings and effectiveness of interventions.

Figure 6–5 Sample of a standardized care plan based on the nursing diagnosis of pain.

Disadvantages. Using standardized care plans can be limiting because it is rare that all of the client's specific problems will be addressed by one standardized care plan. If the care plan is not appropriately individualized it will not be specific to the client's needs.

Computerized

The basic elements of care plan systems—nursing diagnoses, outcomes, and interventions—are also present in computer-generated plans. The plan of care may be prepared at a terminal in the client's room or in a central location. Once data are validated and entered, a printed version may be generated daily, on each shift, or on demand. There are a number of mechanisms by which care plans are generated. Three commonly used systems are (1) standardized plans based on the medical diagnosis, (2) standardized plans based on the nursing diagnosis, and (3) individually constructed plans.

Medical Diagnoses. In these systems, the computer provides the nurse with nursing diagnoses, outcomes, and nursing interventions commonly associated with the medical diagnoses. These are very similar to the printed standardized care plans discussed earlier. The nurse who is formulating the plan selects the appropriate items from the standardized data base. Additional diagnoses, outcomes, and interventions may be entered to reflect other concerns of the client.

Nursing Diagnoses. Other computerized systems are more directly associated with the specific nursing diagnoses identified at the time of the detailed nursing assessment. The computer lists each diagnosis, and the nurse defines outcomes and nursing interventions by selecting from a menu of appropriate choices. The nurse may add other specific outcomes and interventions for an individual client, if appropriate.

Individually Constructed. In these systems, the nurse develops the care plan in a fashion similar to that used in a manual individualized plan. You are not prompted to focus on specific diagnoses but use a menu to select those diagnoses, outcomes, and interventions that apply to the individual client. Additional outcomes or interventions not identified in the menu may also be added when necessary.

Most computerized care-planning systems facilitate frequent updating of the plan. The nurse identifies problems that have been resolved, and they are eliminated from the plan. Other options may include (1) revision of diagnoses, outcomes, and interventions to reflect the changing status of the client, and (2) addition of new diagnoses, outcomes, and interventions. Printed care plans, which are a permanent part of the medical record, document the client's progress as reflected by the changing plan of care.

More sophisticated programs compare the client's data with a list of defining characteristics for specific nursing diagnoses. If the client's data match the defining characteristics, the program will display the nursing diagnosis. You have the option of choosing the displayed diagnosis or rejecting it and selecting another. If the displayed diagnosis is accepted, the system will present expected outcomes and interventions that would be applicable. You choose the appropriate outcomes and interventions or enter the individualized ones.

Advantages. The advantages of computerized care plans include the following:

1. Computerized care plans increase the potential for accurate and thorough documentation of the delivery of care. The computer identifies specific nursing approaches listed on the plan and prompts the nurse to document the outcome of the intervention. This process also encourages frequent review of the plan as well as modification, when appropriate.
2. Preparation of a computer-generated care plan from a standardized plan takes less time than handwriting an individualized care plan.

3. The computerized plan can be designed to determine the staffing needs of the unit.
4. Plans that are prepared on a printer are easy to read.
5. Automated care-planning consistently uses a systematic method to develop care plans, thereby decreasing the possibility of error.
6. Utilizing computer-assisted planning permits the identification of common nursing diagnoses for research and planning purposes.

Disadvantages. Along with the many advantages, some disadvantages do exist and include the following:

1. Adequate numbers of computers must be available to the nursing staff. If sufficient hardware is not available because of cost or space considerations, the care-planning process will become more difficult.
2. Errors that occur in computerized nursing care plans may be harder to detect. Nurses have a tendency to lend more credence to computer printouts than they would to handwritten records.
3. The computer may develop a care plan that may be logically consistent but is not applicable to a client.

Multidisciplinary Care Plans

In long-term care, rehabilitation, psychiatric, and drug and alcohol detoxification units, it is common for the care plan to include the contributions of other disciplines in addition to nursing. These plans may be structured to identify the client's problem (rather than using only nursing diagnosis terminology), outcomes, and interventions. Typically the plans are developed and revised in multidisciplinary team conferences. As appropriate, the client or significant other is present to offer contributions and to validate the acceptability of the plan of care.

Critical paths are a new form of multidisciplinary plan of care that emerged in the late 1980s. The critical path is a structured document that defines the outcomes and interventions for each day of the hospitalization. These documents are a tool used in case management. Case management is a method of organizing and directing the client through a hospitalization by identifying a critical path that should be followed. For example, there may be a critical path for a client who has had a total hip replacement. This plan will suggest tests, diet, treatments, consults, activity, teaching, and discharge planning that should be performed each day. In some settings the nursing diagnosis and daily outcomes are included on the critical path. This document serves as a multidisciplinary plan of care.

Advantages

1. The care of the client is strengthened by the communication that occurs when several disciplines share their perceptions.
2. Critical paths have resulted in cost savings and increased satisfaction of clients and health care professionals.

Disadvantages

1. The development of critical paths is time-consuming because it is typically done by a multidisciplinary team who must achieve agreement.
2. There is some resistance to critical paths. They are called "cookbook medicine" by those who fear that individualization of care is lost in this system.

SUMMARY

The development of nursing interventions is the third stage of the planning phase of the nursing process. Nursing interventions define the activities that assist the client in achieving desired outcomes.

Nursing interventions are developed through a scientific approach and include date, signature, precise action verbs, specific aspects of interventions, and modifications in standard therapy. The registered nurse is responsible and accountable for the development of nursing interventions.

The fourth stage of the planning phase consists of documentation of the plan. Care plans may be individualized, standardized, computerized, or multidisciplinary. Much time is wasted when care plans are not developed. New forms of plans of care are expected to emerge as health care delivery continues to change.

1. The introductory paragraph is about

____

____

2. List the boldface headings.

____

____

____

____

____

3. List the key words in the selection.

____

____

____

4. Are there any graphic aids in the selection?

____

5. What is this selection about?

____

____

• VOCABULARY CHECK

Directions. Below are 10 words taken from the key words section of this chapter. Circle the letter of the best definition from the four choices.

1. Impending
- **a** dependent on others
- **b** about to occur
- **c** independent of others
- **d** about to finish

2. Sterile
a filled with living microorganisms
b resembling the sternum
c pertaining to steroids
d free from living microorganisms

3. Extraneous
a unrelated
b related
c necessary
d crucial

4. Ostomy
a inflammation of the inner ear
b closure of an orifice
c hardening of the bones
d formation of artificial opening

5. Delegate
a to remove
b to dismiss
c to appoint
d to appreciate

6. Regimen
a the natural renewal of a structure
b regulated activity designed to achieve certain ends
c an instrument used for measuring the refractive power of the eye
d the backward or returning flow

7. Locus
a an insect
b a point
c a split
d a passage

8. Irrigate
a to wash a body cavity or wound using water or fluid
b to release pressure in a specific area
c to react to an external or internal stimulus
d to cause a physical or psychological disorder

9. Document
a to check on a chart
b to prove with verbal evidence
c to support with written information
d to disprove a medical theory

10. Dressing
- **a** medicinal substance taken orally
- **b** a daily routine of postoperative exercise
- **c** a feeding tube to collect specimens from the duodenum
- **d** materials used for protecting a wound

• CRITICAL THINKING LOG

List the strategies you learned in this chapter.	Select the strategy that is most useful for your school success.	How can you apply this strategy to your nursing studies?

• SUMMARY

Prereading strategies involve previewing the chapter before your actual reading. Read the title, introduction, summary, and headings. Look up the meanings of italicized words and examine all graphic aids.

The five prereading strategies presented in this chapter will help you to get started, stay involved, and organize, concentrate on, and comprehend the information in your textbooks.

CHAPTER 3

Monitoring Your Comprehension

• OBJECTIVE

To become aware of when you are reading without comprehension and to learn five monitoring strategies to regain understanding.

• KEY WORDS

Pay attention to the key words, which are listed on the following page. They are underscored the first time they appear in this chapter. Try to determine the meaning of these words from the surrounding words in the passage. If you need further help, use your dictionary or the glossary in the back of this book.

Look up the medical terminology in your medical dictionary or the glossary. As you read the exercises in this chapter, write additional words you need to learn in the spaces provided.

GENERAL VOCABULARY	MEDICAL TERMINOLOGY
clarify	basophil
incorporated	cognitive

maladaptive	coping
miscommunication	corticosteroids
monitoring	excitation
moral	hormones
multitude	immunosuppressive
schema	neuron
summarize	permeability
visualize	superego
________________	________________
________________	________________
________________	________________
________________	________________

• MONITORING

An important strategy for improving your concentration is monitoring. When you monitor your comprehension, you are continually asking yourself if you understand what you're reading. Depending on the complexity of the material, you may have to do this every sentence, paragraph, section, or page. When you monitor your comprehension, you become immediately aware of when you are not understanding your textbook. When you monitor your comprehension, you become an active reader rather than a passive one. You become involved with and part of the material rather than just looking at words and remaining removed from your reading selection. Good readers constantly ask, "Am I comprehending?" When the answer is no, and they become alert to the fact that they are not understanding, active readers have various monitoring strategies to correct the situation. These strategies are used to regain understanding. An explanation of five useful strategies to monitor comprehension follows.

• FIVE STRATEGIES TO MONITOR COMPREHENSION

Monitoring Strategy No. 1: Reread

When active readers become aware that they do not understand what they are reading, the strategy they most commonly use is simply to reread the portion they did not understand. Often on a second reading, complex information becomes clear. If need be, don't hesitate to reread aloud. This practice in itself can help <u>clarify</u> the content.

EXERCISE 3–1

Directions. Read the following passage from Ignatavicius, et al., *Medical Surgical Nursing* (p. 1084; underscores added). Then reread, noting how much more you understood with the second reading. Try rereading the passage aloud to see if this strategy further helps your comprehension.

The basic unit of the nervous system is the neuron. When a neuron receives an impulse from another neuron, the effect may be excitation or inhibition as well as conduction of the impulse. Each neuron has:

- A cell body, or soma
- A short branching process called a dendrite
- A single axon

Dendrites may have many branches or few. Each dendrite synapses with another cell body, axon, or dendrite and brings information to the cell body from other neurons. The dendritic process can also be described as an afferent pathway; the dendrite receives an impulse from another neuron and carries that impulse to the cell body.

Did your second reading help you understand the passage better? Yes ____________ No ____________

Was rereading aloud helpful? Yes ____________ No ____________

Remember to reread passages so that you can better understand complex textbook readings.

Monitoring Strategy No. 2: Summarize

When reading nursing texts, you will often encounter technical information that may prove challenging. Sentences may be long, and sometimes the material will appear to be poorly organized. When you read complex text information, your best strategy is to summarize the passage. To summarize, you look only for the main idea and important details (see Chapters 8 and 9) and rewrite them in your own words, a shorter version of the original. Depending on the length of the selection, you can do this as brief margin notes right in the textbook or you can summarize in your notebook. In any case, by summarizing and rewriting complex information in your own words, you simplify the material into ideas that you understand—a first step to learning new information.

EXAMPLE 3–1

Directions. Below is an excerpt from the nursing text by Ignatavicius, et al., *Medical Surgical Nursing* (p. 106; underscores added). Following that is a summary of this passage. Notice that only the main points were included in the summary, and the writer's own words were used to rewrite the selection.

Coping is any behavioral or cognitive activity that is used to deal with stress. If an event is perceived as taxing or dangerous, coping should occur. The concept of coping implies that most people do not remain passive and allow events to happen; rather they react. The reactions to a stress-provoking event can be either to use the problem-solving approach to change the event (problem-focused coping) or to change emotional reactions to the event (emotion-focused coping). Coping strategies vary from person to person and event to event. It is thought that individuals generally use coping strategies that they have found successful in the past. If a strategy is not successful in the current situation, others may be considered.

Summary
Coping is what we do to deal with a stressful situation. When someone is coping, they are not passive but instead are actively trying to deal with the situation. There are two general types of coping: problem-focused coping and emotion-focused coping. The use of these two strategies differs from person to person and situation to situation; however, we tend to use coping strategies that worked for us in the past.

EXERCISE 3–2

Directions. In the space provided, summarize the following paragraph from the nursing text by Arnold and Boggs (p. 556; underscore added). Remember to keep it brief. Focus on the main idea and important details. Paraphrase, using your own words.

A professional nurse is called upon daily to communicate with other professionals in some type of written format. Written communication has several advantages over other forms of communication. Written text provides a potentially permanent record of information and may diminish miscommunication. The natural tendency to distort verbal messages or forget components over time is alleviated when there are written records to refer to, particularly when the topic being discussed is complex or when the communication is directed at larger groups of people.

SUMMARY

____

____

____

____

____

Monitoring Strategy No. 3: Defining New Words

At times, reading a specific nursing passage is difficult because you do not know the meanings of general vocabulary words or medical terminology. The best method for correcting this situation is to look up the words in the dictionary or textbook glossary (see Chapter 6). Looking up unknown words in a dictionary or glossary, although time-consuming, will lead you to an accurate and precise definition. Understanding vocabulary is an important factor in comprehending your nursing textbook.

EXERCISE 3–3

Directions. In this exercise taken from Ignatavicius, et al., *Medical Surgical Nursing* (p. 440; underscore added), write the meanings of any unknown words in the space provided. Use your dictionary or glossary to obtain a precise definition.

Of all the leukocytes, basophils are the smallest and the rarest. They are derived from myeloid stem cells and are released from the bone marrow after a short maturation period. Even though they are rare, basophils are associated with the obvious signs and symptoms that often accompany inflammation. Basophils contain enormous numbers of cytoplasmic granules.

UNKNOWN WORD	MEANING
1. ______________	______________________________
2. ______________	______________________________
3. ______________	______________________________
4. ______________	______________________________
5. ______________	______________________________
6. ______________	______________________________
7. ______________	______________________________
8. ______________	______________________________
9. ______________	______________________________
10. ______________	______________________________

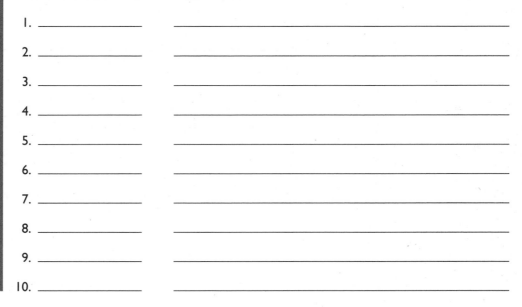

Monitoring Strategy No. 4: Visualization

Another major reason for poor reading comprehension is lack of concentration. This inability to focus on textbook selections may account for the greatest degree of reading problems in nursing schools. Many factors can cause concentration problems, but primarily they fall into two categories: internal distractions and external distractions. **Internal distractions** are elements within ourselves that won't let us concentrate, such as hunger, personal problems, and headaches. **External distractions** are elements outside ourselves that won't let us concentrate, such as radio sounds, a noisy little brother, or too warm a room.

Regardless of the reasons for poor concentration, in nursing school you are expected to understand your textbook. One good strategy for overcoming poor concentration is to visualize what you are reading. When you visualize, you create a mental picture of what you are reading—like a television picture in your mind. As you read each sentence, you adjust the mental image you have, either adding new information or somehow changing the picture to fit each new fact as you read it. In Figure 3–1 pay close attention to the handwritten notes above the printed line. This is one reader's description of what she visualized as she read the passage.

medicine tubes — *chemical messages*
Corticosteroids are adrenocortical hormones used in the treatment of many immunologically mediated diseases, neoplasms, and several neurologic and endocrine disorders. Corticosteroids
wiping out redness — *stop sign in the immune system* — *swollen and red*
have both anti-inflammatory and immunosuppressive effects. They inhibit inflammation by
walls of veins — *road block* — *flying little circles*
stabilizing the vascular membrane decreasing permeability, thereby blocking the migration and
calling of troops
mobilization of neutrophils and monocytes.

Figure 3–1 How one reader visualized a particular passage from Ignatavicius, et al. (p. 531).

EXERCISE 3–4

Directions. As you read the following passage from the nursing textbook by Varcarolis (p. 13; underscores added), try to visualize what you are reading and make adjustments to your image according to any new facts provided. As in the previous example, write what you visualize above the line.

The superego consists of two subsystems: the conscience and the ego-ideal. What parents view as improper and what they punish the child for doing become incorporated into the child's conscience. The conscience refers to the capacity for self-evaluation and criticism. When moral codes are violated, the conscience punishes the person by instilling guilt. A maladaptive example of this behavior is seen in the extreme condition of depression, in which people berate themselves cruelly for minor actions and trivial shortcomings.

Monitoring Strategy No. 5: Research

The best way to learn new information is by having old information or a framework on which to add the new facts. This framework is called a schema and constitutes background information to which you add new knowledge. Many times, the reason you lose comprehension while reading your nursing textbook is that you have insufficient schema or background knowledge on the subject. A solution to this problem may be as simple as reading an encyclopedia entry or consulting another textbook or a nursing journal to get a different perspective on the same subject. Whatever means you choose, once you build up your background knowledge of a difficult subject, your reading comprehension on this subject will improve.

EXERCISE 3–5

Sometimes you need additional information to understand your textbook readings. It's important for you to know which resource material to consult when researching a topic.

Directions. Below is a list of topics you will encounter in nursing school. In the space next to the topic, write whether you would find the best additional information in a general encyclopedia, general nursing textbook, or nursing journal.

1. Latest information on caring for patients with diabetes ______________________

____

2. Human sexuality ______________________

____

3. General description of the eye ______________________

____

4. Writing a care plan ______________________

____

5. Newest technique for helping clients with eating disorders ______________________

____

6. Cell structure ______________________

____

• USING MONITORING STRATEGIES FOR LONGER PASSAGES

When you are actively reading your nursing textbook and you realize that you are not understanding what you have read, you may need to use one, some, or all of the five monitoring strategies discussed in this chapter. Figure 3–2 is an excerpt from the nursing textbook by Arnold and Boggs (p. 190). Above the lines are handwritten notes describing examples of the strategies used. Read carefully, paying close attention to the various ways one reader used these five strategies to monitor comprehension.

reread

Culturally specific modes of emotional expression can sometimes confuse as well as clarify the meaning of a verbal message. The vocal emphasis given to certain sounds and tone

the use of pitch to convey meaning

modulations is in part culturally determined. In some cultures sounds are punctuated, whereas in others sounds have a lyrical or singsong quality. Contrast, for example, the vocalizations of

I see the different ethnic neighborhoods in New York City — *Changes in loudness of voice*

an Oriental client with that of a German or Spanish client. The vocal inflections are quite

Note: Research more about spoken languages

different. Nurses need to orient themselves to the characteristic voice tones associated with different cultures to avoid being distracted by them in the process of communication.

Summary: In order to understand foreign speaking clients, nurses must be familiar with how different languages sound and are spoken.

Figure 3–2 Various ways one reader used the five strategies to monitor comprehension in a passage from Arnold and Boggs (p. 190).

EXERCISE 3–6

Directions. Read the following exercise taken from the nursing textbook by Arnold and Boggs (pp. 205–206). Using the method demonstrated in the previous example, indicate above the printed line the use of the monitoring strategies described in this chapter:

1. Reread
2. Summarize
3. Define new words
4. Visualize
5. Research

When the client makes choices the nurse finds hard to accept, it can have a strong impact on communication. The alcoholic who persists in drinking and the HIV-positive mother who continues to get pregnant discourage the nurse's investment in communicating with these clients. Watching a client make choices that indicate the client has given up also makes therapeutic conversations difficult. For example, an 80-year-old woman with multiple health problems requiring nursing home care may be hard to motivate. Why should she live? Likewise, the teenager suddenly rendered a paraplegic in an auto accident may not want to engage in rehabilitation. So much has been lost that, from the client's perspective, there is little reason to try. Working with clients who have given up is a communication challenge for the nurse. At such times, it is important to remember the ethical principle of autonomy governing all aspects of the relationship. It is essential interpersonally to meet and respect clients where they are rather than trying to change them.

• QUESTION TO MONITOR COMPREHENSION

As mentioned in the beginning of this chapter, the first responsibility of good readers is to become aware of when they are losing comprehension. They do this simply by continually asking themselves whether they are comprehending. To help you get accustomed to doing this, the following question appears throughout the remaining chapters to remind you to monitor your comprehension:

Comprehending? Yes ___ No ___

When you see this question, please check the response that most accurately reflects how well you understand what you have just read. If the answer is yes, continue reading. If the answer is no, go back and use any of the five strategies to monitor comprehension that you feel will be most helpful. Then continue reading.

• VOCABULARY CHECK

Directions. Below are 10 words taken from the key words section of this chapter. Circle the letter of the best definition from the four choices.

1. Schema
a a devious plan
b part of the care plan
c a mental code
d diagnosis of an illness

2. Basophil
a part of the cell nucleus of a plant or animal
b structure of plant cell that contains chlorophyll
c structure outside the cell nucleus
d any structure stained readily with basic dyes

3. Miscommunication
a talking across a great distance
b unfinished communication
c failure to communicate clearly
d communicating clearly

4. Coping
a contending with difficulties in an effort to overcome them
b feeling closed in, shut in, or removed from a situation
c not having difficulties or major responsibilities
d being unable to solve or deal with problems independently

5. Visualize
a to dream or fantasize
b to see an object in reality
c to hear a sound in reality
d to see or form a mental image

6. Hormones
a chemical transmitters produced by bones
b chemical transmitters produced by cells
c electricity produced by cells
d electricity produced by the movement of bones

7. Summarize
a covering the main points succinctly
b describing in complete detail
c reviewing the client's progress
d describing the client's progress

8. Permeability
a being permanent
b ability to be stable
c passage of a substance
d containment of a substance

9. Moral
a relating to principles of right and wrong
b relating to religious feelings or sentiments
c disposed to feel good or bad
d message at the beginning of every folk tale

10. Neuron
a connection between nerve cells
b chemical transmission of nerves
c gap between nerve cells
d the actual nerve cell

• CRITICAL THINKING LOG

List the strategies you learned in this chapter.	Select the strategy that is most useful for your school success.	How would you apply this strategy to your nursing studies?

• SUMMARY

In this chapter you learned to become aware of when you are losing comprehension while you are reading. You learned five monitoring strategies to help improve your comprehension:

1. Reread
2. Summarize
3. Define new words
4. Visualize
5. Research

You were also introduced to the question that will be used throughout the book to help you monitor your comprehension.

Comprehending? Yes ___ No ___

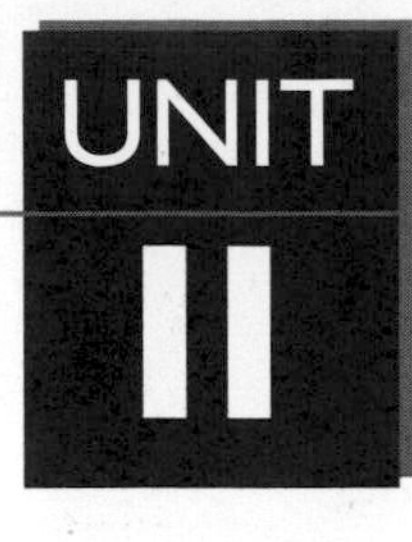

VOCABULARY DEVELOPMENT

A well-developed vocabulary, both for medical and for general terminology, is an important asset that will help you through nursing school. A good vocabulary not only will make comprehending your textbook easier but also will enable you to converse better with both patients and colleagues.

This unit will give you strategies for defining unknown words encountered in your textbooks and lectures. Chapter Four, "Word Parts," will teach you to analyze prefixes, roots, and suffixes for meanings. Chapter Five, "Using Context Clues," will show you how to use surrounding words to figure out the meaning of an unknown word. Chapter 6, "Dictionary, Glossary, and Thesaurus," will instruct you in the use of the dictionary and glossary for obtaining definitions of unknown words and the thesaurus for choosing a more precise word. Finally, Chapter 7, "Word Bank," will suggest a system for memorizing the meanings of unknown words once you have obtained the definitions.

After completing Unit 2, you will have many techniques that will help you define and remember unknown words. Once these words become familiar enough to be part of your everyday speech, you will be well on your way to greater nursing school success.

CHAPTER 4

Word Parts

• OBJECTIVE

To learn the definition of unknown general vocabulary and medical terminology by analyzing roots, prefixes, and suffixes (word parts).

• KEY WORDS

Pay attention to the following key words, which are underscored the first time they appear in this chapter. Try to determine the meaning of these words from the surrounding words in the passage. If you need further help, use your dictionary or the glossary in the back of this book.

Look up the medical terminology in your medical dictionary or the glossary. As you read the exercises in this chapter, write additional words you need to learn in the space provided.

MEDICAL TERMINOLOGY	GENERAL VOCABULARY
agoraphobia	word parts
anti-inflammatory	prefix
appendicitis	pregnant
cardiovascular	pressure
endocrine	purification
hemoglobin	root
hysterectomy	socialism
prematurity	suffix

somatic	transmit
tonsillectomy	unilateral
______________________	______________________
______________________	______________________
______________________	______________________

• INTRODUCTION TO WORD PARTS

Part of the experience of being a nursing student is encountering new and unfamiliar words in your nursing textbooks. One of the most efficient ways of unlocking the definitions of these words is by analyzing the meanings of the word parts that make up the structure of the word. This technique is useful for both medical and nonmedical vocabulary. Once you have mastered the meanings of a relatively small number of word parts, you will be able to analyze the meanings of thousands of words.

• TYPES OF WORD PARTS

Many words in the English language consist of two or more of these word parts: prefix, root, and suffix.

A **prefix** is a word part that comes at the beginning of the word. Its function is to change the meaning of the basic portion of the word. For example, "dislike" (the opposite of like) and overprotect (to protect too much).

The **root** is the main part of the word and provides the basic meaning of the word. For example, dis***like*** and over***protect***.

The **suffix** is located at the end of the word and serves two purposes: to change the meaning of the root and to alter the part of speech. For example, dislikeable (not able to be liked) and overprotective (tending to guard too much). Originally, "dislike" was a verb, but when the "able" suffix was added, it became an adjective. Similarly, "overprotect" is a verb, but adding the suffix "ive" changes it to an adjective.

EXAMPLE 4–1

Look at the following word:

mature

You know that "mature" means being fully developed.

Now look at the word below:

premature

In this example, a word part has been added before the main part, or root, of the word. This word part is a prefix and has its own meaning—"before." Combining the meaning of "pre" with that of "mature" you get a new definition: "before being fully developed."

Next consider the last example:

prematurity

Now you have added a word part after the root. This word part is the suffix, and it refers to "the state of." So adding up all the meanings of the word parts:

pre = before
mature = fully developed
ity = state of

you arrive at the full definition of the words, "the state before being fully developed," the meaning of "prematurity." Also note that "premature" is an adjective and "prematurity" is a noun.

• WORD PART ANALYSIS IS NOT ALWAYS APPLICABLE

The technique of analyzing word parts can be used on many of the unknown words you will see in your nursing textbooks. However, you should be cautioned that what may seem to be a word part may in reality be the main part of the word. Consider pregnant and pressure. Both words begin with "pre," but in each case the "pre" is part of the root.

To avoid this type of error, memorize or at least familiarize yourself with the most common prefixes, roots, and suffixes.

Table 4–1 lists the 20 most frequently used prefixes, roots, and suffixes, followed by their definitions and examples of how the word parts are used. The starred (*) entries suggest word parts with a medical use.

EXERCISE 4–1

Directions. In Table 4–1 under the heading "Definition of Example," write the meanings of the example words. Consult a dictionary or glossary, if necessary.

EXERCISE 4–2

Directions. In Table 4–1 under the column labeled "Your Example," write another example of a word with the same prefix, root, or suffix as that on the line. If necessary, use your dictionary or glossary.

Comprehending? Yes ___ No ___

EXERCISE 4–3

Directions. In the blank spaces numbered *21 to 25* in Table 4–1 write in any additional prefixes, roots, or suffixes you may encounter in your readings. Refer back to this table as a quick reference to help you to analyze word parts.

TABLE 4–1 Prefixes, Roots, Suffixes

		Definition	Example	Definition of Example	Your Example
Prefix					
1	anti	against	anti-inflammatory		
2	*dys	bad, difficult	dysfunction		
3	*endo	within	endocrine		
4	ex	out	exhale		
5	fore	before, in front of	foresight		
6	*hem, hemato	relating to the blood	hemoglobin		
7	*hydra, hydro	relating to water	hydrocephalus		
8	*hyper	over, above, beyond	hyperactive		
9	*hypo	under	hypodermic		
10	*idio	relating to the individual organ, distinct	idiomuscular		
11	inter	between	interstate		
12	mal	poor, bad	malpractice		
13	*micro	small	microscope		
14	*neuro	nerve	neurobiology		
15	non	not	nonviable		
16	*ortho	straight, normal	orthodontia		
17	retro	backward	retroactive		
18	semi	half	semicircle		
19	sub	under	subconscious		
20	tele	distant, far	television		
21					
22					
23					
24					
25					
Root					
1	*arteri, arterio	artery	arteriosclerosis		
2	*arthro, arthr	joint	arthritis		
3	*cardi, cardio	heart	cardiovascular		
4	dem, demo	people	democracy		
5	*derm, dermo	skin	dermatologist		
6	fac, fact	make, do	factory		
7	geo	earth	geology		
8	*gyne	woman	gynecology		
9	later	side	unilateral		
10	mit, miss	send	transmit		
11	*nephro, nephr	kidney	nephritis		
12	neur, neuro	nerve	neurology		
13	*oste, osteo	bone	osteoporosis		
14	*path	disease	pathology		
15	port	carry	transport		
16	*psych	mind	psychology		
17	*soma	body	somatic		
18	spec, spect	to look at	spectator		
19	ven, veno	vein	venous		
20	vers	turn	reversible		
21					
22					
23					
24					
25					

TABLE 4–1 Prefixes, Roots, Suffixes *(Continued)*

		Definition	Example	Definition of Example	Your Example
Suffix					
1	able, ible	capable of	reachable		
2	ation	act of	purification		
3	*cide	causing death	pesticide		
4	*cyte	cell	blastocyte		
5	*ectomy	excision	tonsillectomy		
6	er, or, ant	person who	actor		
7	ful	full of	dreadful		
8	graph	picture or record	cardiograph		
9	gram	instrument that records	cardiogram		
10	ism	doctrine	socialism		
11	*itis	inflammation of	appendicitis		
12	*meter	measure of	centimeter		
13	ology	study of	biology		
14	*oplasty	plastic surgery	rhinoplasty		
15	*osis	condition of	psychosis		
16	*ostomy	opening	colostomy		
17	*phobia	fear	agoraphobia		
18	rupt	break, burst	interrupt		
19	scope	see	telescope		
20	*tomy	cutting	hysterectomy		
21					
22					
23					
24					
25					

*Affixes with a medical use.

EXERCISE 4–4

Directions. The following selection is from the Matteson and McConnell nursing textbook (pp. 706–707). Analyze the root and any prefix or suffix of the underscored words and write the definition in the margin near the word. The first definition has been added for you. If necessary, check your dictionary or glossary for correct meanings.

The act of forestalling

Postinjury Phase. Ideally, accidental injuries should be prevented, but in some instances this simply is not possible. Therefore nurses should attend to optimizing postinjury prevention efforts, to minimize the long-range effects of an injury. Many communities have emergency call systems, such as "Lifeline," that allow older people at risk of falling ready access to postfall assistance. The systems work by activating a central emergency call board (such as in an emergency room) when the client pushes a button. These buttons are generally small and may be worn on light clothing. Other alternatives include daily checking systems, in which neighbors, friends, or family phone the older person each day.

An example of a fall-related injury prevention protocol developed for a nursing home is shown on this page. It includes both preinjury and postinjury interventions to reduce injury.

Evaluation
Criteria for evaluation of nursing care for those with potential for injury are:

1. What is the incidence of injury in the target client population? How does it compare with national averages?
2. What is the incidence of *functional* impairment *attributable* to injury in the client population?
3. Are the patients assessed for potential for specific injuries: fall-related injury, other trauma, burns, poisoning?
4. Are steps taken to reduce the at-risk individual's likelihood of sustaining injury?
5. Is the client's lifestyle adversely affected by the injury prevention program?
6. What is the cost of the injury prevention program to the individual, family, and facility or agency?

NONCOMPLIANCE
Definition and Scope of Problem
Noncompliance is a term with many definitions and connotations. Even leading experts on nursing diagnosis offer quite different definitions. Carpenito defines noncompliance as "personal behavior that deviates from health-related advice given by health care professionals." Gordon defines it as "failure to participate in carrying out the plan of care *after indicating initial intention* to comply." The North American Nursing Diagnosis Association has developed yet another definition: "A person's informed decision not to adhere to a therapeutic recommendation." Compliance is a concern of nurses because the goal of compliance is improved health status. Despite inconsistencies in definition, there is widespread agreement that achieving compliance is problematic in many different categories of patients. Research on compliance shows that noncompliance is found in patients of all ages, social classes, and ethnic groups; it is found in all types of health care delivery systems and in patients whose symptoms vary from nonexistent to life-threatening.

Noncompliance is most often seen in the community setting, where patients have greater control over their daily routines and are more likely to have competing demands on their time. In institutional settings there are fewer opportunities for noncompliance because many self-care activities are either closely supervised or done for the patient.

The extent of noncompliance by the elderly is thought to be high by some observers, with medication noncompliance rates averaging about 50 percent. However, variations in the definition of noncompliance used in studies and measurement difficulties make accurate estimates of the extent of this problem among the elderly difficult to obtain.

Most of the compliance literature focuses on younger adults. Sackett and Snow's review of 31 compliance studies shows that one third of the studies specifically exclude the elderly, and only 2 of 31 are specific to this population. Much of what we know about compliance in the elderly has been extrapolated from studies of age-heterogeneous groups with specific chronic diseases, such as diabetes and hypertension. The literature that considers the elderly as a discrete group calls attention to sensory deficits and memory impairment as two important contributors to noncompliance.

• VOCABULARY CHECK

Directions. Following are 10 words taken from the key word section of this chapter. Circle the letter of the best definition from the four choices.

1. Socialism
   - a the state of being with others
   - b the system of government in the United States
   - c a method by which people are made ready to partake in group activities
   - d a system in which there is no private ownership

2. Agoraphobia
   - a fear of open and public places
   - b fear of spiders
   - c fear of close spaces
   - d fear of germs

3. Transmit
   - a to exchange between individuals
   - b to carry from place to place
   - c to send from one person to another
   - d to change the shape of

4. Cardiovascular
   - a pertaining to a device measuring heart function
   - b pertaining to the lungs and heart
   - c pertaining to the lungs
   - d pertaining to the heart and blood vessels

5. Tonsillectomy
   - a treatment of tonsils
   - b excision of tonsils
   - c infection of tonsils
   - d pertaining to tonsils

6. Unilateral
   - a done by one person or party
   - b single-handed
   - c partial functioning
   - d pertaining to an element in the universe

7. Endocrine
   - a part of blood constituents
   - b pertaining to heart-lung functioning
   - c pertaining to hormonal secretion
   - d part of the kidneys and their output

8. Prefix
   - a a word part found at beginning and end of the word
   - b a word part forming the base of the word
   - c a word part attached at the end of a word
   - d a word part attached to the beginning of a word

9. Somatic
- **a** pertaining to the body
- **b** pertaining to the stomach
- **c** pertaining to the ego
- **d** pertaining to the nervous system

10. Pregnant
- **a** immediate period right after delivery of unborn young
- **b** the unborn young
- **c** containing unborn young within the body
- **d** the egg containing unborn young

• CRITICAL THINKING LOG

List the strategies you learned in this chapter.	Select the strategy that is most useful for your school success.	How can you apply this strategy to your nursing studies?

• SUMMARY

In this chapter you have learned a new method for defining unknown general vocabulary and medical terminology: analyzing word parts. You learned the functions of the following word parts:

- Prefix—a part added to the beginning of the root word that changes its meaning
- Root—the main part of the word
- Suffix—a part added to the end of the root word that changes the meaning of the word and part of speech

You have become familiar with the definitions of these word parts and have had practice learning the meanings of new words by analyzing word parts.

CHAPTER 5

Using Context Clues

• OBJECTIVES

In this chapter you will learn to use familiar words to figure out the meaning of unknown medical and nonmedical words and to recognize and apply five types of context clues.

• KEY WORDS

Pay attention to the following key words, which are underscored the first time they appear in this chapter. Try to determine the meanings of these words in the passage. If you need further help, use your dictionary or the glossary in the back of this book.

Look up the medical terminology in your medical dictionary or the glossary. As you read the exercises in this chapter, write additional words you need to learn in the space provided.

MEDICAL TERMINOLOGY	GENERAL VOCABULARY
aspirate	adventitious
chronic	approximate

enzymes
exocrine
lethargy
neologisms
pancreas
pharmacology
schizophrenia
secrete
syndrome
____
____
____

complication
disruption
secrete
limitation
manipulates
obstacle
precise
verify
____
____
____
____

• DEFINING CONTEXT CLUES

A major obstacle to good reading comprehension is not knowing the meanings of key words. This is especially true for nursing students, who are required to know the meanings of both medical terminology and general vocabulary. One way to arrive at an approximate definition of a word is to use context clues.

EXERCISE 5–1

Directions. Look at the following passage from Lehne (p. 3) and try to fill in the missing words.

If you are typical of the students for whom this book was ____________ , by this time in your life you have spent 15 or more ____________ in school and have probably asked yourself, "What's the purpose of all this ____________ ?" In the past your question may have lacked a satisfying ____________ . Happily, now you have one: You have undergone all that education to prepare yourself to ____________ pharmacology.

By looking at the entire passage, you should have filled in the words "written," "years," "education," "answer," and "study." What you have done is to use familiar or known words in the sentence to figure out the unknown word. This is what is meant by using the context to arrive at the meaning of an unknown word. The advantage of this process is that you do not have to interrupt the flow of your reading to consult the dictionary for the meaning of a new word.

However, there is a limitation in the use of this strategy when reading nursing texts. When you use context clues, you can arrive at an approximate meaning of a word, in other words, a guess. Although this may be sufficient for general vocabulary, precise definitions are necessary for medical terminology. Therefore, use context when possible, but always refer to a medical dictionary or glossary to verify definitions of medical terms. Consider the following example.

EXAMPLE 5–1

Two major cellular bodies within the pancreas have separate functions: exocrine and endocrine (Ignatavicius and Bayne, p. 1494).

Even if you consider the entire sentence, no amount of guessing would allow you to arrive at a definition of exocrine (digestive enzymes) or endocrine (internal secretions) that would be sufficiently precise for your nursing studies. Therefore, first use context clues to help you understand both nonnursing and nursing terms, but always double-check the meaning of medical vocabulary by using your medical dictionary or glossary.

• FIVE TYPES OF CONTEXT CLUES

Reading a nursing text can be challenging, especially when you are confronted with unknown words. However, many of these words are defined within the text if you know how to use context clues to look for the definitions. Nursing students should be able to recognize and use five basic types of context clues:

1. Direct definitions
2. Appositives
3. Antonyms
4. Examples
5. Surrounding sentences

Direct Definitions

Read the following sentence and see whether you can determine the meaning of the boldface term.

EXAMPLE 5–2

For clarity, one might use **paraphrasing:** that is, one might restate in newer and fewer words the basic content of a client's message. (Varcarolis, p. 118)

You can see that the definition for "paraphrasing"—restate in newer and fewer words the basic content of a client's message—is found right in the sentence. This sentence where the unknown word is first encountered also supplies the definition. Here are a few more examples of direct definition.

EXAMPLE 5–3

1. **Empathy** is the ability to feel for and with another and to understand the other's experience. (Varcarolis, p. 198)
2. **Suppression** is the conscious denial of a disturbing situation or feeling. (Varcarolis, p. 204)
3. **Primary gain** refers to the anxiety relief resulting from the use of defense mechanisms and symptom formation. (Varcarolis, p. 311)

EXERCISE 5–2

Directions. Read each sentence and write a definition in your own words for each boldface word or phrase. Use the direct definition context clue to help you arrive at the meaning.

1. This ability to recognize self versus nonself, which is necessary so that healthy body cells are not destroyed along with the invaders, is called **self-tolerance.** (Ignatavicius et al., p. 434)

   ____

   ____

2. **Agoraphobia** is fear and avoidance of being in open spaces from which escape may be difficult. (Varcarolis, p. 314)

   ____

   ____

3. **Clang associations** is the stringing together of words because of their rhyming sounds, without regard to their meaning, such as "Good luck, buck, chuck, duck" or "red, bed, said, ted, led." (Varcarolis, p. 472.)

   ____

   ____

4. This reality checking of thoughts, feelings, and actions with others Sullivan calls **consensual validation.** (Varcarolis, p. 495.)

   ____

   ____

5. **Neologisms** are words a person makes up that have special meaning for the person. (Varcarolis, p. 501)

   ____

   ____

Appositives

Read the following sentence, paying attention to the boldface term.

EXAMPLE 5–4

Platelets demonstrate a reduced ability to **aggregate** (clump together) and secrete substances important for blood clotting. (Ignatavicius et al., p. 313)

You may have noticed that next to the boldface term was a word in parentheses that had the same meaning as *aggregate*—"clump together." This type of context clue is an appositive, a word or phrase next to, or in apposition to, the unknown word that should help you figure out the meaning of the word. Read the following examples and note that the appositives are usually set off by the word "or," parentheses, commas, or dashes.

EXAMPLE 5–5

1. Respiratory failure may follow quickly as a complication of laryngeal edema and suffocation or lower airway bronchoconstriction causing hypoxemia (insufficient oxygenation of blood) and hypercapnia (increased carbon dioxide in blood). (Ignatavicius, p. 533)
2. Vertebral fractures, called wedge fractures, produce acute episodes of sharp pain. (Matteson et al., p. 176)
3. Dissociative amnesia, or **psychogenic amnesia,** the most common dissociative disorder, differs from ordinary forgetfulness because the extent of the disturbance is much greater. (Varcarolis, p. 358)

EXERCISE 5–3

Directions. Read the following sentences and circle the appositive for the boldface word or phrase.

1. Individuals suffering from **dissociative fugue,** or psychogenic fugue physically travel away from their homes and jobs. (Varcarolis, p. 358)
2. **Dysthymia** (depressive neurosis) is mild to moderate in degree and characterized by a chronic depressive syndrome that is usually present for many years. (Varcarolis, p. 423)
3. At times, the nurse may try to **decipher** or decode the client's messages and begin to understand the client's feelings and needs. (Varcarolis, p. 501)
4. A person's declining intellect often leads to emotional changes, lack of self-care, and finally, to **hallucinations** and **delusions**—that is, psychotic symptoms brought on by organic changes. (Varcarolis, p. 556)
5. The client experiencing urticaria initially reports **pruritus** (itching), followed by the appearance of wheals. (Ignatavicius, p. 535)

Antonyms

Read the following sentence and try to determine the meaning of the boldface word.

EXAMPLE 5–6

Harry Stack Sullivan believed that anxiety resulted from **interpersonal** conflicts rather than from an intrapsychic process. (Varcarolis, p. 198)

In this sentence, "interpersonal" means "between people," the opposite of "intrapsychic," which means "inside one's mind." The clue words "rather than" alert the reader to the use of an antonym as a context clue for determining vocabulary meaning. Antonyms are opposites. By recognizing some connecting words—such as "rather than," "or," "but," "however," "are not" and "neither . . . nor"—the reader will become aware of the use of antonyms as context clues.

EXAMPLE 5–7

Following are a few more examples of using antonyms as context clues.

1. Drugs "are not" **magic bullets:** they are simply **chemicals.** (Lehne, p. 60)
2. The **relaxation response,** identified by Herbert Benson, "is the opposite of" the **fight-or-flight response.** (Varcarolis, p. 196)
3. An adventitious crisis is **not a part of everyday life** "but" is **unplanned and accidental.** (Varcarolis, p. 237)

EXERCISE 5–4

Directions. Read the following sentences and circle the antonyms of the boldface words. Look for a possible connecting term that will help you find the antonyms.

1. Effective feedback is **specific** rather than general. (Arnold and Boggs, p. 225)
2. Instead of **wooing** the nurse, as does the seducer, the passive-aggressor manipulates in ways that push the nurse away. (Varcarolis, p. 383)
3. Silence is **not the absence of communication**; silence is a specific channel for transmitting and receiving messages. (Varcarolis, p. 121)
4. Talking is highly individualized: some find the telephone a **nuisance,** whereas others believe they cannot live without it. (Varcarolis, p. 121)
5. It doesn't **occur in a vacuum** but is shaped by the situation in which the interaction occurs. (Arnold and Boggs, p. 195)

Examples

Read the following sentence and notice how the examples in the surrounding words help you to define the unknown word in boldface.

EXAMPLE 5–8

Acute anxiety may be seen in performers before a concert. For example, Barbra Streisand admits to experiencing acute anxiety before live concerts. Patients preparing for surgery often experience acute anxiety. The death of a loved one can stimulate acute anxiety when there is a great *disruption* in one's life. (Varcarolis, p. 196)

The examples given—"seen in performers in concert," "Barbra Streisand experiencing acute anxiety," "patients preparing for surgery" and "death of a loved one"—allow you to define the term "acute anxiety" as an extreme feeling caused by a life-change or loss. Such examples or illustrations allow you to arrive at definitions of unknown words. The details when considered all together help you to approximate word meanings.

Notice how the italicized examples help you define the unknown boldface words in the following sentences:

EXAMPLE 5–9

1. The **honeymoon stage** is characterized by *kindness and loving behaviors*. The *abuser feels remorseful and apologetic* and may *bring presents, make promises, and generally tell the victim how much she or he is loved and needed.* (Varcarolis, p. 261)
2. Particularly disturbing to clients are the **intrusive symptoms,** such as *nightmares, flashbacks, and memories of traumatic events.* (Varcarolis, p. 318)
3. A depressive syndrome frequently accompanies other **psychiatric disorders,** such as schizophrenia, psychoactive substance dependence disorder, or *eating disorders.* (Varcarolis, p. 423)

You can apply this strategy in the following exercise.

EXERCISE 5–5

Directions. Read the following sentences and determine the meaning of the boldface words or phrases from the examples given in the context of each sentence or sentences. In your own words, write the definition in the space provided.

1. Complaints of <u>lethargy</u> and fatigue can result in **psychomotor retardation.** Movements are extremely slow, facial expressions are decreased, and the gaze is fixed. (Varcarolis, p. 429)

   Definition ______________________________

2. Depression and fatigue can be important indications of various **medical disorders** such as hepatitis, mononucleosis, multiple sclerosis, and cancer. (Varcarolis, p. 423)

   Definition ______________________________

3. **Values indicators** are attitudes, beliefs, feelings, worries, or convictions. (Arnold and Boggs, p. 148)

   Definition ______________________________

4. Posture, rhythm of movement, and gestures accompanying a verbal message are other **nonverbal behaviors** associated with the overall process of communication. (Arnold and Boggs, p. 191)

   Definition ______________________________

5. **Therapeutic communication** is a specified form of dialogue that is descriptive, problem focused, and supportive of the client's strength. (Arnold and Boggs, p. 200)

   Definition ______________________________

Surrounding Sentences

Read the following short passage and notice how the surrounding sentences provide the context for helping you determine the meaning of the boldface unknown word.

EXAMPLE 5–10

An **arthrocentesis** is a common diagnostic procedure used for clients with joint involvement. It may be done at the bedside or in a physician's office or clinic. After administering a local anesthetic, the physician inserts a large-gauge needle into the joint, usually the knee, to *aspirate* a sample of synovial fluid, which may also relieve pressure. The fluid is analyzed by use of tests .... (Ignatavicius, p. 480)

The first sentence in the above paragraph tells you in general terms what an arthrocentesis is. The subsequent sentences provide further information about the meaning of arthrocentesis. Each sentence adds to your understanding of this medical term. Once you have finished reading the entire passage, you have a working idea of what the unknown word means. Sometimes, then, it is necessary to read the sentences preceding and following an unknown word in order to glean the greatest meaning of the unfamiliar word.

EXERCISE 5–6

Directions. Below are passages taken from nursing textbooks. Underline all the context clues in the surrounding sentences that will help you figure out the meanings of the boldface words.

1. **Serum sickness** is a complex of symptoms that occurs after the administration of foreign serum or certain drugs. It is caused by collection of immune complexes in the walls of vessels in the skin, joints, and the glomeruli of the kidney. The most common causes of serum sickness today are penicillin and related drugs and some horse serum antitoxins. (Ignatavicius, p. 537)
2. **Impulsiveness** is an action that is abrupt, unplanned, and directed toward immediate gratification. Thinking things over or considering the effects of the action on others does not occur. These clients have a history of unpredictable and hasty decisions. Frustration is poorly tolerated and often precipitates an impulsive response. A client's impulsive behavior has been described as erratic, self-serving, and thoughtless. In certain situations, the antisocial client's impulsive behavior is able to generate fear and aggression in others. (Varcarolis, p. 383)
3. Bandler and Grindler (1975) offer a different approach to the study of communication in their conceptual model, defined as **neurolinguistic programming** (NLP). This conceptual model focuses on the way a person takes in and internally processes verbal information. According to these theorists, people make sensory-based interpretations about the realities they observe. (Arnold and Boggs, p. 18)
4. Nurses learn about themselves through self-reflection and the feedback of others. **Self-reflection** is a mental process by which we are able consciously to examine the meaning of our motives and actions. It is a mental faculty available only to humans. (Arnold and Boggs, p. 70)
5. The roles people assume represent an effort to influence the judgments of others about their self-concept. As a result, they emphasize certain parts of the self-concept and suppress those aspects they consider less desirable. Jung calls this public expression of self the **"persona."** The persona represents all the surface masks a person wears to bridge the gap between the inner self and society's expectations of the self. (Arnold and Boggs, p. 131)

• CONTEXT CLUES AND THE NURSING STUDENT

When reading textbooks, you must determine when context helps you find the meaning of an unknown word and when context clues are not giving you the information you need. In nursing books, much of the medical terminology is defined for you in the text by direct definition. The other context clues—antonyms, appositives, examples, and surrounding sentences—also help you learn the meanings of many general vocabulary words and medical terms. However, while it may be appropriate to approximate meanings for general vocabulary, medical terminology calls for precise meanings. When there are no clues in the context or when the clues do not help you to find exact definitions for medical terms, it is time to turn to the glossary of the textbook, general dictionary, or a medical dictionary. Through practice you will learn to assess when you can use context to define words and when you need to use a glossary, dictionary, or medical dictionary.

EXERCISE 5–7

Directions. Read the following selection from the Matteson and McConnell nursing textbook (pp. 183–186). Seventeen words are in boldface. Fill in the chart at the end of the selection to indicate which word meanings you derived from context and/or which definitions came from a glossary, dictionary, or medical dictionary. The first is done for you.

Rheumatoid Arthritis

Rheumatoid arthritis is a chronic, **systemic, progressive** disease of unknown origin. The onset of the disease can occur at any age, but it usually begins between the ages of 20 and 60, peaking between 35 and 45. The **prevalence** of the disease rises with each decade, the largest incidence occurring after age 60. Women are affected two to three times more frequently than men, and there seems to be a familial tendency toward the disease. Onset is more common in the spring, especially during March. Although the cause is unknown, most scientists believe that it is associated with **immune** (antigen-antibody) factors, called **rheumatoid factors,** in the bloodstream (Vaughan, 1980; Hamerman, 1986).

The disease generally begins with inflammation of the **synovial membrane,** which later thickens and adheres to the **adjacent** margins of the **articular cartilage.** The thickened synovium, or **pannus,** is composed of fibrous tissue containing chronic inflammatory cells. The pannus erodes the cartilage and underlying bone, forming either **adhesions** between the opposing surfaces of the joint or cysts within the spaces of the bone (Barnes, 1980) (Fig. 7–12). Small peripheral joints are usually affected symmetrically, especially the hand, wrist, knee, ankle, elbow, and shoulder. Affected joints in the hands are usually **proximal** (metacarpophalangeal) rather than **distal** (distal interphalangeal) as in osteoarthritis (Bluestone, 1980).

Systemic involvement in rheumatoid arthritis is characteristic of the disease; the tendon sheaths, bursae, and connective tissues of the heart, lungs, pleura, and arteries are affected. Manifestations of systemic involvement include peripheral neuropathy, leg ulcers, anemia, enlarged spleen, leukopenia, pleuritis, and pericarditis. Rheumatoid nodules, a diagnostic feature of the disease, are subcutaneous masses located over the pressure points of the body such as the elbows, occiput, sacrum, and heel (Barnes, 1980).

Rheumatoid arthritis is characterized by bony fusion and limited motion of the joints, pain, swelling, and deformity. Initial symptoms include pain and stiffness of involved joints, malaise, and fatigue. Early morning stiffness lasting more than one-half hour is diagnostically significant. Pain or movement may be relieved by rest early in the disease, but later pain may occur spontaneously, even at rest. In the elderly, pain or limitation of movement in the shoulders is more common. Synovitis and synovial effusion produce swelling, warmth, tenderness, edema, and a "boggy" feeling around the joints. A phenomenon called "spindle fingers" results from swelling of the interphalangeal joints (Fig. 7–13). Limited motion is due to synovial effusions, muscle spasms, and contractures. Flexion contractures, which are due to the dominance of flexor muscles, and fibrosis of the joint capsule, ligaments, and tendons produce joint deformities of the knees, hips, elbows, and toes. Ulnar deviation of the metacarpophalangeal joints, "swan-neck" deformity, **boutonniere** (button-hole) deformity, and flexion deformities of the knee are most common (Figs. 7–14 to 7–17) (Gordon et al., 1981; Stevens, 1983).

Laboratory studies show an increase in sedimentation rate and gamma globulin level and the presence of the rheumatoid factor, which occurs in 75 per cent of cases within 2 years after the onset of the disease. Aspirated synovial fluid is inflamed with an increased white blood cell count. X-rays show erosion of the articular margins.

The course of the disease is marked by **remissions** and **exacerbations** in a downhill, stepwise progression. In younger persons the disease tends to have a slower, more insidious onset than in older persons. In people over 60, the symptoms are acute, explosive, and widespread; however, the duration is shorter, and there is a greater chance for improvement.

In general, the prognosis of the disease is more favorable under the following conditions:

1. Onset in persons over forty
2. Duration less than 1 year
3. Acute onset
4. Asymmetrical distribution or limited to one joint
5. Absence of rheumatoid nodules or radiographic changes
6. Absent or low titer of rheumatoid factor

Older persons who are males, who have had good joint function, one period of remission, good muscle conditioning, and normal body weight are most likely to have a good prognosis (Giansiracuso and Kantrowitz, 1982). Table 7–6 compares rheumatoid arthritis with osteoarthritis (Hamerman, 1986).

Treatment of older persons with rheumatoid arthritis is similar to that in the young: client and family education, psychological support, general rest, local rest (**splinting**), analgesic and anti-inflammatory medications, physical therapy, occupational therapy, and surgery. Problems with treatment may arise in elderly people who find it difficult to stay ambulatory and remain independent, who have difficulty tolerating supports and braces, or who tolerate drugs poorly (Brewerton, 1979). The aged experience more muscle weakness and atrophy, progressive bone loss, and a greater tendency toward flexion contractures than the young, so that **judicious** use of range of motion exercises, isometric exercises for muscle strengthening, and joint splinting is crucial to promote mobility and independence. Although it is important to avoid immobilization in the elderly, rest and splinting are imperative during flare-ups to enhance the action of anti-inflammatory medications and to prevent further damage to the joint. Rest and immobility of inflamed joints actually speed recovery and do not result in permanent loss of joint function as one might assume. Gentle range of motion exercises one to two times per day provide enough exercise to maintain function (Sack, 1980a).

Drug treatment for all persons with rheumatoid arthritis is aimed toward relief of pain and suppression of inflammation. Because the elderly metabolize drugs differently and because they may have accumulated a variety of chronic health problems, they are more susceptible to side effects and toxicities of the analgesic and anti-inflammatory agents. The most frequently used drugs for elderly arthritics include the following:

1. Nonsteroidal anti-inflammatory drugs
   Salicylates (aspirin)
   Ibuprofen (Motrin)
   Fenoprofen calcium (Nalfon)
   Naproxen (Naprosyn)
   Sulindac (Clinoril)
   Indomethacin (Indocin)
   Phenylbutazone (Butazolidin)
2. Slow-onset agents: Anti-malarials (Aralen, Plaquenil)
   D-Penicillamine (Cuprimine)
   Gold sodium thiomalate (Myochrysine)
   Cytotoxic/immunosuppressive agents
3. Corticosteroids
4. Simple analgesics: Salicylates (aspirin)
   Acetaminophen (Tylenol)
   Codeine

Doses for these drugs are generally lower for older clients, and the goal is to use as few as possible. Major side effects are gastrointestinal disturbances and a potential for gastric ulcer; antacids help to minimize these effects when taken concurrently (Barnes, 1980; Sack, 1980b).

WORD	Definition	Context	Glossary	Dictionary	Medical Dictionary
1. systemic	Referring to entire body		√	√	√
2. progressive					
3. prevalence					
4. immune					
5. rheumatoid factors					
6. synovial membrane					
7. adjacent					
8. articular cartilage					
9. pannus					
10. adhesions					
11. proximal					
12. distal					
13. boutonniere					
14. remissions					
15. exacerbations					
16. splinting					
17. judicious					

• VOCABULARY CHECK

Directions. Below are 10 words taken from the key word section of this chapter. Circle the letter of the best definition from the four choices.

1. Aspirate

a to remove fluid
b to inject fluid
c to remove solids
d to inject solids

2. Obstacle

a something that one accomplishes
b something that one achieves
c something that impedes progress
d something that aids progress

3. Pharmacology
a the study of agriculture
b the study of drugs
c the process related to establishing pharmacies
d the process for filing drug-related insurance

4. Approximate
a to accept as satisfactory
b to reject as unacceptable
c to be specific
d to come close

5. Secrete
a to produce and discharge a substance
b to hold in strict confidence
c to add the presence of a sweetener
d to provide nourishment

6. Verify
a to flower or bud
b serving to eliminate parasites
c to sign one's name to a document
d to establish the truth or reality of

7. Syndrome
a an assortment of symptoms causing a common health problem
b a group of clues that leads to a diagnosis
c symptoms of a disease thought to be incurable
d only those symptoms that can be treated

8. Adventitious
a pertaining to exciting occurrences
b coming from outside of the normal place
c referring to a superior advantage
d referring to a heralded event

9. Disruption
a an explosion in the natural world
b a tearing apart of an external limb or internal organ
c the spewing forth of noxious gases or fumes
d something that stops the normal course of an event

10. Lethargy
a an abnormal degree of fatigue
b a disease of the nervous system
c a high degree of energy
d a disease of the smooth muscles

• CRITICAL THINKING LOG

List the strategies you learned in this chapter.	Select the strategy that is most useful for your school success.	How can you apply this strategy to your nursing studies?

• SUMMARY

In this chapter you have learned that it is possible to figure out the meanings of unknown words by using the familiar, neighboring words that surround the new term. This is called using context clues. Five examples of context clues were given:

1. Direct definitions
2. Appositives
3. Antonyms
4. Examples
5. Surrounding sentences

The most common type of context clue used in nursing texts is direct definition. Use direct definition and the other types of context clues whenever possible to help you determine word meanings.

You were also made aware of the possible limitations of context clues. Context clues may not provide a precise enough definition for medical terminology, or the sentence or passage may not contain any context clues.

Therefore, when you need further help in finding word meanings, consult a glossary, dictionary, or medical dictionary.

CHAPTER 6

Dictionary, Glossary, and Thesaurus

• OBJECTIVES

To become familiar with the format of the dictionary, glossary, and thesaurus and to learn the way these references can teach the meanings of new words.

• KEY WORDS

Pay attention to the following key words, which are underscored the first time they appear in this chapter. Try to determine the meaning of these words in the passage. If you need further help, use your dictionary or the glossary in the back of this book.

Look up the medical terminology in your medical dictionary or the glossary. As you read the exercises in this chapter, write additional words you need to learn in the space provided.

MEDICAL TERMINOLOGY	GENERAL VOCABULARY
afibrinogenemia	antonyms
afterbirth	collegiate

bulimia nervosa
cyrtometer
gynecology
hematoma
incision
myxedema
myxorrhea
pathogen
scleroma
____
____
____

diacritical marks
etymology
glossary
pronunciation
specialized
synonyms
thesaurus
unabridged
____
____
____
____

• USING OTHER SOURCES TO DEFINE WORDS

In the two previous chapters (Chapter 4, "Word Parts" and Chapter 5, "Using Context Clues"), you learned ways of defining unknown words encountered in your readings without the use of references such as the dictionary. When you use these vocabulary strategies, you do not have to disturb your concentration by stopping to refer to another source. In some instances, however, analyzing word parts and interpreting context clues will not be sufficient. For example, the word may not have a word part, the surrounding words may not suggest the meaning of the unknown word, or the word may be an unknown medical term that requires a precise definition. In these cases you will have to take a momentary break from reading to consult an additional source. Depending on the situation, this may be a dictionary (either collegiate or medical), a glossary, or a thesaurus.

• DICTIONARY

Dictionaries are indispensable to your experience as a nursing student. Most nursing schools require that you buy a medical dictionary, such as Miller and Keane's *Encyclopedia and Dictionary of Medicine, Nursing, and Allied Health.* This type of dictionary is a specialized dictionary because it focuses on terminology from a particular profession or field—in this case, health care.

The next type of dictionary that is necessary for your success as a nursing student is a hard-cover collegiate dictionary for general terminology. This dictionary should be used at home and kept in your study area for quick availability.

The last kind of dictionary to buy is a paperback version of a collegiate dictionary. You need a dictionary in this handy form so you can carry it with you to classes and refer to it when necessary. Make sure the paperback dictionary you buy is a complete edition of the hard-cover dictionary, not a shortened version. Otherwise, you may find when you go to look for a word that the entry is not there.

At times you may need to consult an unabridged dictionary in the library. The unabridged dictionary contains most words and is the most complete dictionary.

Purpose of the Dictionary

Many people think that the dictionary is useful only for learning the meaning of an unknown word. However, the dictionary holds a wealth of other information. Consider some of these further uses:

- *Syllabication.* By reading the main entry you can see how many syllables a word has and where to divide the word at the end of a line.
- *Pronunciation.* By knowing how to use the pronunciation guide, you can find out how to pronounce the word accurately.
- *Parts of speech.* By consulting the appropriate abbreviation within the entry, you can determine the part of speech.
- *Etymology.* By looking at the first line in the entry, you can learn the origin of the word and the year it was first encountered in written form.
- *Spelling.* By checking both the beginning and end of the entry, you can see the correct spelling of the entry and in some instances the variations in spelling when suffixes are added.
- *Synonyms and antonyms.* At the end of the entry you may encounter other words that have meanings similar or opposite to the entry word.

Reading a Dictionary Entry

To use the dictionary skillfully, you must be familiar with the various parts of the entry. Below is an entry taken from *Webster's Ninth New Collegiate Dictionary* (p. 609). The different parts have been numbered:

1. 2. 3. 4. 5.

in·ci·sion \in-'sizh-ən\ *n* (15c) **1** **a** : a marginal notch (as in a leaf) **b** : CUT, GASH; *specif* : a wound made esp. in surgery by incising the body **2** : an act of incising something **3** : the quality or state of being incisive

We will examine each of these parts of the entry more closely:

1. The *main entry* or *entry word* is usually printed in boldface. The letters of the word can be set undivided, divided by one or more spaces or, as in this example, divided by hyphens. These divisions tell how many syllables the word has. In the above example, the entry has how many syllables? ____________________

2. The *pronunciation* is placed next to the main entry and is separated from it by backslashes (\\). Later in the chapter we will explain the use of the pronunciation guide. Write the pronunciation of the entry word. ____________________

3. The *part of speech* follows the pronunciation and is usually abbreviated in the following manner:

   adj = adjective
   adv = adverb
   conj = conjunction
   interj = interjection
   n = noun
   prep = preposition
   pron = pronoun
   vb = verb
   vt = transitive verb
   vi = intransitive verb

   In our example the entry word is what part of speech? ____________________

4. The *date* tells the earliest recorded use of the word in English. In many entries this is preceded by the *etymology* or origin of the word, that is, the language where the word is believed to have originated and what the word looked like in its original form. Some abbreviations found in the etymology are as follows:

OE = Old English
ME = Middle English
L = Latin
G = Greek
F = French

In our example entry, the word was first encountered in which century? ____________________

5. The rest of the entry provides the *definitions* of the word. If the word has more than one meaning, the definitions are numbered. Sometimes the definition of the word has two or more shades of meaning or senses. If this is so, the definition is subdivided by letters. In our example, how many definitions are there? ____________________

Which definition has different senses? ______________________________

Comprehending? Yes ___ No ___

Locating an Entry

The dictionary is designed to help you find an entry as efficiently as possible. Interrupting your reading for several minutes to hunt for a word will discourage you from using the dictionary as a vocabulary builder. Because the dictionary entries are listed in alphabetical order, your first step is to make sure you know the order of the letters in the alphabet so you can quickly locate your word. That means that if the word you are looking for begins with a letter toward the end of the alphabet, you need not begin with "A" and go through the entire alphabet to get an approximate idea of where your word is located. You also must understand how to alphabetize up to the third, fourth, and fifth letters of the word. For various reasons, many students have to review alphabetical order. Once you are proficient in using alphabetical order, you will be able to work with your dictionary more skillfully.

EXERCISE 6–1

Directions. Below is a list of medical terms. In the space provided, write these words in alphabetical order.

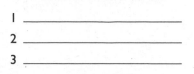

MEDICAL TERMS	ALPHABETICAL ORDER
1 hematoma	1 ____________________
2 peripheral	2 ____________________
3 carcinogen	3 ____________________

4 perioperative 4 ______________________
5 menopause 5 ______________________
6 sinusitis 6 ______________________
7 nematodes 7 ______________________
8 cardiac 8 ______________________
9 hemophilia 9 ______________________
10 peritonitis 10 ______________________

Comprehending? Yes ___ No ___

Guide Words

The dictionary provides a handy tool to make locating an entry easier for you—*guide words,* which are printed at the top of a dictionary page. In the sample page from *Webster's Ninth New Collegiate Dictionary* shown opposite, you can see there are two boldface words, or guide words. (Other dictionaries may have one guide word on the left-hand page and another on the facing page). The guide words in this example are "Caterpillar" and "caucus." This tells you that every word that falls alphabetically between "Caterpillar" and "caucus" appears on this page. You will find the page of your entry much faster by focusing on the guide words than by glancing over each page.

EXERCISE 6–2

Directions. Below in the left-hand column are guide words taken from Miller and Keane's *Encyclopedia and Dictionary of Medical, Nursing and Allied Health.* In the right-hand column are entries taken from the same dictionary. In the space provided in the center, write the number of the guide words that would be found on the page where the entry appears. The first one is done for you.

GUIDE WORDS		ENTRIES
1 myoplasm/myxedema	8	scleroma
2 globulinuria/glomerulus	____	cyrtometer
3 bulbous/burn	____	myotomy
4 dissociative disorders/distortion	____	pathogen
5 myxedema/myxovirus	____	glomerulitis
6 afibrinogenemia/agammaglobulinemia	____	scolex
7 cyclomethycaine/cyst	____	myxorrhea
8 sclerogenous/sclerosis	____	bulimia nervosa
9 pathobiology/pathway	____	afterbirth
10 scleroskeleton/scoliosis	____	distillation

Comprehending? Yes ___ No ___

Caterpillar *trademark* — used for a tractor made for use on rough or soft ground and moved on two endless metal belts

cat·er·waul \'kat-ər-,wȯl\ *vi* [ME *caterwawen*] (14c) **1** : to make a harsh cry **2** : to quarrel noisily — **caterwaul** *n*

cat·fac·ing \'kat-,fā-siŋ\ *n* (1940) : a disfigurement or malformation of fruit suggesting a cat's face in appearance

cat·fish \-,fish\ *n* (1612) : any of numerous usu. stout-bodied large-headed fishes (order Ostariophysi) with long tactile barbels

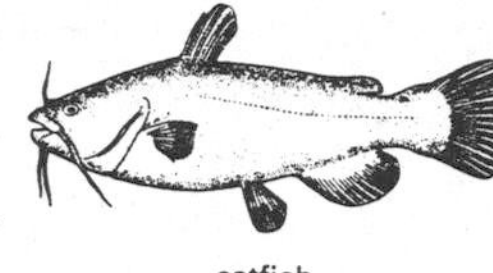
catfish

cat·gut \-,gət\ *n* (1599) : a tough cord made usu. from sheep intestines

cath- — see CATA-

Cath·ar \'kath-,är\ *n, pl* **Cath·a·ri** \'kath-ə-,rī, -,rē\ *or* **Cathars** [LL *cathari* (pl.), fr. LGk *katharoi*, fr. Gk, pl. of *katharos* pure] (1637) : a member of one of various ascetic and dualistic Christian sects flourishing in the later Middle Ages teaching that matter is evil, and professing faith in an angelic Christ who did not really undergo human birth or death — **Cath·a·rism** \'kath-ə-,riz-əm\ *n* — **Cath·a·rist** \-rəst\ *or* **Cath·a·ris·tic** \,kath-ə-'ris-tik\ *adj*

ca·thar·sis \kə-'thär-səs\ *n, pl* **ca·thar·ses** \-,sēz\ [NL, fr. Gk *katharsis*, fr. *kathairein* to cleanse, purge, fr. *katharos*] (1803) **1** : PURGATION **2 a** : purification or purgation of the emotions (as pity and fear) primarily through art **b** : a purification or purgation that brings about spiritual renewal or release from tension **3** : elimination of a complex by bringing it to consciousness and affording it expression

[1]**ca·thar·tic** \kə-'thärt-ik\ *adj* [LL or Gk; LL *catharticus*, fr. Gk *kathartikos*, fr. *kathairein*] (1612) : of, relating to, or producing catharsis

[2]**cathartic** *n* (1651) : a cathartic medicine : PURGATIVE

cat·head \'kat-,hed\ *n* (1626) : a projecting piece of timber or iron near the bow of a ship to which the anchor is hoisted and secured

ca·thect \kə-'thekt, ka-\ *vt* [NL *cathexis*] (1925) : to invest with mental or emotional energy

ca·thec·tic \kə-'thek-tik, ka-\ *adj* [NL *cathexis*] (1927) : of, relating to, or invested with mental or emotional energy

ca·the·dra \kə-'thē-drə\ *n* [L, chair — more at CHAIR] (15c) : a bishop's official throne

[1]**ca·the·dral** \kə-'thē-drəl\ *adj* (13c) **1** : of, relating to, or containing a cathedra **2** : emanating from a chair of authority **3** : suggestive of a cathedral

[2]**cathedral** *n* (1587) **1** : a church that is the official seat of a diocesan bishop **2** : something that resembles or suggests a cathedral ⟨higher education has been . . . the secular ~ of our time — David Riesman⟩

ca·thep·sin \kə-'thep-sən\ *n* [Gk *kathepsein* to digest (fr. *kata-* cata- + *hepsein* to boil) + E *-in*] (1929) : any of several intracellular proteinases of animal tissue that aid in autolysis in some diseased conditions and after death

cath·er·ine wheel \,kath-(ə-)rən-\ *n, often cap C* [St. *Catherine* of Alexandria †ab307 Christian martyr] (15c) **1** : a wheel with spikes projecting from the rim **2** : PINWHEEL 1 **3** : CARTWHEEL 2

cath·e·ter \'kath-ət-ər, 'kath-tər\ *n* [LL, fr. Gk *kathetēr*, fr. *kathienai* to send down, fr. *kata-* cata- + *hienai* to send — more at JET] (1601) : a tubular medical device for insertion into canals, vessels, passageways, or body cavities usu. to permit injection or withdrawal of fluids or to keep a passage open

cath·e·ter·iza·tion \,kath-ət-ə-rə-'zā-shən, ,kath-tə-rə-\ *n* (1849) : the use of or introduction of a catheter (as in or into the bladder, trachea, or heart) — **cath·e·ter·ize** \,kath-ət-ə-,rīz, ,kath-tə-\ *vt*

ca·thex·is \kə-'thek-səs, ka-\ *n, pl* **ca·thex·es** \-,sēz\ [NL (intended as trans. of G *besetzung*), fr. Gk *kathexis* holding, fr. *katechein* to hold fast, occupy, fr. *kata-* + *echein* to have, hold — more at SCHEME] (1922) : investment of mental or emotional energy in a person, object, or idea

cath·ode \'kath-,ōd\ *n* [Gk *kathodos* way down, fr. *kata-* + *hodos* way — more at CEDE] (1834) **1** : the negative terminal of an electrolytic cell — compare ANODE **2** : the positive terminal of a primary cell or of a storage battery that is delivering current **3** : the electron-emitting electrode of an electron tube — **ca·thod·ic** \ka-'thäd-ik\ *or* **cath·od·al** \'kath-,ōd-ᵊl\ *adj* — **ca·thod·i·cal·ly** \-i-k(ə-)lē\ *or* **cath·od·al·ly** \-ē\ *adv*

cathode ray *n* (1880) **1** : one of the high-speed electrons projected in a stream from the heated cathode of a vacuum tube under the propulsion of a strong electric field **2** : a stream of cathode-ray electrons

cathode–ray tube *n* (1905) : a vacuum tube in which cathode rays usu. in the form of a slender beam are projected on a fluorescent screen and produce a luminous spot

cath·o·lic \'kath-(ə-)lik\ *adj* [MF & LL; MF *catholique*, fr. LL *catholicus*, fr. Gk *katholikos* universal, general, fr. *katholou* in general, fr. *kata* by + *holos* whole — more at CATA-, SAFE] (14c) **1** : COMPREHENSIVE, UNIVERSAL; *esp* : broad in sympathies, tastes, or interests **2** *cap* **a** : of, relating to, or forming the church universal **b** : of, relating to, or forming the ancient undivided Christian church or a church claiming historical continuity from it; *specif* : ROMAN CATHOLIC — **ca·thol·i·cal·ly** \kə-'thäl-i-k(ə-)lē\ *adv* — **ca·thol·i·cize** \kə-'thäl-ə-,sīz\ *vb*

Cath·o·lic \'kath-(ə-)lik\ *n* (15c) **1** : a person who belongs to the universal Christian church **2** : a member of a Catholic church; *specif* : ROMAN CATHOLIC

Catholic Apostolic *adj* (1837) : of or relating to a Christian sect founded in 19th century England in anticipation of Christ's second coming

ca·thol·i·cate \kə-'thäl-ə-,kāt, -'thäl-i-kət\ *n* (ca. 1847) : the jurisdiction of a catholicos

Catholic Epistles *n pl* (1582) : the five New Testament letters including James, I and II Peter, I John, and Jude addressed to the early Christian churches at large

Ca·thol·i·cism \kə-'thäl-ə-,siz-əm\ *n* (1613) **1** : the faith, practice, or system of Catholic Christianity **2** : ROMAN CATHOLICISM

cath·o·lic·i·ty \,kath(-ə)-'lis-ət-ē\ *n, pl* **-ties** (1704) **1** *cap* : the character of being in conformity with a Catholic church **2 a** : liberality of sentiments or views ⟨~ of viewpoint — W. V. O'Connor⟩ **b** : UNIVERSALITY **c** : comprehensive range ⟨the ~ of subjects represented by the press's trade list — *Current Biog.*⟩

ca·thol·i·con \kə-'thäl-ə-,kän\ *n* [F or ML; F, fr. ML, fr. Gk *katholikon*, neut. of *katholikos*] (15c) : CURE-ALL, PANACEA

ca·thol·i·cos \kə-'thäl-i-kəs\ *n, pl* **-i·cos·es** \-kə-səz\ *or* **-i·coi** \-'thäl-ə-,kȯi\ *often cap* [LGk *katholikos*, fr. Gk, general] (1625) : a primate of certain Eastern churches and esp. of the Armenian or of the Nestorian church

cat·house \'kat-,hau̇s\ *n* (1931) : a house of prostitution

cat·ion \'kat-,ī-ən\ *n* [Gk *kation*, neut. of *katiōn*, prp. of *katienai* to go down, fr. *kata-* cata- + *ienai* to go — more at ISSUE] (1834) : the ion in an electrolyzed solution that migrates to the cathode; *broadly* : a positively charged ion

cat·ion·ic \,kat-(,)ī-'än-ik\ *adj* (ca. 1920) **1** : of or relating to cations **2** : characterized by an active and esp. surface-active cation ⟨a ~ dye⟩ — **cat·ion·i·cal·ly** \-i-k(ə-)lē\ *adv*

cat·kin \'kat-kən\ *n* [fr. its resemblance to a cat's tail] (1578) : a usu. long ament densely crowded with bracts

cat·like \'kat-,līk\ *adj* (1600) : resembling a cat; *esp* : STEALTHY ⟨with ~ tread, upon our prey we steal —W. S. Gilbert⟩

cat·mint \-,mint\ *n* (13c) : CATNIP

cat·nap \-,nap\ *n* (1823) : a very short light nap — **catnap** *vi*

cat·nap·per *or* **cat·nap·er** \'kat-,nap-ər\ *n* [[1]*cat* + *-napper* (as in *kidnapper*)] (1942) : one that steals cats usu. to sell them for research

cat·nip \-,nip\ *n* [[1]*cat* + obs. *nep* (catnip), fr. ME, fr. OE *nepte*, fr. L *nepeta*] (1712) **1** : a strong-scented mint (*Nepeta cataria*) that has whorls of small pale flowers in terminal spikes and contains a substance attractive to cats **2** : something very attractive

cat–o'–nine–tails \,kat-ə-'nīn-,tālz\ *n, pl* **cat–o'–nine–tails** [fr. the resemblance of its scars to the scratches of a cat] (1665) : a whip made of usu. nine knotted lines or cords fastened to a handle

ca·top·tric \kə-'täp-trik\ *adj* [Gk *katoptrikos*, fr. *katoptron* mirror, fr. *katopsesthai* to be going to observe, fr. *kata-* cata- + *opsesthai* to be going to see — more at OPTIC] (1774) : of or relating to a mirror or reflected light; *also* : produced by reflection — **ca·top·tri·cal·ly** \-tri-k(ə-)lē\ *adv*

cat rig *n* (1867) : a rig consisting of a single mast far forward carrying a single large sail extended by a boom — **cat–rigged** \'kat-'rigd\ *adj*

CAT scan \'kat-, ,sē-,ā-'tē-\ *n* [computerized axial tomography] (1975) : an image made by computerized axial tomography

CAT scanner *n* (1975) : a medical instrument consisting of integrated X-ray and computing equipment and used for computerized axial tomography

cat's cradle *n* (1768) **1** : a game in which a string looped in a pattern like a cradle on the fingers of one person's hands is transferred to the hands of another so as to form a different figure **2** : INTRICACY ⟨the socioreligious *cat's cradle* of small Greek communities — *Times Lit. Supp.*⟩

cat's–eye \'kat-,sī\ *n, pl* **cat's–eyes** (1599) **1** : any of various gems (as a chrysoberyl or a chalcedony) exhibiting opalescent reflections from within **2** : a marble with eyelike concentric circles

cat's–paw \'kat-,spȯ\ *n, pl* **cat's–paws** (1769) **1** : a light air that ruffles the surface of the water in irregular patches during a calm **2** [fr. the fable of the monkey that used a cat's paw to draw chestnuts from the fire] : one used by another as a tool : DUPE **3** : a hitch in the bight of a rope so made as to form two eyes into which a tackle may be hooked — see KNOT illustration

cat·sup \'kech-əp, 'kach-; 'kat-səp\ *n* [Malay *kĕchap* spiced fish sauce] (1690) : a seasoned tomato puree

cat·tail \'kat-,tāl\ *n* (1548) : any of a genus (*Typha* of the family Typhaceae, the cattail family) of tall reedy marsh plants with brown furry fruiting spikes; *esp* : a plant (*Typha latifolia*) with long flat leaves used for making mats and chair seats

cat·tery \'kat-ə-rē\ *n, pl* **-ter·ies** (1834) : an establishment for the breeding and boarding of cats

cat·tle \'kat-ᵊl\ *n pl* [ME *catel*, fr. ONF, personal property, fr. ML *capitale*, fr. L, neut. of *capitalis* of the head — more at CAPITAL] (13c) **1** : domesticated quadrupeds held as property or raised for use; *specif* : bovine animals on a farm or ranch **2** : human beings esp. en masse

cattle call *n* (1952) : a mass audition (as of actors)

cattle egret *n* (ca. 1899) : a small white egret (*Bubulcus ibis*) with a yellow bill and in the breeding season buff on the crown, breast, and back that has been introduced into the eastern U.S. from the Old World

cattle grub *n* (1926) : any of several heel flies esp. in the larval stage; *esp* : COMMON CATTLE GRUB

cat·tle·man \-mən, -,man\ *n* (1864) : a man who tends or raises cattle

cattle tick *n* (1869) : a tick (*Boophilus annulatus*) that infests cattle in the southern U.S. and tropical America and transmits the causative agent of Texas fever

cat·tleya \'kat-lē-ə; kat-'lā-ə, -'lē-\ *n* [NL, fr. Wm. *Cattley* †1832 Eng. patron of botany] (1828) : any of a genus (*Cattleya*) of tropical American epiphytic orchids with showy hooded flowers

[1]**cat·ty** \'kat-ē\ *n, pl* **catties** [Malay *kati*] (1598) : any of various units of weight of China and southeast Asia varying around 1⅓ pounds; *also* : a standard Chinese unit equal to 1.1023 pounds

[2]**catty** *adj* **cat·ti·er; -est** (1903) **1** : resembling a cat; *esp* : slyly spiteful : MALICIOUS **2** : of or relating to a cat — **cat·ti·ly** \'kat-ᵊl-ē\ *adv* — **cat·ti·ness** \'kat-ē-nəs\ *n*

cat·ty–cor·ner *or* **cat·ty–cor·nered** *var of* CATERCORNER

cat·walk \'kat-,wȯk\ *n* (1885) : a narrow walkway (as along a bridge)

Cau·ca·sian \kȯ-'kā-zhən, -'kazh-ən\ *adj* (1807) **1** : of or relating to the Caucasus or its inhabitants **2 a** : of or relating to the white race of mankind as classified according to physical features **b** : of or relating to the white race as defined by law specif. as composed of persons of European, No. African, or southwest Asian ancestry — **Caucasian** *n* — **Cau·ca·soid** \'kȯ-kə-,sȯid\ *adj or n*

Cau·chy sequence \kō-,shē-\ *n* [Augustin-Louis *Cauchy* †1857 Fr. mathematician] (1955) : a sequence of elements in a metric space such that for any positive number no matter how small there exists a term in the sequence for which the distance between any two consecutive or nonconsecutive terms beyond this term is less than an arbitrarily small number

[1]**cau·cus** \'kȯ-kəs\ *n* [prob. of Algonquian origin] (1763) : a closed meeting of a group of persons belonging to the same political party or faction usu. to select candidates or to decide on policy; *also* : a group of people united to promote an agreed-upon cause

[2]**caucus** *vi* (1788) : to hold or meet in a caucus

Pronunciation Key

One of the dictionary's functions is to help you pronounce unknown words. You learn pronunciation by consulting the *pronunciation key.* In some dictionaries the pronunciation key can be found at the bottom of each page, in others on the inside front cover, and in still others on a page near the front of the book. Check the dictionary's table of contents if you are having trouble locating the pronunciation key. If you need to buy a new dictionary, you may want to consider one with a pronunciation key at the bottom of each page. This format will help you check pronunciation easily.

Following is the pronunciation key found at the bottom of each page in *Webster's Ninth New Collegiate Dictionary:*

\ə\ **abut** \ᵊ\ **kitten,** F table \ər\ **further** \a\ **ash** \ā\ **ace** \ä\ **cot, cart**
\au̇\ **out** \ch\ **chin** \e\ **bet** \ē\ **easy** \g\ **go** \i\ **hit** \ī\ **ice** \j\ **job**
\ŋ\ **sing** \ō\ **go** \ȯ\ **law** \ȯi\ **boy** \th\ **thin** \th̲\ **the** \ü\ **loot** \u̇\ **foot**
\y\ **yet** \zh\ **vision** \á, k̲, ⁿ, œ, œ̅, ue, ue̅, ʸ\ *see* Guide to Pronunciation

As you can see, it consists of symbols (diacritical marks) and simple words. Parts of it are printed in boldface. Look more closely at one entry:

\ī\ **ice**

This tells you that when you are reading the pronunciation portion of a dictionary entry and you see the symbol ī, you pronounce that "i" as you would say the word "ice." For a further illustration, consider the following:

bīl

Again, this diacritical mark is pronounced like the "i" in "ice." Pronounce the "i" sound, and you come up with the word for liver secretion—bile.

Now look at a more difficult word:

gī̲n-ə̲-kä̲l-ə̲-Jē̲

Referring back to the pronunciation key, try to figure out the pronunciation of the underlined letters.

ī = like the "i" in **ice**
ə = like the "a" and the "u" in **abut**
ä = like the "o" in **cot**
ə = like the "a" and the "u" in **abut**
j = like the "j" in **job**
ē = like the "ea" in **easy**

The word is *"gynecology"*—the branch of medicine that deals with women's health.

EXERCISE 6–3

Directions. Use the pronunciation key above to determine the correct spelling and pronunciation of the following words. Write the word in the space provided.

1. ā-ort-ə ____________________
2. kə-rē-ə ____________________
3. dī-(y)ə-ret-ik ____________________
4. hī-pə-gas-trik ____________________
5. fȧs-fāt ____________________

6. spī-nə bĭ-fed-ə ____________________

7. tĕk-nŏl-ō-jĭst ____________________

8. kŏn-vō-lū-shŭn ____________________

9. dĭs-grăf-ĭ-ă ____________________

10. mer-kū-rē ____________________

Comprehending? Yes ___ No ___

Multiple Definitions

Many medical and nonmedical terms have more than one meaning. When a word has multiple definitions, the individual meanings in the entry will be numbered. It is important that you choose the correct definition for your purpose when you are using the dictionary to determine the meaning of an unknown word. To do this you must consider how the unknown word is used in the sentence. For example, you may read the word "callus" in the following context or sentence:

She got a *callus* on her heel from walking barefoot.

You check your medical dictionary and you see two definitions: 1. localized hyperplasia of the horny layer of the epidermis due to pressure or friction. 2. an unorganized network of woven bone formed about the ends of a broken bone (Miller and Keane, p. 237).

From the sentence, the context clues "heel" and "walking barefoot" let you know that you are not concerned with broken bones, but rather with roughened skin from going shoeless. The first definition is the more appropriate. Again, when searching for the correct definition of an unknown word, make sure the meaning fits the sense of the sentence.

EXERCISE 6–4

Directions. Following are sentences with an unknown word or phrase in boldface. Read the sentence and determine the correct use of the word. Then look up the definition in the page from *Webster's Ninth New Collegiate Dictionary* shown on p. 70. In the blank, write the number of the correct definition.

1. The doctor's **succinct** way of talking made him easy to listen to.

____

2. The child dropped the lemon **sucker** the pediatrician gave him.

____

3. Eventually, he will **succumb** to cancer.

____

1178 success • sudden death

suc·cess \sək-ˈses\ *n* [L *successus*, fr. *successus*, pp. of *succedere*] (1537) **1** *obs* : OUTCOME, RESULT **2 a** : degree or measure of succeeding **b** : favorable or desired outcome; *also* : the attainment of wealth, favor, or eminence **3** : one that succeeds

suc·cess·ful \-fəl\ *adj* (1588) **1** : resulting or terminating in success **2** : gaining or having gained success — **suc·cess·ful·ly** \-fə-lē\ *adv* — **suc·cess·ful·ness** *n*

suc·ces·sion \sək-ˈsesh-ən\ *n* [ME, fr. MF or L; MF, fr. L *succession-, successio*, fr. *successus*, pp.] (14c) **1 a** : the order in which or the conditions under which one person after another succeeds to a property, dignity, title, or throne **b** : the right of a person or line to succeed **c** : the line having such a right **2 a** : the act or process of following in order : SEQUENCE **b (1)** : the act or process of one person's taking the place of another in the enjoyment of or liability for his rights or duties or both **(2)** : the act or process of a person's becoming beneficially entitled to a property or property interest of a deceased person **c** : the continuance of corporate personality **d** : unidirectional change in the composition of an ecosystem as the available competing organisms and esp. the plants respond to and modify the environment ⟨the highlights of the ~ were the weed, grass, and forest communities developed in that order⟩ **3 a** : a number of persons or things that follow each other in sequence **b** : a group, type, or series that succeeds or displaces another — **suc·ces·sion·al** \-ˈsesh-nəl, -ən-ᵊl\ *adj* — **suc·ces·sion·al·ly** \-ē\ *adv*

succession duty *n, chiefly Brit* (1853) : INHERITANCE TAX

suc·ces·sive \sək-ˈses-iv\ *adj* (15c) **1** : following in order : following each other without interruption **2** : characterized by or produced in succession — **suc·ces·sive·ly** *adv* — **suc·ces·sive·ness** *n*

suc·ces·sor \sək-ˈses-ər\ *n* [ME *successour*, fr. OF, fr. L *successor*, fr. *successus*, pp.] (13c) : one that follows; *esp* : one who succeeds to a throne, title, estate, or office

suc·ci·nate \ˈsək-sə-ˌnāt\ *n* (1790) : a salt or ester of succinic acid

suc·cinct \(ˌ)sək-ˈsiŋ(k)t, sə-ˈsiŋ(k)t\ *adj* [ME, fr. L *succinctus*, pp. of *succingere* to gird from below, tuck up, fr. *sub-* + *cingere* to gird — more at CINCTURE] (13c) **1** *archaic* **a** : being girded **b** : close-fitting **2** : marked by compact precise expression without wasted words **syn** see CONCISE — **suc·cinct·ly** \-ˈsiŋ(k)-tlē, -ˈsiŋ-klē\ *adv* — **suc·cinct·ness** \-ˈsiŋt-nəs, -ˈsiŋk-nəs\ *n*

suc·cin·ic acid \(ˌ)sək-ˌsin-ik-\ *n* [F *succinique*, fr. L *succinum* amber + F *-ique* -ic] (ca. 1790) : a crystalline dicarboxylic acid $C_4H_6O_4$ found widely in nature and active in energy-yielding metabolic reactions

succinic dehydrogenase *n* (1942) : an iron-containing flavoprotein enzyme that catalyzes often reversibly the dehydrogenation of succinic acid to fumaric acid in the presence of a hydrogen acceptor and that is widely distributed esp. in animal tissues, bacteria, and yeast — called also *succinate dehydrogenase*

suc·ci·nyl \ˈsək-sən-ᵊl, -sə-ˌnil\ *n* [ISV] (ca. 1868) : either of two groups of succinic acid: **a** : a bivalent group $OCCH_2CH_2CO$ **b** : a univalent group $HOOCCH_2CH_2CO$

suc·ci·nyl·cho·line \ˌsək-sən-ᵊl-ˈkō-ˌlēn, -sə-ˌnil-\ *n* (1952) : a basic compound that acts similarly to curare and is used intravenously chiefly in the form of a hydrated chloride $C_{14}H_{30}Cl_2N_2O_4{\cdot}2H_2O$ as a muscle relaxant in surgery

[1]**suc·cor** \ˈsək-ər\ *n* [ME *succur*, fr. earlier *sucurs*, taken as pl., fr. OF *sucors*, fr. ML *succursus*, fr. L *succursus*, pp. of *succurrere* to run up, run to help, fr. *sub-* up + *currere* to run — more at CURRENT] (13c) **1** : RELIEF; *also* : AID, HELP **2** : something that furnishes relief

[2]**succor** *vt* **suc·cored; suc·cor·ing** \ˈsək-(ə-)riŋ\ (13c) : to go to the aid of : RELIEVE — **suc·cor·er** \ˈsək-ər-ər\ *n*

suc·co·ry \ˈsək-(ə-)rē\ *n* [alter. of ME *cicoree*] (1533) : CHICORY

suc·co·tash \ˈsək-ə-ˌtash\ *n* [of Algonquian origin; akin to Narraganset *msakwatas* succotash] (1751) : lima or shell beans and green corn cooked together

suc·cour \ˈsək-ər\ *chiefly Brit var of* SUCCOR

suc·cu·ba \ˈsək-yə-bə\ *n, pl* **-bae** \-ˌbē, -ˌbī\ [LL, prostitute] (1559) : SUCCUBUS

suc·cu·bus \-bəs\ *n, pl* **-bi** \-ˌbī, -ˌbē\ [ME, fr. ML, alter. of LL *succuba* prostitute, fr. L *succubare* to lie under, fr. *sub-* + *cubare* to lie, recline — more at HIP] (14c) : a demon assuming female form to have sexual intercourse with men in their sleep — compare INCUBUS

suc·cu·lence \ˈsək-yə-lən(t)s\ *n* (1787) **1** : the state of being succulent **2** : succulent feed ⟨wild game subsisting on ~⟩

[1]**suc·cu·lent** \-lənt\ *adj* [L *suculentus*, fr. *sucus* juice, sap; akin to L *sugere* to suck — more at SUCK] (1601) **1 a** : full of juice : JUICY **b** : moist and tasty : TOOTHSOME **c** *of a plant* : having fleshy tissues designed to conserve moisture **2** : rich in interest — **suc·cu·lent·ly** *adv*

[2]**succulent** *n* (1825) : a succulent plant (as a cactus)

suc·cumb \sə-ˈkəm\ *vi* [F & L; F *succomber*, fr. L *succumbere*, fr. *sub-* + *-cumbere* to lie down — more at HIP] (1604) **1** : to yield to superior strength or force or overpowering appeal or desire **2** : to be brought to an end (as death) by the effect of destructive or disruptive forces **syn** see YIELD

[1]**such** \(ˈ)səch, (ˌ)sich\ *adj* [ME, fr. OE *swilc*; akin to OHG *sulīh* such, OE *swā* so — more at SO] (bef. 12c) **1 a** : of a kind or character to be indicated or suggested ⟨a bag ~ as a doctor carries⟩ **b** : having a quality to a degree to be indicated ⟨his excitement was ~ that he shouted⟩ **2** : of the character, quality, or extent previously indicated or implied ⟨in the past few years many ~ women have shifted to full-time jobs⟩ **3** : of so extreme a degree or quality ⟨never heard ~ a hubbub⟩ **4** : of the same class, type, or sort ⟨other ~ clinics throughout the state⟩ **5** : not specified

[2]**such** *pron* (bef. 12c) **1** : such a person or thing **2** : someone or something stated, implied, or exemplified ⟨~ was the result⟩ **3** : someone or something similar : similar persons or things ⟨tin and glass and ~⟩

usage For reasons that are hard to understand, commentators on usage disapprove of *such* used as a pronoun. Dictionaries, however, recognize it as standard; all of the citations upon which our definitions of this word are based are clearly standard.

— **as such** : intrinsically considered : in itself ⟨*as such* the gift was worth little⟩

[3]**such** *adv* (bef. 12c) **1 a** : to such a degree : SO ⟨~ tall buildings⟩ ⟨~ a fine person⟩ **b** : VERY, ESPECIALLY ⟨hasn't been in ~ good spirits lately⟩ **2** : in such a way

[1]**such and such** *adj* (15c) : not named or specified

[2]**such and such** *pron* (1560) : something not specified

[1]**such·like** \ˈsəch-ˌlīk\ *adj* (15c) : of like kind : SIMILAR

[2]**suchlike** *pron* (15c) : SUCH 3

[1]**suck** \ˈsək\ *vb* [ME *souken*, fr. OE *sūcan*; akin to OHG *sūgan* to suck, L *sugere*, Gk *hyein* to rain] *vt* (bef. 12c) **1 a** : to draw (as liquid) into the mouth through a suction force produced by movements of the lips and tongue ⟨~*ed* milk from his mother's breast⟩ **b** : to draw something from or consume by such movements ⟨~ an orange⟩ ⟨~ a lollipop⟩ **c** : to apply the mouth to in order to or as if to suck out a liquid ⟨~*ed* his burned finger⟩ **2 a** : to draw by or as if by suction ⟨when a receding wave ~*s* the sand from under your feet —Kenneth Brower⟩ ⟨inadvertently ~*ed* into the . . . intrigue —Martin Levin⟩ **b** : to take in and consume by or as if by suction ⟨a vacuum cleaner ~*ing* up dirt⟩ ⟨~ up a few beers⟩ ⟨opponents say that malls ~ the life out of downtown areas —Michael Knight⟩ ~ *vi* **1** : to draw something in by or as if by exerting a suction force; *esp* : to draw milk from a breast or udder with the mouth **2** : to make a sound or motion associated with or caused by suction ⟨his pipe ~*ed* wetly⟩ ⟨flanks ~*ed* in and out, the long nose resting on his paws —Virginia Woolf⟩ **3** : to act in an obsequious manner ⟨when they want votes . . . the candidates come ~*ing* around —W. G. Hardy⟩ ⟨~*ed* up to the boss⟩ **4** *slang* : to be extremely objectionable or inadequate ⟨our lifestyle ~*s* —*Playboy*⟩ ⟨people who went said it ~*ed* —H.S. Thompson⟩

[2]**suck** *n* (13c) **1** : a sucking movement or force **2** : the act of sucking

[1]**suck·er** \ˈsək-ər\ *n* (14c) **1 a** : one that sucks esp. a breast or udder : SUCKLING **b** : a device for creating or regulating suction (as a piston or valve in a pump) **c** : a pipe or tube through which something is drawn by suction **d (1)** : an organ in various animals for adhering or holding **(2)** : a mouth (as of a leech) adapted for sucking or adhering **2** : a shoot from the roots or lower part of the stem of a plant **3** : any of numerous freshwater fishes (family Catostomidae) closely related to the carps but distinguished from them esp. by the structure of the mouth which usu. has thick soft lips **4** : LOLLIPOP **5 a** : a person easily cheated or deceived **b** : a person irresistibly attracted by something specified ⟨a ~ for ghost stories⟩ **c** — used as generalized term of reference ⟨see if you can get that ~ working again⟩

[2]**sucker** *vb* **suck·ered; suck·er·ing** \ˈsək-(ə-)riŋ\ *vt* (1661) **1** : to remove suckers from ⟨~ tobacco⟩ **2** : HOODWINK ~ *vi* : to send out suckers

suck in *vt* (15c) **1** : to contract, flatten, and tighten (the abdomen) esp. by inhaling deeply **2** : DUPE, HOODWINK

suck·ing *adj* (bef. 12c) : not yet weaned; *broadly* : very young

sucking louse *n* (ca. 1907) : any of an order (Anoplura) of wingless insects comprising the true lice with mouthparts adapted to sucking body fluids

suck·le \ˈsək-əl\ *vt* **suck·led; suck·ling** \-(ə-)liŋ\ [prob. back-formation fr. *suckling*] (15c) **1 a** : to give milk to from the breast or udder ⟨a mother *suckling* her child⟩ **b** : to nurture as if by giving milk from the breast ⟨was *suckled* on pulp magazines⟩ **2** : to draw milk from the breast or udder of ⟨lambs *suckling* the ewes⟩

suck·ling \ˈsək-liŋ\ *n* (15c) : a young unweaned animal

su·crase \ˈsü-ˌkrās, -ˌkrāz\ *n* [ISV, fr. F *sucre* sugar, fr. MF — more at SUGAR] (ca. 1900) : INVERTASE

su·cre \ˈsü-(ˌ)krā\ *n* [Sp, fr. Antonio José de *Sucre*] (1886) — see MONEY table

su·crose \ˈsü-ˌkrōs, -ˌkrōz\ *n* [ISV, fr. F *sucre* sugar] (1862) : a sweet crystalline dextrorotatory disaccharide sugar $C_{12}H_{22}O_{11}$ that occurs naturally in most land plants, is obtained from sugarcane or sugar beets, and unlike glucose and galactose does not reduce Fehling's solution to produce a colored precipitate

suc·tion \ˈsək-shən\ *n* [LL *suction-, suctio*, fr. L *suctus*, pp. of *sugere* to suck — more at SUCK] (1626) **1** : the act or process of sucking **2 a** : the act or process of exerting a force upon a solid, liquid, or gaseous body by reason of reduced air pressure over part of its surface **b** : force so exerted **3** : a device (as a pipe or fitting) used in a machine that operates by suction — **suc·tion·al** \-shən-ᵊl, -shnəl\ *adj*

suction pump *n* (1825) : a common pump in which the liquid to be raised is pushed by atmospheric pressure into the partial vacuum under a retreating valved piston on the upstroke and reflux is prevented by a check valve in the pipe

suction stop *n* (1887) : a voice stop in the formation of which air behind the articulation is rarefied with consequent inrush of air when articulation is broken

suc·to·ri·al \ˌsək-ˈtōr-ē-əl, -ˈtȯr-\ *adj* [NL *suctorius*, fr. L *suctus*, pp.] (1833) : adapted for sucking; *esp* : serving to draw up fluid or to adhere by suction ⟨~ mouths⟩

suc·to·ri·an \-ē-ən\ *n* [NL *Suctoria*, fr. neut. pl. of *suctorius* suctorial] (ca. 1842) : any of a class (Suctoria) of complex protozoans which have cilia only early in development and in which the mature form is fixed to the substrate, lacks locomotor organelles or a mouth, and obtains food through specialized suctorial tentacles

Su·dan grass \sü-ˈdan-, -ˈdän-\ *n* [the *Sudan*, region in Africa] (1911) : a vigorous tall-growing annual grass (*Sorghum vulgare sudanensis*) widely grown for hay and fodder

Su·dan·ic \sü-ˈdan-ik\ *n* [the *Sudan*] (1925) : the languages neither Bantu nor Hamitic spoken in a belt extending from Senegal to southern Sudan — **Sudanic** *adj*

su·da·to·ri·um \ˌsüd-ə-ˈtōr-ē-əm, -ˈtȯr-\ *n* [L, fr. *sudatus*, pp. of *sudare* to sweat — more at SWEAT] (1756) : a sweat room in a bath

su·da·to·ry \ˈsüd-ə-ˌtōr-ē, -ˌtȯr-\ *n, pl* **-ries** (1615) : SUDATORIUM

sudd \ˈsəd\ *n* [Ar, lit., obstruction] (1874) : floating vegetable matter that forms obstructive masses in the upper White Nile

[1]**sud·den** \ˈsəd-ᵊn\ *adj* [ME *sodain*, fr. MF, fr. L *subitaneus*, fr. *subitus* sudden, fr. pp. of *subire* to come up, fr. *sub-* up + *ire* to go — more at SUB-, ISSUE] (14c) **1 a** : happening or coming unexpectedly ⟨a ~ shower⟩ **b** : changing angle or character all at once **2** : marked by or manifesting abruptness or haste **3** : made or brought about in a short time : PROMPT **syn** see PRECIPITATE — **sud·den·ly** *adv* — **sud·den·ness** \ˈsəd-ᵊn-(n)əs\ *n*

[2]**sudden** *n, obs* (1558) : an unexpected occurrence : EMERGENCY — **all of a sudden** *or* **on a sudden** : sooner than was expected : at once

sudden death *n* (1548) **1** : unexpected death that is instantaneous or occurs within minutes from any cause other than violence ⟨*sudden death* following coronary occlusion⟩ **2** : extra play to break a tie in a sports contest in which the first to go ahead wins

4. A cactus in the hospital is a **succulent** plant.

___

5. The mother will **suckle** her baby.

___

6. The calf will **suckle** the cow.

___

7. Nurse Smith is first in line of **succession** to be dean.

___

8. The chubby man tried to **suck in** his stomach.

___

9. The **suction** on the vacuum tube was broken.

___

10. Her **sudden death** at 30 was alarming.

___

Comprehending? Yes ___ No ___

When analyzing word parts and context clues is not sufficient, having a good collegiate dictionary and a medical dictionary is crucial to your success in learning unknown words. The efficient use of a dictionary enables you to locate the meanings of unknown words effortlessly.

• GLOSSARY

The *glossary* is a collection of key words at the back of some textbooks. As in a dictionary, the entries are listed in alphabetical order, but unlike a dictionary, the glossary usually provides only the definition of the entries. Syllabication, pronunciation, etymology, date of earliest recorded use, and synonyms and antonyms are usually omitted. The advantage of looking up words in the glossary instead of a dictionary is that the glossary is handier and easier to use. Having a collection of key words and definitions in the back of your textbook saves invaluable time when you need to learn a new word. The disadvantage of a glossary, however, is that it is usually limited to definitions of the key terms in the textbook. If you need to learn the meaning of a word that the author hasn't selected as a "key" or "major" word, you will not find it in the glossary. Also, if you need to know more than just the definition of an unknown word, for example, the pronunciation, the glossary may not be useful. However, if your book has a glossary, we recommend that you look there first to define unknown words after word part and context analysis fail.

Group process: The identifiable structural development of the group that is needed for a group to mature. (12)

Group think: Fear of expressing conflicting ideas and opinions because loyalty to the group and approval by other group members has become so important. (12)

Health: A broad concept that is used to describe an individual's state of well-being and level of functioning. (1)

Health teaching: A flexible, person-oriented process in which the helping person provides information and support to clients with a variety of health-related learning needs. (16)

High-risk nursing diagnosis: A state for which the client is at high risk and that is validated by the presence of risk factors (formerly referred to as "potential" diagnosis). (23)

Holistic construct: The unified whole of a person, with each functional aspect of self-concept fitting together, and each single element affecting all other parts. (3)

Homeostasis: A person's sense of personal security and balance. (20)

I–Thou relationship: A relationship in which each individual responds to the other from his or her own uniqueness and is valued for that uniqueness in a direct, mutually respected, reciprocal alliance. (1)

Individuation: Finding and acknowledging all parts of oneself; being true to one's nature. (1)

Informed consent: Assurance that the client fully understands what is happening or is about to happen in his or her health care and knowingly consents to care. (16)

Intercultural communication: Communication in which the sender of a message is a member of one culture and the receiver is from a different culture. (11)

Interpersonal: Between two or more people. (14)

Interpersonal competence: The ability to interpret the content of a message from the point of view of each of the participants and the ability to use language and nonverbal behaviors strategically to achieve the goals of the interaction. (9)

Interpersonal process record: A three-part record of the nurse–client interaction: (1) a written anecdotal record of the client's and the nurse's words as well as their nonverbal behavior; (2) a written analysis of the interaction, identifying communication skills and interventions; and (3) written suggestions for making more effective comments. (23)

Intrapersonal: Within a particular individual. (14)

Intrinsic values: Values that relate to the maintenance of life, such as eating to survive. (7)

Laissez-faire attitude: Allowing others to do as they please without intervening. (7)

Laissez-faire leadership: The style in which the leader provides little or no structure and essentially abdicates leadership responsibilities. (22)

Leadership: Interpersonal influence, exercised in situations and directed through the communication process, toward the attainment of a specified goal or goals. (12)

Leveling: Communication that is healthy and direct. (13)

Linear communication: An activity involving the transmission of messages by a source to a receiver for the purpose of influencing the receiver's behavior. (1)

Lived experience: The personal meaning of an experience as described by the person experiencing it. (3)

Maintenance functions: Group role functions that foster the emotional life of the group. (12)

Medical model of health: Health as the absence of signs and symptoms of disease or injury. (15)

Message: A verbal or nonverbal expression of thoughts or feelings intended to convey information to the receiver and requiring interpretation by that person. (1)

Message competency: The ability to use language and nonverbal behaviors strategically to achieve the goals of the interaction. (9)

Metacommunication: All of the factors that influence how a message is received. (9)

Metaphor: An anecdote in which one idea or object is substituted for another in a way that implies their similarity. (10)

Modeling: The transmission of values by presenting oneself in an attractive manner and living by a certain set of values, hoping that others will follow one's lead; teaching by performing a behavior that another observes. (7, 16)

Moral dilemma: *See* **Ethical dilemma.** (7)

Moral distress: A feeling that occurs when one knows what is "right" but is bound to do otherwise because of legal or institutional constraints. (7)

Moral uncertainty: Difficulty deciding which moral rules (values, beliefs, etc.) apply to a given situation. (7)

Moralizing: The transference of the values of the parents directly onto the child. (7)

Morphostasis: The tendency of a system to want to stay the same. (13)

Motivation: The forces that activate behavior and direct it toward one goal instead of another. (12)

Multiculturalism: A term used to describe a heterogeneous society in which diverse cultural worldviews can coexist with some general characteristics shared by all cultural groups and some perspectives that are unique to each group. (11)

Mutuality: Agreement on problems and the means for resolving them; a commitment by both parties to enhance well-being. (5)

EXERCISE 6–5

Directions. A portion of a glossary taken from a nursing textbook (Arnold and Boggs, p. 568) is shown on page 72. Following are five statements with a term in boldface. Read the statement. Then locate the term in the glossary. In the space provided after the statement, write "T" if the statement is true according to the entry in the glossary and "F" if the statement is false according to the entry in the glossary.

1. **Leveling** is indirect communication. ____________
2. **Individuation** is being true to oneself. ____________
3. **Health** is a specific term that describes how someone behaves. ____________
4. **Homeostasis** refers to balance. ____________
5. **Metaphor** implies similarity. ____________

• THESAURUS

The *thesaurus* is a collection of words and their synonyms (different words that have the same meaning). In most cases the thesaurus is written in dictionary form. Therefore, you would look up an entry the same way you would in your collegiate or medical dictionary. However, instead of giving the definition of a word, the thesaurus groups together all words that have similar meanings. The main purpose of the thesaurus is to aid you in your writing. When you are doing a written assignment, you may find yourself using the same words repeatedly, or you may need a new word with a slightly different meaning. Consulting the thesaurus will help you solve these writing problems.

Reading a Thesaurus Entry

Below is an example of an entry from *Roget's New Pocket Thesaurus in Dictionary Form* (p. 285):

Nurse, N. attendant, medical, RN
(MEDICAL SCIENCE)

Note that the entry word is in boldface type and is followed by the part of speech.

In this example "nurse" is what part of speech?

After this, three synonyms are given for "nurse." The entry ends with a term in capital letters and parentheses (MEDICAL SCIENCE). This is an alternative entry to look up if the original entry does not provide you with the synonym you need.

Once you have acquired a thesaurus, you will find it one of the most valuable references for good writing. Keep it in a convenient place in your study area so it will be available when you need it. Remember to use it when you need a better word choice.

pass, defile, cut, **gap,** neck, gully, passage, gorge.

V. **notch,** nick, mill, score, cut, dent, indent, jag, **scarify,** scallop, gash, crimp; crenelate.

Adj. **notched,** crenate, scalloped, dentate, toothed, **palmate,** serrate, serrated, serriform, **sawlike;** machicolated, castellated.

See also HOLLOW, INTERVAL, PASSAGE. *Antonyms*—See SMOOTHNESS.

---

note, *n.* letter, communication, message (EPISTLE); memorandum (MEMORY); bill, paper money (MONEY); jotting, record (WRITING); commentary, annotation (EXPLANATION).

note, *v.* write, jot down (WRITING); observe, remark, notice (LOOKING); distinguish, discover (VISION).

notebook, *n.* diary, daybook (RECORD).

noted, *adj.* eminent, renowned (FAME).

nothing, *n.* nil, zero, cipher (NONEXISTENCE).

nothingness, *n.* nullity, nihility, void (NONEXISTENCE).

notice, *n.* announcement, proclamation, manifesto (INFORMATION); handbill, poster, circular (PUBLICATION); caution, caveat, admonition (WARNING).

notice, *v.* remark, observe, perceive (VISION, LOOKING).

noticeable, *adj.* conspicuous, marked, pointed (VISIBILITY).

notify, *v.* inform, let know, acquaint (INFORMATION).

notion, *n.* impression, conception, inkling (UNDERSTANDING, IDEA); concept, view (OPINION); fancy, humor, whim (CAPRICE).

notorious, *adj.* infamous, shady, scandalous (DISREPUTE, FAME).

notwithstanding, *adv.* nevertheless, nonetheless, however (OPPOSITION).

nourish, *v.* feed, sustain, foster, nurture (FOOD).

nourishing, *adj.* nutrient, nutritive, nutritious (FOOD).

nourishment, *n.* nutriment, foodstuff, sustenance (FOOD).

nouveau riche (*F.*), *n.* parvenu, *arriviste* (*F.*), upstart (SOCIAL CLASS, WEALTH).

novel, *adj.* fresh, off-beat (*colloq.*), unusual (UNUSUALNESS); original, Promethean (NEWNESS); unique, atypical (DIFFERENCE).

novel, *n.* fiction, novelette, novella (STORY).

novelist, *n.* fictionist, anecdotist (WRITER).

novelty, *n.* freshness, recency, originality; original, *dernier cri* (*F.*), wrinkle (NEWNESS); item, conversation piece (MATERIALITY).

novice, *n.* beginner, tyro, neophyte (BEGINNING, LEARNING); novitiate, postulant (RELIGIOUS COMMUNITY).

now, *adv.* **at this time,** at this moment, at present (PRESENT TIME).

noxious, *adj.* virulent, unhealthy (HARM); unwholesome, pestiferous, pestilent (IMMORALITY).

nozzle, *n.* spout, faucet (EGRESS, OPENING).

nuance, *n.* shade of difference (DIFFERENCE); implication, suggestion (MEANING).

nucleus, *n.* heart, hub, focus (CENTER); meat, pith, principle (PART).

nude, *adj.* stripped, naked, bare (UNDRESS).

nudge, *v.* push, poke, prod (PROPULSION).

nudity, *n.* nakedness, denudation, exposure (UNDRESS).

nuisance, *n.* gadfly, terror, pest (ANNOYANCE).

nullify, *v.* annul, disannul, invalidate (INEFFECTIVENESS).

numb, *adj.* dazed, torpid, stuporous (INSENSIBILITY).

numb, *v.* dull, blunt, obtund (INSENSIBILITY).

number, *n.* amount (QUANTITY); numeral (NUMBER); song (SINGING).

NUMBER—*N.* **number,** symbol, character, numeral, figure, statistic, Arabic number, cipher, digit, integer, whole number, folio, round number; cardinal number, ordinal number, Roman number; decimal, fraction; infinity, googol; numerator, denominator; prime number.

sum, difference, product, quotient; addend, summand, augend; dividend, divisor; factor, multiple, multiplicand, faciend, multiplier; minuend, subtrahend, remainder; total, summation, aggregate, tally; quantity, amount.

ratio, proportion, quota, percentage; progression, arithmetical progression, geometric progression.

power, root, exponent, index, logarithm.

numeration, notation, algorism, cipher, algebra; enumeration, count, tally, census, poll; statistics; numerology.

V. **count,** enumerate, numerate, reckon, tally; count down, tell, tell out (off, *or* down).

page, number, foliate, paginate, mark.

Adj. **numeral,** numerary, numeric, numerical; **numbered,** numerate.

proportional, commeasurable, commensurate, proportionate.

See also ADDITION, COMPUTATION, LIST, MULTITUDE, QUANTITY, TWO, THREE, ETC.

---

numbers, *n.* scores, heaps, lots (MULTITUDE).

numberless, *adj.* countless, innumerable, myriad (MULTITUDE, ENDLESSNESS).

numeral, *n.* symbol, character, figure (NUMBER).

numerical, *adj.* numeral, numerary (NUMBER).

numerous, *adj.* many, multitudinous, abundant (MULTITUDE, FREQUENCE)

nun, *n.* sister, *religieuse* (*F.*), vestal, vestal **virgin** (RELIGIOUS COMMUNITY, UNMARRIED STATE).

nunnery, *n.* convent, abbey, cloister (RELIGIOUS COMMUNITY).

nuptial, *adj.* matrimonial, marital, conjugal (MARRIAGE).

nurse, *n.* attendant, medic, R.N. (MEDICAL SCIENCE).

nurse, *v.* attend, tend, care for (CARE); suck, suckle, lactate (BREAST).

nursery, *n.* day nursery, crèche (CHILD); garden, greenhouse, hothouse (FARMING); cradle, childhood, infancy (YOUTH).

nurture, *v.* feed, nourish, sustain (FOOD); care for, cherish, foster (CARE).

nuthouse (*slang*), *n.* lunatic asylum, madhouse (INSANITY).

nutritious, *adj.* nourishing, wholesome (FOOD, HEALTH).

nutty (*slang*), *adj.* potty (*colloq.*), touched, crazy (INSANITY).

nuzzle, *v.* nestle, snuggle, cuddle (PRESSURE, REST).

nymph, *n.* dryad, hamadryad, hyad (GOD).

nymphomania, *n.* erotomania, andromania (SEX).

O

oaf, *n.* lummox, lout, gawky (CLUMSINESS); boob, nincompoop, blockhead (FOLLY).

oar, *n.* paddle, scull (SAILOR).

oath, *n.* curse, curseword, swearword (MALEDICTION, DISRESPECT); affidavit, deposition (AFFIRMATION); word of honor, vow (PROMISE).

OBEDIENCE—*N.* **obedience,** observance, conformance, conformity, accordance, compliance, docility, servility, subservience, tameness.

[*one who demands obedience*] **disciplinarian, martinet,** authoritarian, precisian.

[*obedient person*] **servant,** minion, myrmidon, slave.

discipline, training; military discipline, blind obedience.

V. **obey,** observe, comply, conform, submit; mind, heed, do one's bidding, follow orders, do what one is told; behave.

discipline, train, **tame;** enforce, compel, force; put teeth in.

Adj. **obedient,** compliant, compliable, observant, law-abiding; dutiful, duteous; orderly, quiet, docile, meek, manageable, tractable, biddable, well-behaved; submissive, servile, subservient, tame.

disciplinary, strict, stern, authoritative, authoritarian.

See also DUTY, FORCE, OBSERVANCE, SLAVERY, SUBMISSION, TEACHING. *Antonyms*—See DISOBEDIENCE, NONOBSERVANCE.

---

obese, *adj.* paunchy, pursy, fat (SIZE).

obey, *v.* observe, comply, submit (OBEDIENCE).

object, *n.* thing, article, commodity (MATERIALITY); matter, phenomenon, substance (REALITY); mission, objective, end (PURPOSE).

object, *v.* demur, protest, remonstrate (OPPOSITION, UNPLEASANTNESS).

objection, *n.* exception, demurral (OPPOSITION); dislike, disesteem (HATRED).

objectionable, *adj.* displeasing, distasteful, unpalatable (UNPLEASANTNESS, HATRED); exceptionable, opprobrious (DISAPPROVAL).

objective, *adj.* impartial, unprejudiced, unbiased (IMPARTIALITY); actual, concrete, material (REALITY).

objective, *n.* mission, object, end (PURPOSE).

object of art, *n.* *bibelot* (*F.*), *objet d'art* (*F.*), curio (ORNAMENT).

object to, *v.* dislike, have no stomach for, be displeased by, protest (HATRED, UNPLEASANTNESS).

obligate, *v.* indebt, bind, astrict (DEBT).

EXERCISE 6–6

Directions. On page 74 are copies of pp. 284 and 285 from *Roget's New Pocket Thesaurus in Dictionary Form.* Read the following short passage with words in boldface. After referring to the thesaurus pages, choose a better word for each boldface word and print it above the boldface term. Make sure the part of speech for the synonym matches the original word. The first word is done for you.

jot down

The nurse drew out her notebook from the desk in the station. She wanted to **note** some of the happenings she **noticed** during her shift. In particular the **nurse** wanted to object to some of the **objectionable** occurrences on the floor. However, she wanted to be **objective,** so the **objective** of her observation would not be to **object** to the other nurse, but to get him to change his **notions** on what it is to **nurse** a patient.

• VOCABULARY CHECK

Directions. Below are 10 words taken from the key words section of this chapter. Circle the letter of the best definition from the four choices.

1. Unabridged
- **a** condensed
- **b** complete
- **c** inaccurate
- **d** unfinished

2. Incision
- **a** sharp tooth
- **b** foolish ideas
- **c** a knife
- **d** a surgical cut

3. Collegiate
- **a** referring to college
- **b** referring to a column
- **c** referring to a professor
- **d** referring to classrooms

4. Bulimia nervosa
- **a** bile secretions
- **b** an eating disorder
- **c** the endocrine system
- **d** a fear of pregnancy

5. Synonyms
a words that are opposites
b words that sound the same but have different meanings
c words that are contradictory
d different words that mean the same

6. Myxorrhea
a flow of mucus
b flow of blood
c flow of hormones
d flow of fluids

7. Antonyms
a words that are opposites
b words that sound the same but have different meanings
c words that are contradictory
d different words that mean the same

8. Pathogen
a study of blood diseases
b factor following path of oxygen in lungs
c disease-producing agent
d path of blood circulation

9. Specialized
a designed for one particular purpose
b having been put to a specific use
c related to the unconventional
d written in a unique way

10. Gynecology
a branch of medicine that deals with women's health
b the inner reproductive organ of a flower
c the study of women's roles in medicine
d the philosophy that deals with women's rights

• CRITICAL THINKING LOG

List the strategies you learned in this chapter.	Select the strategy that is most useful for your school success.	How can you apply this strategy to your nursing studies?

• SUMMARY

Using word-part analysis and context clues as tactics for learning unknown words can be helpful but may not be appropriate in all instances. It may be necessary to consult a dictionary, glossary, or thesaurus for help with new words. A collegiate dictionary is particularly useful for learning pronunciation, parts of speech, etymology, word meaning, and in some cases synonyms and antonyms. A medical dictionary is best for helping you with specialized vocabulary encountered in nursing school. The glossary of a textbook is convenient for finding the meanings of key words in the textbook. The thesaurus is helpful for choosing a better word for your writing. All these references are invaluable to your task of building a better vocabulary for nursing school success.

CHAPTER 7

Word Bank

• OBJECTIVE

To learn a method for remembering the definitions of new words.

• KEY WORDS

Pay attention to the following key words, which are underscored the first time they appear in this chapter. Try to determine the meaning of these words from the surrounding words in the passage. If you need further help, use your dictionary or the glossary in the back of this book. As you read the exercises in this chapter, write additional words you need to learn in the space provided.

GENERAL VOCABULARY

arbitrary	reinforce
conversely	repertoire
deposit	variety
flexibility	______________
idioms	______________
maximize	______________
portable	______________

• ENCOUNTERING UNKNOWN WORDS

In nursing school you encounter many unknown words, both medical and general. During lectures and clinical experiences you constantly hear new terms and phrases. As you read your textbooks, for both nursing and liberal arts courses, you come across more unfamiliar words. Even when socializing and conversing with your fellow nursing students, you hear words and expressions you do not understand. When this happens, do not ignore these new terms but instead indicate the words you need to learn.

• INDICATING UNKNOWN WORDS

During lectures, copy any unknown words from the board and mark them with a question mark (?). This signal will indicate that you should look these words up later in a dictionary or glossary. Similarly, when you are reading your textbooks, place a question mark over any unknown vocabulary terms. When you finish reading that section, take a brief break and check the definitions of the unknown words in your dictionary or glossary. Even when you are with your friends in nursing school, you should not be embarrassed to ask them to explain the meanings of any expressions you do not understand. Remember that you all have the same goal—increasing your vocabulary to maximize your nursing school success. Carry a small notebook with you so you can jot down new expressions and idioms.

• REMEMBERING NEW WORDS

Once you have the meaning of a new word, write the definition in your lecture notes, textbook margin, or notebook. This will ensure that you have a record of the word meaning. But this written note won't be sufficient to help you learn and remember the word. To learn a new medical term or general vocabulary word, you must have a strategy to help you memorize its meaning. This method should allow you to visualize the word repeatedly to reinforce the learning until you can remember the word and it becomes a natural part of your speaking and reading repertoire.

• CREATING YOUR WORD BANK

An excellent means of learning new words is to create a word bank. To do this, buy a package of index cards on which one side is ruled and the other side blank.

On the blank side, clearly write the unknown word. You may find it helpful to write the pronunciation underneath the word. Use a pronunciation key that you understand, either one you make up yourself or one copied from a dictionary. Make sure that the pronunciation key you use will help you say the word correctly.

On the ruled side of the index card, write the precise definition of the word. Underneath the definition, use the word in a sentence, either your own or one copied from the textbook. This way, when you refer to the card later, you will be reminded of how the word is actually used. See Figure 7–1.

What you have created is a flashcard with which you can practice new words over and over again. The word is on one side of the flashcard, and its definition is on the other side. The first advantage of the word bank is that it is personalized. These are words that you decide you need to know, not some arbitrary list of words assigned to you by an instructor.

The second advantage of the word bank is that it is portable. Put a rubber band around your cards and you can carry them anywhere. You can use the cards to practice learning new words anytime, on the subway to nursing school, during a lunch break, or while waiting for a doctor's appointment. At home you should "deposit" your words in a file or container to which you can add more new words as you encounter them.

A third advantage of the word bank is its variety. Try to be creative in its use. For instance, show yourself the word side and quiz yourself by supplying the definition. Or

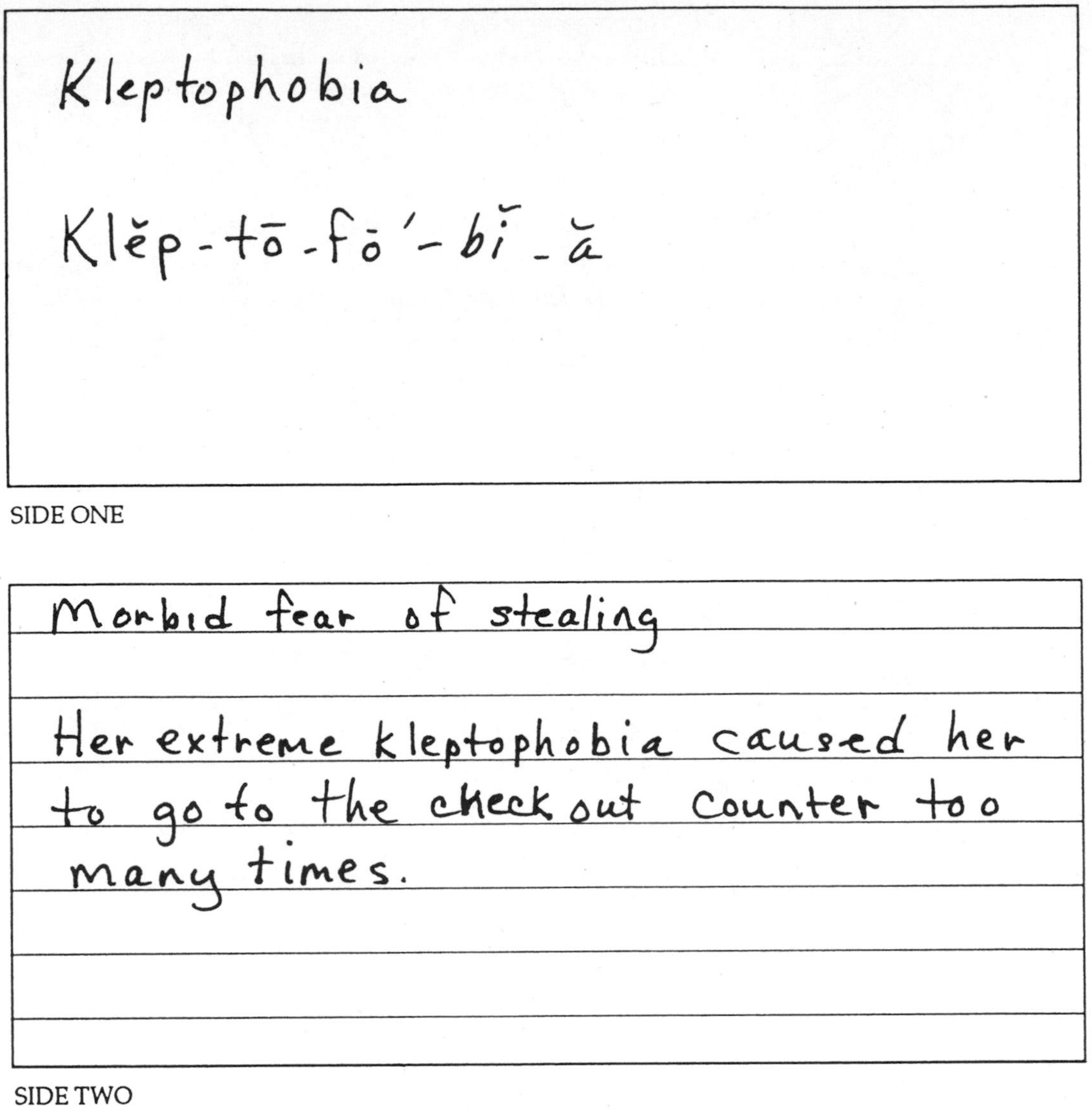

Kleptophobia

Klĕp-tō-fō′-bĭ-ă

SIDE ONE

Morbid fear of stealing

Her extreme kleptophobia caused her to go to the check out counter too many times.

SIDE TWO

Figure 7–1 Sample item for word bank.

conversely, look at the definition and try to recall the correct word. Be imaginative. Create games that will help you memorize the meanings of these words as pleasantly as possible. Learning vocabulary does not have to be a chore.

The last advantage of the word bank is its flexibility. The index card format allows you to group the words according to your needs. For instance, you can place all the new terms learned in a lecture on pediatrics with any other pediatric terms you came across when reading in your textbook on the same subject. You can also separate words you have learned very well from those that still need more work or that you don't know at all.

Considering the simplicity of making a word bank and all of its advantages, this is one of the richest ways of developing vocabulary appropriate for nursing school. Use your word bank daily and you will be wealthier for it.

EXERCISE 7–1

Directions. From this textbook or any of your other books, choose 25 words you don't know. Create the beginning of a word bank, using the example in the illustration. Practice learning these words by following the suggestions from this chapter or invent your own ways of learning the meanings of unknown words.

• VOCABULARY CHECK

Directions. Below are 10 words taken from the key words section of this chapter. Circle the letter of the best definition from the four choices.

1. Arbitrary
- **a** pertaining to judging or determining
- **b** pertaining to settling a controversy
- **c** pertaining to sale of securities
- **d** pertaining to individual preference or convenience

2. Deposit
- **a** to place in safekeeping
- **b** to remove from authority
- **c** to build railroads
- **d** to testify under oath

3. Idioms
- **a** ideas related to a specific field
- **b** people who are not bright
- **c** language peculiar to a people or class
- **d** specific grammars

4. Portable
- **a** pertaining to a seaport
- **b** capable of being carried
- **c** the ability to dock a ship
- **d** stationary

5. Repertoire
- **a** a drama series
- **b** a list or supply of capabilities
- **c** constant repetition
- **d** a series of tricks or stunts

6. Conversely
- **a** ability to talk on a social level
- **b** ability to change or adapt
- **c** able to carry from place to place
- **d** reversed in order, relation, or action

7. Flexibility
 a capability of making a brief movement
 b ability to strike with a light motion
 c ability to lengthen or strengthen
 d capability to adapt to new requirements

8. Maximize
 a to relate a proverb
 b to adjust the upper jaw
 c to make the most of
 d to make the least of

9. Reinforce
 a to make someone bend to one's will
 b to strengthen by additional assistance
 c to create again in a more permanent manner
 d to act in a decisive way

10. Variety
 a having different forms
 b having similar forms
 c having possession of the truth
 d having ability to change

• CRITICAL THINKING LOG

List the strategies you learned in this chapter.	Select the strategy that is most useful for your school success.	How can you apply this strategy to your nursing studies?

• SUMMARY

In this chapter you were reminded to indicate any new words you come across while listening to class lectures, reading your textbooks, or talking with classmates. Techniques for indicating unknown words include marking these words with a question mark indicating the words you need to learn. You can look up these words in the dictionary or glossary to get their precise meanings. So that you will remember these words and make them a natural part of your vocabulary, you were taught how to make a word bank using index cards and how to use these cards to increase your word knowledge.

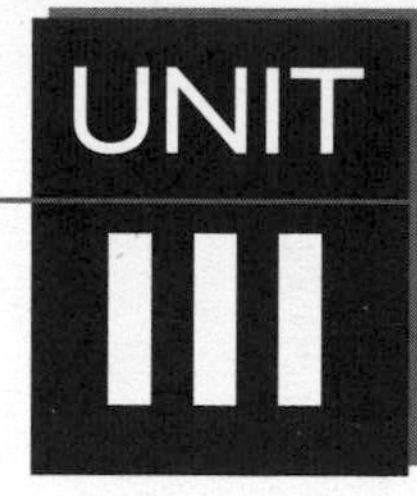

UNIT III READING COMPREHENSION

One of your major responsibilities in nursing school is to read and comprehend your textbooks with ease. Unless you have this ability, your reading assignments will take a long time to complete and will seem incomprehensible. Unit III, "Reading Comprehension," introduces the skills that will help you read the information in your textbooks with greater understanding and efficiency.

Chapter 8, "Topics and Main Ideas," teaches you to focus on the subject and main point of a passage. Chapter 9, "Details," helps you to identify the important facts that relate to the main idea. Chapter 10, "Paragraph Organization," illustrates how following patterns of organization will help you to concentrate on, comprehend, and retain textbook organization.

Once you have mastered the strategies for organizing textbook information, you can read and comprehend your nursing textbooks with less effort and greater clarity. Improved reading comprehension thus depends on your ability to organize ideas. Unit III, "Reading Comprehension," provides the comprehension strategies needed for success in nursing school.

CHAPTER 8

Topics and Main Ideas

• OBJECTIVE

To learn to identify the topics and main ideas in textbook material as an aid to concentration and comprehension.

• KEY WORDS

Pay attention to the following words, which are underscored the first time they appear in this chapter. Try to determine the meaning of these words in the passage. If you need further help, use your dictionary or the glossary. As you read the exercises in this chapter, write additional words you need to learn in the spaces provided.

MEDICAL TERMINOLOGY	GENERAL VOCABULARY
affect	assert
Alzheimer's disease	autonomy
asthma	gestures

diaphoresis	mandates
edema	objective
generativity	ombudsmen
hypotension	retirement
inguinal hernia	shrugging
nitroglycerin	spiritual
pallor	validation
______________	______________
______________	______________
______________	______________
______________	______________

• IMPROVING CONCENTRATION

You may find your mind wandering while reading your textbooks. Staying focused is sometimes difficult. Reading with a purpose gives direction to your reading. Your objective should be to find the topics and main ideas. Check yourself as you read. As you do exercises, pay attention to your reading attention span. Did you concentrate throughout the chapter? Did you have any concentration problems? If so, where? Looking for the topics and main ideas keeps you involved with your reading. Keep track of your reading concentration. Stay on task and use identifying the topics and main ideas as a strategy to improve your reading concentration and comprehension.

• FINDING THE TOPIC

The topic of a reading selection is its subject. It is *who* or *what* is being talked about. You should identify the topic as the first step toward comprehending the content of any reading selection. The topic is the general subject, and the details in the reading passage fit under it. Practice finding the topic in lists of words.

EXAMPLE 8–1

sight senses hearing touch smell

Which of the items in this series is the *topic?* The answer is *senses.* All the other items—hearing, touch, smell, and sight—are specific senses that fit under this general topic.

EXERCISE 8–1

Directions. Select the topic in each list of words:

1. pointing ______________________
   gestures
   nodding
   shrugging
   waving

2. inspection ______________________
   auscultation
   palpation
   percussion
   examination

3. systems ______________________
   respiratory
   gastrointestinal
   cardiovascular
   neurologic

4. rough ______________________
   smooth
   leathery
   thin
   texture

5. depth ______________________
   measurements
   color
   description
   odor

Comprehending? Yes ___ No ___

You have now practiced putting specific details under a general topic. Identifying the topic is a first step to finding the *main idea* in any reading selection. Look for the topic when reading paragraphs or longer selections. Ask *who* or *what* the selection is about.

• SELECTING THE CORRECT TOPIC

The following exercise will help you to choose the correct topic. When determining the topic of a passage, your answer choice should cover the information in the passage. In other words, do not select answer choices that are:

- *Too broad.* The answer covers more than what is discussed in the passage.
- *Too narrow.* The answer reflects a detail of the passage and does not cover the entire topic.
- *Not mentioned.* The answer is not discussed in the passage.

EXAMPLE 8–2

Directions. Read the following selections and state whether each answer choice is too broad, too narrow, not mentioned, or the correct topic.

The preschool years lay the groundwork for moral and spiritual development. Most theorists believe that children are initially amoral, or without knowledge of right and wrong. They learn morals (or mores) from significant others, peers, television, books, and so on. Spiritual beliefs come from teachings by significant others and formal or informal religious training, and are highly related to moral development. Feedback (both positive and negative) from significant others, as well as individual cognitive development, influences a child's moral and spiritual development. Young children tend to rely on authority figures for information about good and bad. If mother says it, it must be right. They also evaluate their own behavior by the consequences. If they were punished, the behavior must have been wrong. Therefore, young children may engage in behaviors if they know they will not be caught. If not punished, the behavior is not wrong. (Bolander, 3rd ed., p. 201)

a Preschool years of children
b Children's moral and spiritual development during preschool years
c Feedback from significant others
d Discipline problems during preschool years

Choice **a** is too broad. More can be said about play-age years than is discussed in this passage. Choice **b** is correct; it most precisely defines the ideas in the passage. Choice **c** is just one detail in the passage, so it is too narrow. Choice **d** is not discussed in this passage.

• IDENTIFYING THE TOPIC IN PARAGRAPHS

EXERCISE 8–2

Directions. Read the following paragraphs and state whether each answer choice is too broad, too narrow, not mentioned, or the correct topic.

1. Adolescence is marked by profound changes, not only in accelerated physical growth but also in cognitive ability, social expectations, and personality development. As a result, the adolescent faces many choices that distinguish adolescence as a unique stage in human development on the way to independence. (Bolander, 3rd ed., p. 210)

   a Accelerated physical growth during adolescence
   b Changes during adolescent years
   c Stress of early childhood
   d Adolescent years

2. The developmental stage associated with middle adulthood is Erikson's stage of generativity versus stagnation. Generativity implies productivity and creativity for self as well as others. Generative people expand interests and responsibilities. They are involved and accept leadership roles in their careers, communities, social and religious activities, politics, and cultural and artistic efforts. They are concerned with creating something that will be

lasting and worthwhile for future generations. The generative person has a sense of parenthood and takes pride in guiding the next generation. This means caring about children as well as assisting them to become independent young adults. (Bolander, 3rd ed., pp. 229–230)

a Creativity
b Problems during retirement years
c Definition of generativity
d Life's work during adult years

3. Adolescents experiment with alcohol and drugs for many reasons. They may feel insecure or anxious, and drugs give them confidence by releasing some inhibitions. Others may feel more mature by engaging in "adult" behaviors or may be rebelling against their parents. While many parents feel that using a substance once is considered an experiment, we know that "once" with some of these substances can kill. Many famous actors and actresses are now appealing to youths to discourage experimenting with crack cocaine even once. Drug abuse by minors may be a sign of some deeper psychologic disturbance and should be identified as soon as possible so treatment options can be explored. (Bolander, 3rd ed., p. 214)

a Substance abuse
b Substance abuse by health professionals
c Reasons for teenage involvement with substance abuse
d Releasing inhibitions in teenagers

4. Deciding to become parents usually depends on whether or not the young adults have accomplished their developmental tasks. Pregnancy and parenthood also depend on adequate physical, psychologic, and social development that allows the couple to deal with the requirements of this developmental period. Having children outside of marriage is not as taboo as it once was. When young women get pregnant today, they have many choices. It is not unusual for a young woman to choose to raise her child alone and not be disowned by her parents, as might have happened years ago. (Bolander, 3rd ed., p. 221)

a Choices about pregnancy
b Raising children alone
c Pregnancy
d Birth control to avoid pregnancy

5. Many people look forward to retirement with relief. They have never found fulfillment in their work and now no longer have to endure the constraints of full-time employment. They now have an opportunity for choices. Probably the most powerful factors in retirement satisfaction are health status, sufficient income, and the option to continue working if one wants to. (Bolander, 3rd ed., p. 240)

a Satisfaction during retirement
b Difficulty during work
c Difficulty when fired from a job
d Satisfaction

Comprehending? Yes ___ No ___

EXERCISE 8–3

Directions. Read the following selections and establish the correct topic by asking yourself *who* or *what* the selection is about.

1. While assessing a client, the nurse accumulates a large volume of data. The nurse may find it extremely difficult to manage this volume in total. The classification process begins following the nursing assessment and allows the nurse to develop more manageable categories of information. It also stimulates discrimination between data, which helps the nurse to focus on data that are pertinent to the client's needs. (Iyer et al., 3rd ed., p. 96)

The topic is ______________________________

2. The final step in data processing is validation. In this phase, the nurse attempts to verify the accuracy of the data interpretation. This is most often accomplished through direct interaction with the client or significant other(s), consultation with other health care professionals, or comparison of data with an authoritative reference. (Iyer et al., 3rd ed., p. 102)

The topic is ______________________________

3. The ability to formulate a nursing diagnosis is dependent on an accurate and complete data base. Several factors may interfere with the collection of data. These may include communication problems, withholding information, and distractions or interruptions. (Iyer et al., 3rd ed., p. 106)

The topic is ______________________________

4. Even when the nurse and client speak the same language, either may use language that confuses the other. The client's age, environment, or cultural background may involve the use of expressions that are foreign to the nurse. (Iyer et al., 3rd ed., p. 106)

The topic is ______________________________

5. It is now recommended that nurses carry their own malpractice insurance policies in addition to whatever coverage may be provided by their employer. One of the reasons for having personal insurance is the need for coverage for actions outside of the employment setting, such as private duty nursing and giving advice to neighbors. Some nurses believe that if they are covered by an employer's policy and money is paid out on a claim, the employer's insurance company will try to collect this sum from the nurse. This is a misconception and is untrue. Insurance companies work hard to maintain a good relationship with those they insure and are not interested in trying to obtain a nurse's assets. (Iyer et al., 3rd ed., p. 330)

The topic is ______________________________

Comprehending? Yes ___ No ___

• FINDING THE TOPIC AS AN AID TO CONCENTRATION

Many students find it difficult to concentrate while reading textbooks. They have problems maintaining their focus. Establishing the topic of a reading selection will help you to concentrate on the passage.

EXERCISE 8–4

Directions. Read the following selection and establish the precise topic to help you concentrate while reading.

Four types of data are collected by the nurse during assessment: subjective, objective, historical, and current. A complete and accurate data base usually includes a combination of these types. (Iyer et al., 3rd ed., p. 36–38)

Subjective data might be described as the individual's perspective of a situation or a series of events. This information cannot be determined by the nurse independent of interaction or communication with the individual. Subjective data are frequently obtained during the nursing history and include the client's perceptions, feelings, and ideas about self and personal health status. Examples include the client's descriptions of pain, weakness, frustration, nausea, or embarrassment. Information supplied by sources other than the client—e.g., family, consultants, and other members of the health care team—may also be subjective if based on the individual's opinion rather than substantiated by fact.

In contrast, objective data consist of observable and measurable information. This information is usually obtained through the senses—sight, smell, hearing, and touch—during the physical examination of the client. Examples of objective data include respiratory rate, blood pressure, presence of edema, and weight.

During the assessment of a client, you must consider both subjective and objective findings. Frequently, these findings substantiate each other, as in the case of John Thomas, the client whose incision opened three days after surgery. The subjective information provided by Mr. Thomas, "feels like my stitches are popping," was validated by the nurse's objective findings: pallor, diaphoresis, hypotension, and protrusion of the bowel through the incision.

Example. You observe Peggy Malletts crying as she stands in front of the nursery two days after the premature delivery of her first child. You suggest that Peggy seems "upset," and the client validates that she is "afraid that her baby might die."

Here, the objective data you observe (crying) is substantiated by subjective data obtained from the client (feelings of fear).

At times, subjective and objective data may be in conflict.

Example. Casey Smithson is a 15-year-old client in your eating disorders clinic. She is 5 ft, 5 in. tall and weighs 82 lb. Her blood pressure is 80/50, her pulse rate is 62, and her skin is dry with little turgor. Casey looks malnourished; however, when you ask her how she is feeling, she pinches a fold of skin and replies, "Fat! Look at this roll—I just have to lose weight."

Clearly, your objective data—height, weight, vital signs, and appearance—are in conflict with the client's subjective expression of feeling "fat." Therefore you must discuss your findings with the client in an effort to resolve the discrepancy.

Another consideration when describing data concerns the element of time. In this context, data may be either historical or current (Bellack and Bamford, 1984). Historical data consist of situations or events that have occurred in the past. These data are particularly important in identifying the client's normal health patterns and in determining past experiences that may impact on the client's current health status. Examples of historical data might include previous hospitalizations or surgery, ECG results, normal elimination patterns, or chronic diseases.

Example. As a community health nurse, you visit John Kelly, age 62, at his home to teach him how to change a dressing on his abdominal burn. When you begin writing out the directions for him, the client says, "I can't read. I left school after the first grade to help my father on the farm."

In this case, John's educational background (historical data) influences your assessment of his ability to follow written instructions for changing his dressing.

In contrast, current data refer to events that are occurring now. Examples might include blood pressure, vomiting, or postoperative pain. These data are particularly important in your initial assessment and in reassessments to compare current information with previous data to determine the client's progress.

Example. Kelly O'Keefe, age 5, is admitted for tonsillectomy. In the immediate postoperative period, her pulse rate ranges from 90 to 108. Four hours later, the nurse observes that Kelly is swallowing frequently and her pulse rate is 124.

In this situation, current data (pulse rate 124) and frequent swallowing substantiate the existence of a problem (bleeding) when compared with historical data (pulse rate 90 to 108).

For the data base to be complete, you should collect all four types of data. Subjective and objective data provide specific information regarding the client's health status and help to identify problems. Additionally, current and historical data assist in this process by establishing time frames or usual behavioral patterns.

The topic is ______________________________

Comprehending? Yes ___ No ___

• DETERMINING THE MAIN IDEA

Once you have learned to identify the topic, you can next identify the main idea in a reading selection. The main idea answers the question, "What is being said about the topic or subject?"

Finding the main idea is an important method for understanding what you read. Consider the following example.

EXAMPLE 8–3

Long-term care (LTC) units are areas within or adjacent to the hospital in which clients have chronic illnesses or health problems requiring constant care and rehabilitation. Examples are rehabilitation and chronic disease units. Some hospitals also offer a skilled nursing facility (SNF), or nursing home, as part of the in-hospital system. In long-term care units, some clients can learn how to help themselves, whereas other clients are at their optimal level of wellness, which must be maintained. (Ignatavicius and Bayne, 2nd ed., p. 20)

As you just learned, to determine the topic of a passage you ask the question, "*Who* or *what* is this passage mostly about?" In this example you would answer, "Long-term care units." To find the main idea you must further develop the topic. You do this by asking a second question, "What is the most important point that is being made about the topic?" The answer to this second question is the main idea. Look again at the preceding example. We said the topic of this passage was **long-term care units.** What is the most important point being made about rehabilitation centers? The most important point being made about long-term care units is that **they provide care to patients with chronic illness or who need long term constant care.** Which sentence in the example states this? Look again at the first sentence. "Long-term care (LTC) units are areas within or adjacent to the hospital in which clients have chronic illnesses or health problems requiring constant care and rehabilitation." The first sentence in this passage is the main idea sentence.

Read the following examples, keeping in mind the two questions for determining the topic and the main idea:

1. Who or what is this passage mostly about? = topic
2. What is the most important point that is being made about the topic? = main idea

The topic is shown in the margin, and the main idea is boldface in the examples here.

EXAMPLE 8–4

Mental patients' rights

1. **Some states, recognizing mental patients' inability to assert their own rights effectively in the psychiatric setting, have developed ombudsmen programs for mental patients.** State law in California mandates an independent patient advocate, and New York provides for mental health legal services. Both programs assure that patients' constitutional rights are protected and that their expressed interests are represented. (Varcarolis, 2nd ed., p. 51)

Trust between nurse and client

2. **Clients can also jeopardize the trust a nurse has in them.** Sometimes, clients may "test" a nurse's trustworthiness. They may try to send the nurse on unnecessary errands or talk endlessly about superficial topics. As long as nurses recognize testing behaviors and set clear limits on their role and the client's role, it is possible to develop trust. (Arnold and Boggs, 2nd ed., pp. 109–110)

Formulating outcomes with client's input

3. **After nursing diagnoses are established, outcomes are formulated with the client's input.** The involvement of the client in outcome development increases the potential for individualization of nursing interventions. Likewise, after nursing interventions are formulated, they are reviewed with the client. Frequently, clients will participate more actively in their care if their ideas have been solicited. Many clients, as consumers, are demanding a greater say in discussions about health care and are assuming a more active role in making these decisions. (Iyer et al., 3rd ed., p. 191)

EXERCISE 8–5

Directions. Read each of the short passages below. In the space provided indicate the topic and write the main idea. Remember to ask the following questions:

1. Who or what is this passage mostly about? = topic
2. What is the most important point that is being made about the topic? = main idea

1. The three major types of angina pectoris are stable (classic) angina, unstable (crescendo, preinfarction, progressive) angina, and variant (Prinzmetal's) angina. These types differ with regard to severity and frequency of attacks, refractoriness of the pain, and typical precipitants of the pain. Stable angina, the most common type, is usually precipitated by physical exertion or emotional stress, lasts 3 to 5 minutes, and is relieved by rest and nitroglycerin. In all types of angina, the pain usually occurs in the retrosternal area; may or may not radiate; and is described as heaviness or a pressing, squeezing, burning, or choking sensation. (Ulrich, 3rd ed., p. 330)

   Topic: ______________________________

   Main Idea: ______________________________

2. Care for a client with dementia, especially Alzheimer's disease, requires a great deal of patience, creativity, and maturity. The needs of such a client can be enormous for nursing staff and for families who care for their loved ones in the home. As the disease progresses, so do the needs of the client and the demands on the caregivers, staff, and family. (Varcarolis, 2nd ed., p. 562)

   Topic: ______________________________

   Main Idea: ______________________________

3. Churches and other religious institutions serve the elderly in many ways. In addition to their primary role of providing organized worship, they sponsor many activities that bring elderly together with their peers as well as with younger people. Clergypersons, rabbis, and other spiritual leaders are often excellent counselors, and other members of the congregation or religious group are often willing to help older members in time of trouble. (Ignatavicius and Bayne, 2nd ed., p. 76)

   Topic: ______________________________

   Main Idea: ______________________________

4. *Autonomy* is an important component of person-centered communication. Applying this concept means that the nurse leaves decision making to the client whenever possible and supports the client's decision unless there is a chance harm will be done to the client or others. With a clear understanding of the person's needs, the nurse recommends treatment options and gives the client sound reasons for the recommendations. It is up to the client to decide whether or not to follow the recommendations. Control and decision making are left in the client's hands in an interdependent nurse-client relationship. (Arnold and Boggs, 2nd ed., p. 82)

   Topic: ______________________________

   Main Idea: ______________________________

5. Initially, nurses working with antisocial clients may find them charming and intelligent. After a while, nurses react with frustration and anger when these individuals resist or defy their assistance. As clients continue to test the limits of the treatment program or to manipulate others, including the staff, nurses experience increased anger, disappointment, helplessness, and despair. It is sometimes difficult to understand how a person who is reasonably intelligent repeatedly gets into trouble with family, friends, employers, and the law. Crimes include theft, embezzlement, forgery, robbery, rape, and other acts of violence. Often, the nurse's response when hearing about these crimes is moralistic condemnation and contempt. (Varcarolis, 2nd ed., p. 382)

   Topic: ______________________________

   Main Idea: ______________________________

Comprehending? Yes ___ No ___

• LOCATING THE MAIN IDEA

In the preceding examples and exercises, the main idea was located at the beginning of each passage. The main idea sentence was the first sentence in each passage, followed by details or examples. However, this will not always be the case. The main idea sentence can be found in several places in the passage besides the beginning. Look at some of these other places. In the following examples, the topic is written in the space provided and the main idea sentence is in boldface type.

End of the Passage

Sometimes the main idea sentence is the last sentence of the paragraph. When this is so, the writer begins the paragraph with details and the main idea sentence at the end draws together all the facts.

EXAMPLE 8–5

Although expression of emotion can occur verbally, it is more often and more truly communicated nonverbally through facial expression and behaviors such as smiling, laughing, frowning, striking out, and crying. Specific physiological changes in the body such as a quickening of the heartbeat, blushing, headache, muscle tension, or relaxation accompany the experience and expression of strong emotion. **Thus, there is a close connection between physical and emotional expressions of personal identity.** (Arnold and Boggs, 2nd ed., p. 59)

Topic: *Nonverbal expressions of emotion*

Middle of the Passage

Another place to look for the main idea sentence is in the middle of the passage. Often writers begin a passage with interesting facts or details to capture the reader's interest. Then they insert the main idea sentence and finally end the selection with more details to support the main idea.

EXAMPLE 8–6

Biofeedback can be an effective treatment when obvious signs of stress, such as headaches, high blood pressure, muscle tension, and heart palpitations, occur frequently, are debilitating, or may be dangerous. **Biofeedback works by training the client to reverse the subtle changes that lead to a somatic, or physical, response.** For instance, if a headache is the result of muscle tension in the forehead, the client can be trained to relax that tension before a headache results. (Ignatavicius and Bayne, 2nd ed., p. 114)

Topic: *Biofeedback as an effective treatment*

Beginning and End of the Passage

In some cases the main idea is found both at the beginning and at the end of the paragraph. As shown in the first examples introducing the main idea, the paragraph begins with the general main idea sentence, followed by specific details that support the main idea. However, now the paragraph also ends with a main idea sentence that reiterates or restates in different words the idea or ideas expressed in the first main idea sentence.

EXAMPLE 8–7

Trust, however, can be broken. An alcoholic or abusive parent who is gentle one minute and explodes with anger the next leaves children and others unsure of how the parent will behave. The community health nurse who is inconsistent about keeping client appointments and the pediatric nurse who indicates falsely that an injection will not hurt are jeopardizing client trust. **It is hard to maintain trust when one person cannot depend on another.** (Arnold and Boggs, 2nd ed., p. 109)

Topic: *Difficulty in maintaining trust*

• FINDING THE UNSTATED MAIN IDEA

Many times you will read a paragraph that has no main idea sentence. Instead, the passage will consist of only a series of details, facts, or examples. In this situation it is your responsibility to create the main idea sentence. You use the same strategy you used to find the main idea—asking the two questions:

1. Who or what is this passage mostly about? = topic
2. What is the most important point being made about the topic? = main idea

EXAMPLE 8–8

Calling friends and family on the telephone, encouraging visitors, and socializing with others who are in the hospital may reflect the client's use of social support as a coping strategy. Talking with others about what has occurred may reflect the use of event review. (Ignatavicius and Bayne, 2nd ed., p. 111)

1. Who or what is this passage mostly about? *Patients using coping strategies* = topic
2. What is the most important point being made about coping strategies? Clients use socialization as a coping strategy to deal with illness and hospitalization = main idea sentence

EXERCISE 8–6

Read the following short passages. Determine the topic and write it in the space provided. Underline the main idea. If there is no main idea sentence, create your own in the space provided.

1. It is not unusual for a student or practicing nurse to suspect negligence on the part of a peer. In most states, nurses have a legal duty to report such risks of harm to the patient. It is also very important that the nurse document clear and accurate evidence before making serious accusations against a peer. If the nurse questions a physician's orders or actions, or those of a fellow nurse, it is wise to communicate these concerns directly to the person involved. If the risky behavior continues, the nurse has an obligation to communicate these concerns to a supervisor, who should then intervene to ensure that the patient's rights and well-being are protected. If a nurse suspects a peer of being chemically impaired or practicing irresponsibly, the nurse has an obligation to protect not only the rights of the peer but also the rights of all patients who could be harmed by this impaired peer. If, after the nurse has reported suspected behavior of concern to a supervisor, the danger persists, the nurse has a duty to report the concern to someone at the next level of authority. It is important to follow the channels of communication in an organization, but it is also important to protect the safety of the patients. If the supervisor's actions or inactions do not rectify the dangerous situation, the nurse has a continuing duty to report the behavior of concern to the appropriate authority, such as the state board of nursing. (Varcarolis, 2nd ed., p. 59)

Topic: ______________________________

Unstated main idea: ______________________________

____

2. Silence is used to accent an important point in a verbal communication. By pausing briefly after presenting a key idea and before proceeding to the next topic, the nurse encourages the client to notice the most important elements of the communication. Brief silence following an important verbal message dramatizes the significance of the nurse's statement. (Arnold and Boggs, 2nd ed., pp. 219–220)

Topic: ______________________________

Unstated main idea: ______________________________

3. Approximately 10% to 20% of the adult asthmatic population suffer from extrinsic asthma, i.e., asthma that is caused by allergenic exposure (e.g., to pollens, molds, dust, or animal dander). Extrinsic asthma results in bronchoconstriction, edema, and increased mucus production. Approximately 50% of adult asthmatics have intrinsic asthma, which is precipitated by nonallergenic factors, such as viral infection, exercise, cold, cigarette smoke, changes in temperature or humidity, gasoline fumes, and paint fumes. Emotional stress seems to exacerbate an attack but may not have a primary etiologic role. In some adults, both allergenic and nonallergenic factors may trigger asthma attacks. (Ignatavicius and Bayne, 2nd ed., p. 536)

Topic: ______________________________

Unstated main idea: ______________________________

4. Taking responsibility for oneself increases with age. In later childhood, most children become better able to work verbally with the nurse. It still is important to prepare responses carefully and to anticipate problems, but the child is capable of expressing feelings and ventilating frustration more directly through words. (Arnold and Boggs, 2nd ed., p. 425)

   Topic: ____

   Unstated main idea: __________________________________

5. A person who is depressed sees the world through "gray-colored" glasses. Staff and others often observe that posture is poor; the client may look older than his or her stated age. Facial expressions reflect sadness and dejection, and the person may have frequent bouts of weeping. Conversely, a client may say that he or she is unable to cry. Feelings of hopelessness and despair are readily reflected in the person's affect. (Varcarolis, 2nd ed., p. 428)

   Topic: ____

   Unstated main idea: __________________________________

Comprehending? Yes ____ No ____

• READING WITH A PURPOSE

You can now focus on the topic and main idea as aids to concentration when doing textbook assignments. You will be reading with a purpose, which is to create and locate the topic and main idea. Reading with a purpose reduces distractions and helps you to focus on what you are reading.

EXERCISE 8–7

Read the following excerpt from a nursing textbook (Iyer et al., 3rd ed., pp. 341–343). Think about the topic and underline the main idea of each paragraph. Then, in the space provided, write the topic and main idea of the entire reading.

1. The nurse is often placed in the role of client advocate in order to protect the rights of clients. An *advocate* is one who protects the rights of another. You act as a client advocate in many ways, including obtaining resources or information for the client, contacting the physician when there is a change in the client's condition, or lobbying for improved health care. While it is important for the nurse to understand the points contained in the Code for Nurses, the nurse needs more substance in order to make ethical decisions. Ethical theories describe approaches for resolving dilemmas commonly faced by nurses. "Philosophers, beginning with Socrates, Plato, and Aristotle, have for centuries attempted to answer two major questions of ethics: What is the meaning of right and of good? What ought I to do?" Ethical theories help answer these questions.
2. There are two major ethical theories used to help nurses resolve health care dilemmas: deontology and utilitarianism. The *deontologic* approach states that the rightness or wrongness of actions is determined by how the interventions conform to a rule. For instance, breaking a promise to a client would be considered wrong. Deontologists use rules

because they are right, irrespective of the consequences they may produce in a particular situation. When the nurse makes a moral judgment in one given situation, the nurse will make the same judgment in any similar situation regardless of time, place, and persons involved.

3. One of the flaws with this approach is that most situations have extenuating circumstances. For example, in some instances it would be better to break than to keep a promise: You may be asked to keep a promise not to reveal that the client has brought a quart of whiskey to the hospital. After thinking it over, you realize that it is better to break the promise so that you can protect the client from the consequences of consuming alcohol while being treated in the hospital.
4. The *utilitarian* approach states that actions are right or wrong on the basis of the consequences of the actions. This philosophy defines "good as happiness or pleasure and right as maximizing the greatest good and least amount of harm for the greatest number of persons. This position assumes that one can weigh and measure harm and benefit and come out with the greatest possible balance of good over evil for most people."
5. Utilitarians focus on the results of actions rather than on their motivations. According to this approach, the nurse would weigh the consequences of telling the truth. Other factors may take priority, such as the nurse's own survival or the continuation of the system for the benefit of future clients. In this case the nurse may not tell the truth in preference to other interests that promote greater happiness. This view is quite different from the deontologic position, which would maintain that the nurse must tell the truth without exception.

Topic: ______________________________

Main idea: ______________________________

____

____

____

Comprehending? Yes ___ No ___

• VOCABULARY CHECK

Directions. Below are 10 words taken from the key words section of this chapter. Circle the letter of the best definition from the four choices.

1. Pallor
   a redness of skin
   b faint condition
   c lack of iron
   d paleness of skin

2. Spiritual
   a concerned with secular values
   b concerned with religious values
   c concerned with good health
   d concerned with material values

3. Hypotension
   - **a** raised blood pressure
   - **b** lowered blood pressure
   - **c** elevated stress
   - **d** reduction of stress

4. Retirement
   - **a** withdrawal from one's position or occupation
   - **b** disability insurance for nonworkers
   - **c** the state of disliking work
   - **d** condition of aging

5. Asthma
   - **a** a vaccine to prevent sexually transmitted disease
   - **b** a condition caused by spasmodic contraction of the bronchi
   - **c** a serious but never fatal disease
   - **d** a cure for a chronic illness

6. Assert
   - **a** to reply with vigor
   - **b** to argue in a passive manner
   - **c** to state or declare positively
   - **d** to take back a statement

7. Nitroglycerin
   - **a** a heart attack caused by stress and overexertion
   - **b** an allergic reaction to medicine
   - **c** a medically useful chemical that is also well known as an explosive
   - **d** a potentially addictive sleeping pill prescribed for insomnia

8. Autonomy
   - **a** self-directing freedom
   - **b** to be dependent on others
   - **c** rule by a monarchy
   - **d** rule by a governing board

9. Inguinal hernia
   - **a** hernia occurring in the groin
   - **b** hernia surgery
   - **c** a treatment for hernia
   - **d** hernia occurring in the stomach

10. Gestures
   - **a** the expressing of inner thoughts as a means of communication
   - **b** the use of motions of the limbs or body as a means of expression
   - **c** the use of colorful speech as a means of expression
   - **d** the use of hidden actions as a means of miscommunication

• CRITICAL THINKING LOG

List the strategies you learned in this chapter.	Select the strategy that is most useful for your school success.	How can you apply this strategy to your nursing studies?

• SUMMARY

You have learned that the first step toward reading comprehension is identifying the precise topic. The topic answers the question, "Who or what is being talked about in the selection?" Your statement of the topic should not be too broad or too narrow. It should cover the subject discussed in the passage. Focusing on the topic will help you to concentrate on your textbook assignments.

You have also learned that the most important point being made about the topic is the main idea. The main idea sentence can be found in any of the following locations in the passage:

- The beginning
- The end
- The middle
- The beginning and end
- Unstated—you create your own main idea

Finding the topic and main idea in your reading will help you to concentrate on and comprehend the most essential information in your nursing textbooks.

CHAPTER 9

Details

• OBJECTIVE

To learn how details relate to the main idea, how to distinguish between important and unimportant details, and how to recognize five types of details:

- Data
- Cause
- Procedure
- Example
- Description

• KEY WORDS

Pay attention to the following key words, which are underscored the first time they appear in this chapter. Try to determine the meaning of these words from the surrounding words in the passage. If you need further help, use your dictionary or the glossary in the back of this book.

Look up the medical terminology in your medical dictionary or the glossary. As you read the exercises in this chapter, write additional words you need to learn in the space provided.

MEDICAL TERMINOLOGY	GENERAL VOCABULARY
benign	abuse
cancer	anonymity
DNA	core
hyponatremia	elaborate
immune system	exacerbation
medulla	feedback
midbrain	major
mutations	minor
remission	overwhelmed
spinal cord	support
______________________	______________________
______________________	______________________
______________________	______________________

• GETTING THE FACTS

Looking through your nursing textbook, you have undoubtedly noticed how much information is to be found on each page. Perhaps your initial reaction is one of feeling overwhelmed. You may ask yourself: Which of these facts am I supposed to learn? How does one fact relate to another fact or to the main idea of the passage? How will these facts help me to understand the information in this textbook?

Learning what facts, or *details,* are all about will assist you in many ways. First, your reading comprehension will improve once you see how details relate to the bigger picture, or *main idea,* of a selection. Second, your textbook note-taking and highlighting will improve once you know which details are important. Third and most important, you will be able to study more efficiently so you will do better on your nursing school exams.

• HOW DETAILS RELATE TO THE MAIN IDEA

The function of all details in any passage is to support the main idea. This means that the details will further describe or elaborate on the important point that the main idea is making. The role of details is to help you grasp or visualize more fully what the main idea is stating.

Consider this statement taken from a nursing textbook: All types of people may be involved in helping individuals in crisis. (Varcarolis, p. 241)

Certainly this is an interesting statement and, in itself, serves as the main idea of the paragraph. But it leaves out a lot of information: Who are these people who help others in crisis? How do these people help others in crisis? By reading the rest of the paragraph from the same nursing textbook, which provides the details, you get answers to these questions:

For example, people from various professional backgrounds are trained in crisis intervention—police, teachers, welfare workers, clergy, social workers, psychologists, as well as nurses. Crisis intervention is often practiced unwittingly by people without formal training such as bartenders, concerned bystanders, friends and neighbors. People can play a crucial role in the successful resolution of a crisis by responding spontaneously with concern and caring. (Varcarolis, p. 241)

By reading the details of this passage you can see how details support and give greater scope to the main idea.

• MAJOR AND MINOR DETAILS

Although the role of details is to support the main idea, giving a greater understanding of the essential point of the passage, not all details do so in the same way. Some important, or major, details relate directly to the main idea, as explained above. However, there are other, less important details that do not relate directly to the main idea but instead support or describe a major detail. These details are minor details. Below is a diagram that illustrates these relationships:

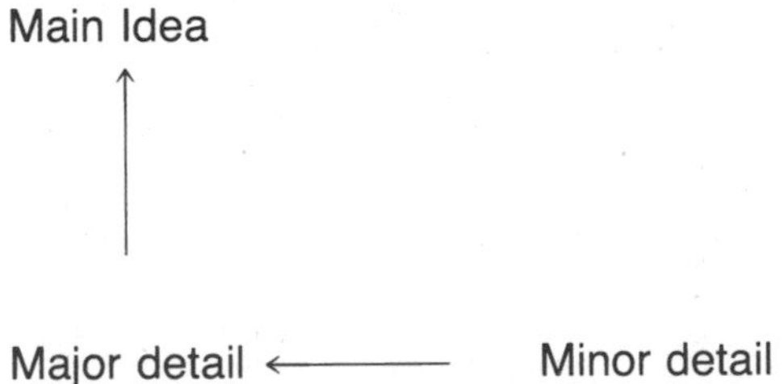

EXAMPLE 9–1

Read the following paragraph from a nursing text. The main idea is in boldface type.

Several theories have been developed to explain the complexity of pain. Early theories emphasized the recognition of specific pathways of pain transmission. Later theories attempted to uncover the complexity of central processing of pain in specific areas of the brain. More recently, the concept of pain-modulating network was introduced. This concept describes the various links and connections in the spinal cord and brain, specially the medulla and the midbrain. The identification of chemical mediators involved in the pain response, has helped in an understanding of pain transmission and perception. (Ignatavicius and Bayne, p. 120)

Following are two diagrams of how the major and minor details from this passage relate to the main idea. The diagrams help you visualize how the major details support the main idea and how the minor details support the major details. You will see in a concrete way how details are organized.

GENERAL DIAGRAM

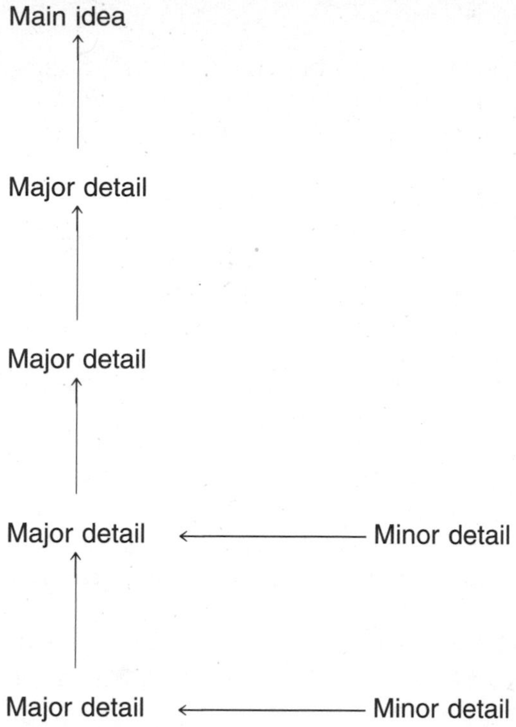

Main idea

↑

Major detail

↑

Major detail

↑

Major detail ← Minor detail

↑

Major detail ← Minor detail

DETAILS DIAGRAM

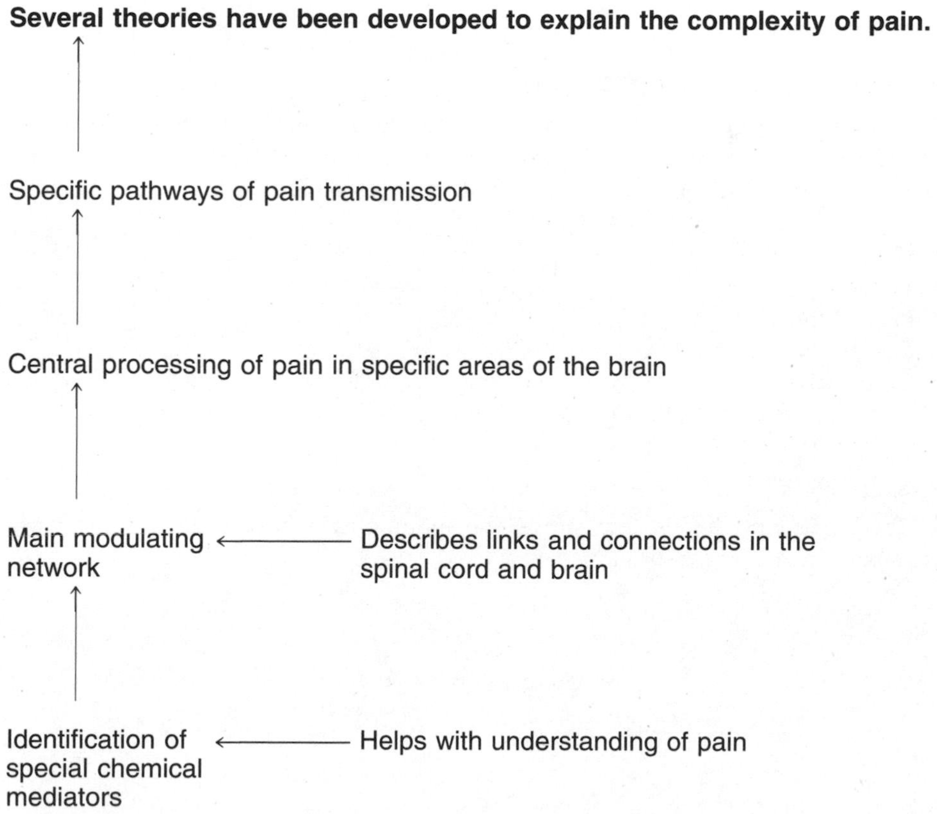

Several theories have been developed to explain the complexity of pain.

↑

Specific pathways of pain transmission

↑

Central processing of pain in specific areas of the brain

↑

Main modulating network ← Describes links and connections in the spinal cord and brain

↑

Identification of special chemical mediators ← Helps with understanding of pain

EXERCISE 9–1

Directions. Read the following paragraph on multiple sclerosis (MS) from a nursing textbook. Study the general diagram, then create a details diagram based on the ideas in the selection. Do this in the space provided.

Four types of MS are seen:

- Benign
- Exacerbation-remission
- Chronic relapsing, or progressive
- Chronic progressive, or combined

Of clients with MS, 20% have the benign type. Those with benign MS present with few episodes of mild attacks; there is minimal or no disability.

The classic picture of the exacerbation-remission type occurs in 25% of the cases of MS and is characterized by increasing frequent attacks. The course of the disease may be mild or moderate, depending on the degree of disability.

Chronic relapsing, or progressive, MS occurs most frequently. It is characterized by the absence of periods of remissions. Progressive, cumulative symptoms and deterioration occur during several years.

Chronic progressive, or combined, MS is similar to chronic relapsing MS, but its initial presentation is more insidious. At some point, it converts to a progressive course without periods of remission. (Ignatavicius et al., p. 1198)

Comprehending? Yes ___ No ___

• FIVE TYPES OF DETAILS

Details, both major and minor, support the main idea in different ways. These details relate to and elaborate on the main idea in their own unique fashion. What results are five different styles of paragraphs. The five types of details are:

- Data
- Cause
- Procedure
- Example
- Description

Data

Data details are details that prove the main idea. These details consist of facts with numbers, percentages, or statistics.

GENERAL DIAGRAM

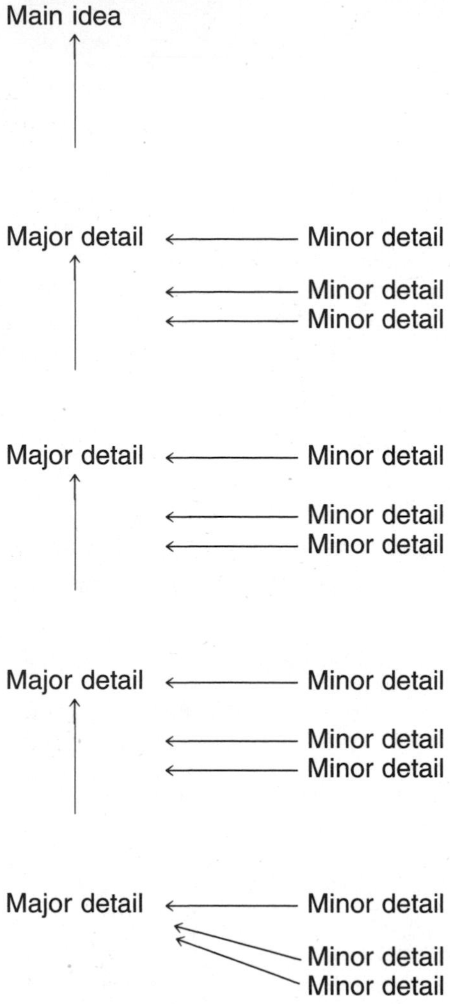

Main idea
↑

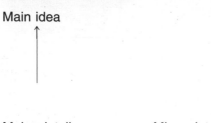

Major detail ← Minor detail
↑ ← Minor detail
← Minor detail

Major detail ← Minor detail
↑ ← Minor detail
← Minor detail

Major detail ← Minor detail
↑ ← Minor detail
← Minor detail

Major detail ← Minor detail
← Minor detail
← Minor detail

DETAILS DIAGRAM

EXAMPLE 9–2

Read the example below from a nursing text and pay attention to the boldface data details.

Because interpersonal abuse occurs most often within families, it is not easy to document the actual incidence or prevalence of this problem. It has been estimated that **half of all Americans** have experienced violence in their families. Battering is the single largest cause of injury to women in the United States. . . . Between 1976 and 1987, the number of reports of child abuse and neglect increased **225%**. . . . Abuse of infants is one of the leading causes of postneonatal mortality. . . . It has been estimated that over **1 million older Americans annually,** or **more than one in 10 elderly persons** living with a family member, are mistreated. (Varcarolis, p. 256)

Cause

Cause details are details that explain why something is happening or has happened. They give reasons and answer the question, "Why?"

EXAMPLE 9–3

Read the following excerpt, especially noting the boldface cause details.

Advancing age is probably the single most significant risk factor relating to the development of cancer. Of all cancers, fifty percent occur in people older than 65 years. The higher cancer incidence in this age group may reflect **lifelong accumulation of DNA mutations, that result in cell transformation and cancer. The body may no longer be able to repair these mutations,** as it did in the early years. **The effectiveness of the immune system, especially cell-mediated immunity is also reduced in the elderly population.** (Ignatavicius and Bayne, p. 557)

Procedure

Procedure details are details that explain how something is done. These details give you directions for doing an action.

EXAMPLE 9–4

Pay attention to the boldface procedure details in this next example.

Use of the written process record is an effective but time-consuming process. To obtain maximum benefit from this learning tool, the nurse needs **to record a series of several nurse-client interactions, conduct a self-analysis and obtain feedback for each** interaction from a reader. Confidentiality must be maintained at all times to protect the client and the therapeutic nature of the nurse-client relationship. Anonymity **can be ensured on the process record by using only client initials rather than full names and by omitting identifying demographic information.** (Arnold and Boggs, p. 557)

Examples

Example details are those that illustrate the main point of the paragraph. These details provide illustrations of the main idea to give you a greater understanding of the essence of the passage. They sometimes appear in list form.

EXAMPLE 9–5

Look at the following paragraph and note that the example details are in boldface type.

Abusive families also include those with abuse in **gay and lesbian relationships, sibling abuse, and parental abuse by children, as well as those in which spouse, child, and elder abuse occurs.** Violence against **children, women, and the elderly** is declared to be wrong, but violence is acceptable in **television, in movies and even in schools.** Such a double message makes it nearly impossible to make inroads against violence in America. (Varcarolis, p. 256)

Description

Description details are details that help you to visualize the main thought of the paragraph. Description details provide a picture that enables you to comprehend the core elements of the paragraph.

EXAMPLE 9–6

Consider the following selection with description details in boldface type.

Hydration is defined as the normal state of fluid balance. . . . **A normally hydrated adult is alert, has moist eyes and mucous membranes, has a urinary output appropriate for the amount of fluid ingested (with a specific gravity of urine of approximately 1.015) and has an adequate state of skin hydration as measured by skin turgor.** (Ignatavicius et al., p. 260)

EXERCISE 9–2

Below are ten main ideas. The names of different types of details are written in parentheses after each main idea. In the space provided, create your own example for each type of detail.

1. More young people are being killed in motorcycle accidents.

   (Data) ______________________________

2. A student's attention span may be affected by his or her diet.

   (Cause) ______________________________

3. Transferring a patient from a bed to a wheelchair should be done cautiously.

   (Procedure) ______________________________

4. There are many causes of depression.

   (Examples) ______________________________

5. The patient presented with the following symptoms.

   (Description) ______________________________

6. The infant mortality rate has risen in urban America.

   (Data) ______________________________

7. More people are suffering from skin cancer.

   (Cause) ____

   ____

   ____

8. Folding bandages is not as difficult as it looks.

   (Procedure) ____

   ____

   ____

9. Different types of people are entering nursing today.

   (Examples) ____

   ____

   ____

10. Beginning at about the age of two, a child's ability to talk begins to change.

    (Description) ____

    ____

    ____

Comprehending? Yes ___ No ___

EXERCISE 9–3

Below is a passage from a nursing textbook. In each paragraph, underline the stated main idea. If the main idea is unstated, create your own in the margin. Underline twice the major details that support the main idea.

Careful attention to the history of a client with a possible infectious disease helps the nurse determine risk factors for infection. The age of a client, history of cigarette smoking or alcohol use, current illness or disease (such as diabetes), past and current medication use, familial predisposition, and poor nutritional status may place the client at increased risk for a number of infectious diseases.

The nurse also determines whether the client has been exposed to infectious agents. A history of recent exposure to someone with similar clinical symptoms or to contaminated food or water, as well as the time of exposure, assists in identifying a possible source for infection. Nurses may find this information helpful for determining the incubation period for the disease and thus for providing a clue to its cause.

Contact with animals, including pets, may facilitate exposure to infection. The nurse asks the client about recent contact with animals at home, at work, or in the course of leisure activities, such as hunting. The nurse also asks the client about recent contact with insects.

The nurse obtains a travel history from the client. Travel to areas both within and outside the client's home country may expose a susceptible client to infectious organisms not encountered in the local community.

A thorough sexual history may reveal sexual behavior associated with increased risk of sexually transmitted diseases. The nurse should obtain a history of intravenous drug use and a transfusion history to assess the client's risk for hepatitis B, hepatitis C, and human immunodeficiency virus (HIV) infections. (Ignatavicius, p. 597)

• VOCABULARY CHECK

Directions. Below are 10 words taken from the key words section of this chapter. Circle the letter of the best definition of the four choices.

1. Benigh
   - **a** not infectious
   - **b** not malignant
   - **c** not genetic
   - **d** not operable

2. Anonymity
   - **a** the state of being irritating
   - **b** the state of being irregular
   - **c** the state of not being named or identified
   - **d** an explanatory note

3. Hyponatremia
   - **a** sodium deficiency in the blood
   - **b** oxygen deficiency in the blood
   - **c** glucose deficiency in the blood
   - **d** iron deficiency in the blood

4. Exacerbation
   - **a** to have one's awareness increased
   - **b** to have one's awareness decreased
   - **c** to make more pleasant, comfortable
   - **d** to make more bitter, severe

5. Medulla
   - **a** the outer edge of an organ
   - **b** the central or inner portion of an organ
   - **c** the middle chamber of the heart
   - **d** the outer portion of the skeletal system

6. Feedback
   - **a** the lower portion of the back
   - **b** regurgitated food
   - **c** insulting responses
   - **d** corrective information

7. Cancer
   - **a** malignant tumor
   - **b** benign tumor
   - **c** combination of malignant and benign tumors
   - **d** infectious disease

8. Overwhelmed
   - **a** ill
   - **b** upset
   - **c** bored
   - **d** tired

9. Remission
   - **a** resubmitting of information
   - **b** diagnosing again, second diagnosis
   - **c** abatement of symptoms of a disease
   - **d** transmission of symptoms of a disease

10. Core
   - **a** outer edges
   - **b** detail
   - **c** central part
   - **d** peripheral element

• CRITICAL THINKING LOG

List the strategies you learned in this chapter.	Select the strategy that is most useful for your school success.	How can you apply this strategy to your nursing studies?

• SUMMARY

In this chapter you learned how supporting details relate to the main idea. You also saw the difference between major and minor details and how you should focus on the major details for note-taking and highlighting in your textbook. You learned a strategy to help you visualize details. Explanations and examples for the following five types of details were given to help you find and understand major details in a passage:

- Data
- Cause
- Procedure
- Example
- Description

Finally, you were given practice locating these five kinds of details and recognizing how these details support the main idea.

CHAPTER 10

Paragraph Organization

• OBJECTIVE

To use paragraph organization as an aid to concentration, comprehension, and retention.

• KEY WORDS

Pay attention to the following key words, which are underscored the first time they appear in this chapter. Try to determine the meaning of these words from the surrounding words in the passage. If you need further help, use your dictionary or the glossary in the back of this book.

Look up the medical terminology in your medical dictionary or the glossary. As you read the exercises in this chapter, write additional words you need to learn in the space provided.

MEDICAL TERMINOLOGY	GENERAL VOCABULARY
angina	assumptions
auscultation	conversion
electro-oculograms	habitual
epidermis	inference

hypertension
melanin
metabolic
myocardial infarction
palpation
percussion
psychological
outcomes
pivotal
proposals
refine
self-directedness
statute
symptoms

______________________ ______________________

______________________ ______________________

______________________ ______________________

• RECOGNIZING PARAGRAPH ORGANIZATION

When authors write textbooks, they often organize their ideas in patterns. If you can learn to recognize these patterns, you will concentrate on and comprehend the author's ideas. Recognizing a familiar pattern makes you part of the author's thinking. You are actively participating in the author's arrangement of the ideas in the text. You will also find it easier to retain textbook information if you associate the ideas with a pattern rather than trying to remember random facts.

• TYPES OF PATTERN

There are varying types of organizational pattern. Both single paragraphs and longer selections can be structured in these patterns. Below are listed the patterns most often found in your nursing textbooks. The description and example of each pattern should help you to recognize these patterns as you read your textbooks.

Chronological (Time Order)

In a chronological pattern, events are presented in sequence. You can recognize this pattern by such words as *first, last, second, later, then, finally, next, ages,* and *dates.*

EXAMPLE 10–1

The First National Conference on Classification of Nursing Diagnosis was held in 1973 and resulted in publication of the first list of approved diagnoses. NANDA evolved from the group formed at the First National Conference and has been in existence in its current form since 1982. Conferences have been held approximately every two years since that time. The members of the organization have continued to develop and refine the list of approved diagnoses. (Iyer et al., 3rd ed., p. 122)

Underline all the words that indicate a time-order pattern.

Cause and Effect

Causes are the reasons for events, while effects are results. Clue words to this pattern are *since, therefore, thus, as a result,* and *consequently.*

EXAMPLE 10–2

Successful nursing care depends as much on the alleviation of mental and emotional suffering as it does on the relief of physical suffering. A person's unmet psychological (mental and emotional) needs can complicate an otherwise uncomplicated illness. Psychologic, social, cultural, and spiritual factors affect not only a person's physiologic well-being but also the ability to respond to treatment and recover from an illness. The connections among body, mind, and spirit are so dynamic and so vital that nurses cannot treat these dimensions of human experience as separate entities without depersonalizing the individual and fragmenting care. (Bolander, 3rd ed., p. 628)

List the word that indicates that the pattern is cause and effect: ________________

____

Comparison-Contrast

Authors look at similarities and differences. Comparisons describe similarities, while contrasts describe differences. Some paragraphs combine comparison and contrast. Comparisons can be recognized by such words as *similarly* or *likewise.* Contrasts can be recognized by such words as *but, on the other hand,* or *however.*

EXAMPLE 10–3

A psychosocial health assessment begins with an interview process that addresses all of the dimensions of an individual. It differs from the traditional medical-surgical history in which you collect only concrete, factual information relevant to the development of symptoms and past medical-surgical conditions. In a psychosocial assessment you also strive to form a picture of the person's unique personality characteristics, including strengths and weaknesses. This picture is subjective and therefore less tangible than assessment of purely physiologic data. A **psychosocial history** is the person's own story told in the person's own words from a personal point of view. The person being interviewed is considered the primary source of data. Valuable information and insight can also be obtained from secondary data sources such as family, friends, previous records, laboratory findings, and other diagnostic tests. (Bolander, 3rd ed., p. 629)

Write the phrase that lets you know that the author is contrasting ideas. __________

____

Simple Listing

In a simple listing pattern the information in a passage will be in the format of a list. The order is not important. Clue words are *and, also,* or *in addition.*

EXAMPLE 10–4

Inspection, palpation, percussion, and auscultation are basic maneuvers used during physical assessment. The sense of smell is also used. (Bolander, 3rd ed., p. 655)

Write the clue word that indicates that this pattern is simple listing. ______________

____

EXERCISE 10–1

Directions. Read each textbook selection and identify the organizational pattern. Write whether each pattern is chronological (time order), cause and effect, comparison-contrast, or simple listing.

1. The actual number of hours a person spends sleeping reflects a balancing of external factors. Employment schedules, social commitments, and societal influences (e.g., the availability of goods and services) are all involved in determining a person's sleep-activity schedule. (Bolander, 3rd ed., p. 951)

The organizational pattern is: ______________________________

2. Sleep is composed of two very distinct types of activity: **rapid eye movement (REM) sleep** and **non–rapid eye movement (non-REM, NREM) sleep.** REM sleep accounts for about 25% of a night's sleep and is characterized by REMs as detected by electro-oculograms and by intense physiologic activation.[5, 9] It is often referred to as active or paradoxic sleep. NREM sleep accounts for about 75% of a night's sleep and is characterized by progressive relaxation. (Bolander, 3rd ed., p. 948)

The organizational pattern is: ______________________________

3. Because of the subjective nature of pain, there exists a need for measurable outcomes that accompany the subjective report of pain relief. For example, "I feel less pain now" is subjective. Objective, measurable data could include the number of times the person was medicated over the past 24 hours. If that number reflects a decrease in medication, then it supports a subjective report of feeling less pain. (Bolander, 3rd ed., p. 978)

The organizational pattern is: ______________________________

4. Aspirin and other antiinflammatory drugs have been found to block the conversion of arachidonic acid into prostaglandin, which results in a decreased nociceptive input to the central nervous system, thus reducing pain. (Bolander, 3rd ed., p. 972)

The organizational pattern is: ______________________________

5. Birthweight generally quadruples by age 2 years, then weight gain slows somewhat. Toddlers gain an average of 4 to 5 pounds between ages 2 and 3 years. Most 2-year-olds are about 3 feet tall and grow another 3 to 4 inches in the next year. By age 3 to 5 years, children grow in a slow, steady pattern. Weight increases at about 5 pounds or less a year. Young children lose that plump baby appearance as their height growth is greater than weight gain, giving them a taller, thinner appearance. All primary (or deciduous) teeth are usually present. (Bolander, 3rd ed., p. 199)

The organizational pattern is: ______________________________

Comprehending? Yes ___ No ___

EXERCISE 10–2

Directions. Read each textbook selection. Identify the organizational pattern. Use this pattern to help you locate the topic, main idea, and major details in each selection.

SKIN STRUCTURE AND FUNCTION

1. Skin, the largest body organ, has three continuous layers: epidermis, dermis, and subcutaneous tissue. The epidermis (most superficial layer) has several layers called strata. The outermost stratum contains dead cells continuously being replaced by cells from deeper layers. Melanin and keratin form in the inner cellular epidermal stratum. Melanin (pigment) provides skin color and protects from ultraviolet sun rays. Keratin contributes to skin acidity.

   The dermis consists of blood vessels, dense connective tissue, nerve fibers, sebaceous (oil) glands and hair follicles. Sebaceous glands are present on all skin surfaces except palms and soles.

   Under the dermis is subcutaneous tissue providing support and blood supply to the dermis. It consists of loose connective tissue, blood and lymph vessels, fat, sweat glands, and hair follicles. (Bolander, 3rd ed., pp. 913–914)

   Organizational pattern: ______________________________

   Topic: ______________________________

   Main idea: ______________________________

   Major details: ______________________________

2. Some people bathe for reasons other than hygiene, e.g., relaxation, therapeutic baths. A warm tub bath can relax and soothe sore tense muscles. For some people bathing is a time for being alone to screen out external stimuli or to relieve generalized tension. For others, bathing is a stimulant to "get started in the morning," e.g., a cool shower to

"get going." In care facilities, wherever possible, maintain an individual's habitual bathing practices. (Bolander, 3rd ed., p. 914)

Organizational pattern: ______

Topic: ______

Main idea: ______

Major details: ______

STATUTORY LAW

3. Statutory law is law created by state legislatures or the United States Congress. State codes and the United States code are contained in multivolume sets of books.

A bill is a proposed new or revised statute. Proposed laws reflect current societal concerns. For example, in the early 1990s, state and federal initiatives in the legislative arena included proposals for revising the health care system. Nurses, as both citizens and health care professionals, have an opportunity to influence the development of statutory law. Two ways to exert this influence are writing or meeting with state legislators or members of Congress. Nurses can support, oppose, or suggest changes in proposed laws. (Bolander, 3rd ed., p. 50)

Organizational pattern: ______

Topic: ______

Main idea: ______

Major details: ______

4. Making nursing diagnoses is an indispensable and high-level intellectual skill that you will develop and practice throughout your professional life. Nursing diagnoses are applicable to all strata of clients. Depending on your area of nursing, you will apply nursing diagnostic skills to individuals, families, groups, or even entire communities.

Because the nursing diagnosis culminates the assessment phase, it is the pivotal step in the nursing process. Without accurate nursing diagnoses, there is no point in progressing to the other stages of the nursing process, for there will be no basis for planning care or intervention or for evaluating the outcome of nursing intervention.

Today it is recognized that diagnosis is *not* the exclusive domain of the physician or even of health care professionals. If a diagnosis is "essentially an inference about a state that is undesirable," then lawyers, social workers, police detectives, and auto mechanics all make diagnoses. Clearly, nurses share with these experts from other fields the common diagnostic skills associated with uncovering problems and finding their cause, such as gathering facts, organizing data, analysis of data, seeking patterns, and stating conclusions. It is the drawing and stating of conclusions that has relevance to our present discussion of diagnosis.

NURSING DIAGNOSIS DEFINED AND EXPLORED

Nursing diagnosis is a complex concept to define. Nursing diagnoses are *not* medical diagnoses, although there are similarities between the two. Nursing diagnoses are *similar* to medical diagnoses in that the same basic methods underlie both processes: obtaining the person's history, performing the physical examination, organizing the data base, and analyzing the data obtained. Both nurses and physicians need similar skills to make diagnoses: communication skills, physical assessment skills, observational skills, and intellectual skills.

On the other hand, nursing diagnoses *differ* from medical diagnoses in their focus and consequently in their specific goals and objectives. Physicians are primarily involved in diagnosing disease and its underlying pathologic processes. Physicians examine people to learn the source of their symptoms and the metabolic, chemical, or pathologic structural changes resulting from the disorder.

A physician may examine a person with chest pain and formulate a medical diagnosis of myocardial infarction (heart attack). The nurse may assess the same person and identify several nursing diagnoses. These diagnoses could relate to specific problems or responses such as pain, fear, ineffective denial, and so on.

Both medical and nursing diagnoses are necessary and valid. To develop a person's total diagnostic picture, nurses and physicians must work together as well as independently. Also, they must communicate their findings to one another.

The North American Nursing Diagnosis Association (NANDA)—an organization formed in the 1980s to promote the development of and education about nursing diagnosis)—has identified three types of nursing diagnoses: actual, high-risk, and wellness diagnoses. In 1990, NANDA accepted a definition of an actual nursing diagnosis. (Bolander, 3rd ed., p. 130)

Organizational pattern: ______________________

Topic: ______________________

Main idea: ______________________

Major details: ______________________

5. Identify the organizational pattern in Figure 10–1. (Ingalls and Salerno, p. 120)

Organizational pattern: ______________________

Topic: ______________________

Main idea: ______________________

Major details: ______________________

Comprehending? Yes ___ No ___

EXERCISE 10–3

Directions. Read the following excerpt from a chapter in a nursing textbook (Bolander, 3rd ed., pp. 471–472). As you read, focus on the organizational pattern. Use this pattern to help you concentrate on and comprehend the author's main ideas. Then answer the questions following the selection.

ASSUMPTIONS THAT CHARACTERIZE ADULT LEARNING

Malcolm Knowles, a leading authority on adult learning theory, identified four assumptions that characterize adult learning. These four assumptions assist nurses in planning the teaching of adults. Remember, however, that adults are highly variable and must be treated as individuals.

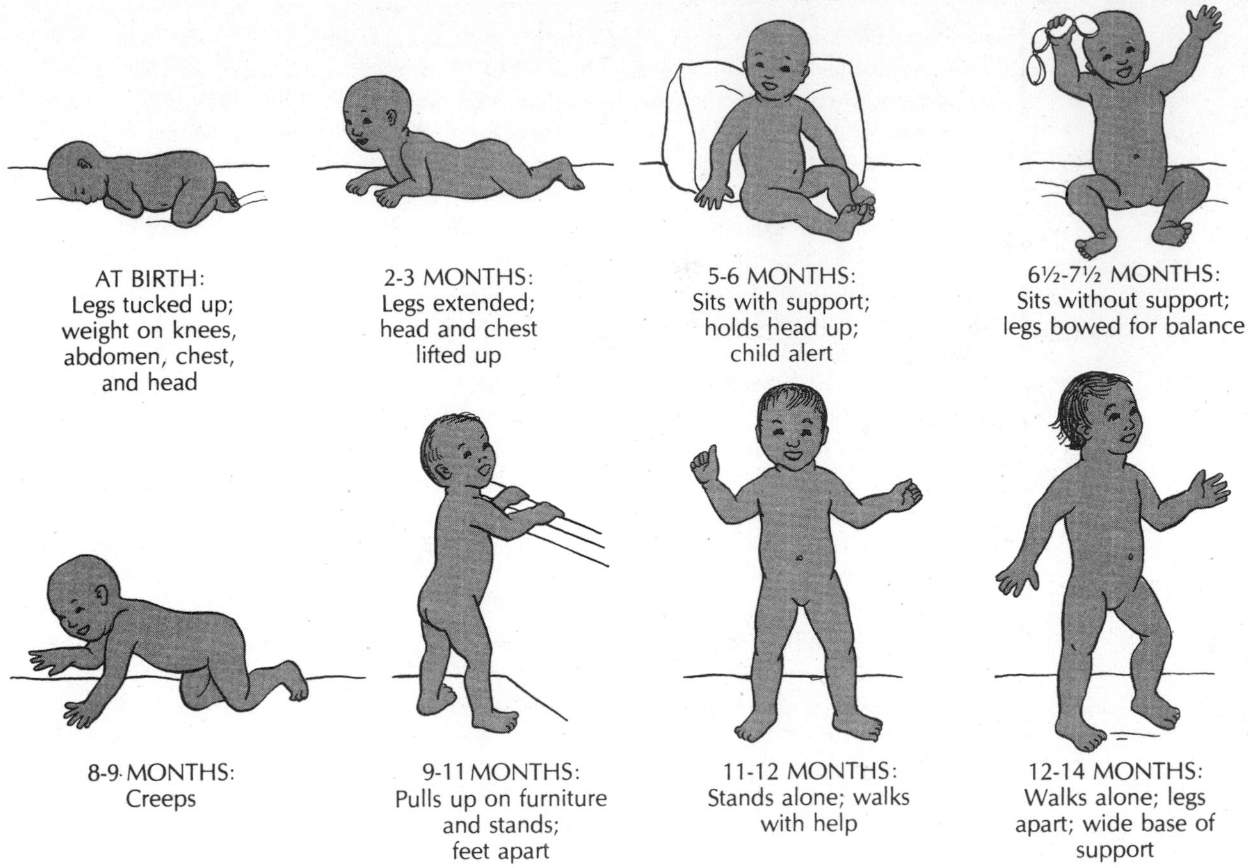

AT BIRTH:
Legs tucked up;
weight on knees,
abdomen, chest,
and head

2-3 MONTHS:
Legs extended;
head and chest
lifted up

5-6 MONTHS:
Sits with support;
holds head up;
child alert

6½-7½ MONTHS:
Sits without support;
legs bowed for balance

8-9 MONTHS:
Creeps

9-11 MONTHS:
Pulls up on furniture
and stands;
feet apart

11-12 MONTHS:
Stands alone; walks
with help

12-14 MONTHS:
Walks alone; legs
apart; wide base of
support

Figure 10–1 Development of infant posture and locomotion. (Adapted from Ingalls, A.J., and Salerno, M.C.: Maternal and Child Health Nursing, 5th ed., St. Louis: The C.V. Mosby Co., 1983.)

Adult Learning Is Self-Directed

The first assumption is that, as individuals mature, they become increasingly *self-directed* regarding learning. Knowles identified those changes in self-concept that take the learner from a state of learning dependency to a state of increasing self-directedness. This self-direction is reflected in adults who first identify their learning needs and then take direct action to acquire the needed knowledge. Consider two adults who want (need) to learn how to use a computer to increase their employment potential. One enrolls in a formal course at a local junior college; the other buys a book on word processing and devises a self-study program that combines reading the book and practicing the skill at the local library using computerized instruction. Both of these adults identified their desire to learn to use the computer and chose a method of study that best suited their own learning style. They exhibited self-directed learning behavior.

Past Experiences Enhance Learning

The second assumption is that the adult learner approaches new learning experiences in light of a *lifetime of accumulated learning.* As adults, "we are what we learn." We define or characterize ourselves in terms of our experiences. This process is quite different from children, who view experiences as something that happens *to* them. The older we become, the more varied (and ingrained) are our learning experiences. Therefore, to facilitate adult learning, we should convey respect for people by making use of their past learning and drawing on their experiences as a resource to enhance present learning.

Adult Learners and Readiness to Learn

Third, the adult learner is often characterized by a *readiness to learn.* For the adult, learning becomes more meaningful as it relates to what the person needs to know to perform effectively in a social role: spouse, parent, nurse, mechanic, professor, and so forth. It is often a challenge to structure health education in terms of developmental readiness to learn. People learn more readily when the information is useful and relevant to them socially, professionally, or personally. Mutual exploration and planning enable you and the adult learner to set learning priorities.

Solving Real-Life Problems

Closely related to readiness to learn is the fourth assumption that adult learning is based on solving *real-life problems* and the necessity for immediate results. This problem-centered orientation to learning is in contrast to the subject-centered orientation typical of a child's learning. Children study mathematics, science, and English because they must in order to pass a test or enter high school, college, or graduate school. Subject-oriented learning has a delayed application.

Adults are more inclined to spend time, effort, and money to obtain knowledge that has *immediate* application to their circumstances. Also, when adults cope ineffectively with some of life's problems, they are motivated to seek new information. People who experience angina that interferes with job performance and activities of daily living, for example, may be motivated to learn how to modify their stress level, lose weight, and stop smoking. The executive who has hypertension may be less motivated to learn these things because the disease process does not presently interfere with job performance. Thus, to spend time performing these activities does not seem relevant to this person's present goals. Your task is to convince the person that performing the healthy behaviors will ultimately lead to a more productive life. On the other hand, the person needs to realize that, by ignoring a serious health problem, complications can develop that may impede work performance altogether (e.g., a stroke). Helping people achieve immediate short-term goals that are positively rewarded reinforces learning. In turn, this success motivates people to continue healthy behaviors.

1. The organization pattern of this selection is
   a. chronological
   b. cause and effect
   c. simple listing
   d. comparison-contrast
2. This selection is mainly about
   a. learning
   b. assumptions about learning
   c. assumptions about adult learning
   d. difficulties adults face when returning to school
3. Adults require
   a. direction from their textbooks
   b. self-direction
   c. no direction
   d. direction from their instructors
4. When adults go back to school, they should
   a. make use of past learning
   b. start a new career
   c. forget information learned in previous courses
   d. learn from their children

5. Adults learn best when they
   a. are forced to go back to school
   b. cram for tests
   c. are in poor health
   d. are ready to learn
6. Adults learn best when the learning is
   a. subject-oriented
   b. problem-centered
   c. delayed
   d. ineffective
7. Adults are motivated to achieve goals which are
   a. immediate
   b. short-term
   c. positively rewarded
   d. all of the above
8. The older we become, our experiences are more
   a. varied
   b. limited
   c. restricted
   d. irrelevant
9. People learn best when information
   a. helps them to escape from life's problems
   b. helps them to forget about priorities
   c. is relevant
   d. is on tape
10. To retain the information in this selection, you should try to remember that the number of points presented by the author is
    a. one
    b. two
    c. three
    d. four

Comprehending? Yes ___ No ___

• VOCABULARY CHECK

Directions. Below are 10 words taken from the key words section of this chapter. Circle the letter of the best definition from the four choices.

1. Metabolic
- **a** the process of the digestion of minerals and vitamins
- **b** nutrients found in the four food groups
- **c** the process of nutrients absorbed into the blood following digestion
- **d** an organ that aids in the digestion of minerals and vitamins

2. Pivotal
- **a** minor
- **b** key
- **c** useless
- **d** detailed

3. Angina
a spasmodic choking
b sharp pain
c heart failure
d an inflammation

4. Proposals
a orders
b suggestions
c changes
d documents

5. Myocardial infarction
a open-heart surgery
b angiogram
c heart attack
d hypertension

6. Statute
a a decision of the jury that changes laws
b a signature needed to verify a document
c a decorative object, usually made of stone or metal
d a law enacted by the legislative branch of a government

7. Hypertension
a low blood pressure
b high blood pressure
c frenetic activity
d extreme anxiety

8. Outcomes
a causes
b external events
c reasons
d results

9. Epidermis
a the outermost layer of the skin
b the innermost layer of skin
c a tough skin or membrane
d a skin disease of the extremities

10. Assumption
a a proven theory or concept
b a mistake in a theory or concept
c the supposition that something is true
d misleading information given in court

• CRITICAL THINKING LOG

List the strategies you learned in this chapter.	Select the strategy that is most useful for your school success.	How can you apply this strategy to your nursing studies?

• SUMMARY

You have learned how to use organizational patterns to improve your concentration and retention. Four patterns which are commonly used in your nursing textbooks are: chronological (time order), comparison-contrast, cause-effect, and simple listing. Use clue words to help you recognize these patterns. Paying attention to organizational patterns will help you to become actively involved with the author's thinking process and enable you to read your textbooks with purpose.

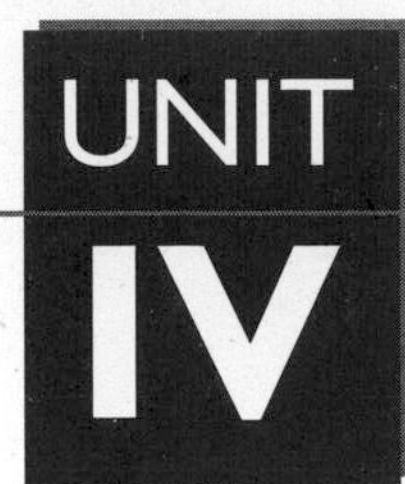

UNIT IV STUDY SKILLS

Learning specific study skills will help you do well in nursing school. Once you have mastered them, the time and effort you put into preparing for exams should produce better results. This unit on study skills will help you learn and practice these techniques. Chapter 11, "Reading the Textbook," will teach you how to read and study from your nursing textbook. Chapter 12, "Graphic Aids," will show you how graphs, pictures, tables, and diagrams can be used to visually reinforce the ideas in the written text. Chapter 13, "Active Listening and Successful Note-Taking," will demonstrate how active listening will help you concentrate on and comprehend information presented during lectures.

Applying the study skills discussed in Unit IV will help you attain better grades. Once you see the positive results, you will be motivated to continue using these study skills to further your academic achievement.

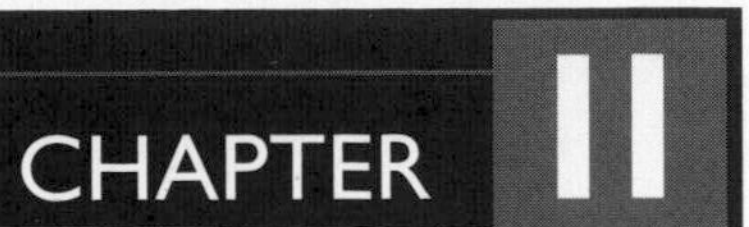

Reading the Textbook

• OBJECTIVE

To learn the active reading strategies required for concentrating on, comprehending, and retaining textbook information.

• KEY WORDS

Pay attention to the following key words, which are underscored the first time they appear in this chapter. Try to determine the meaning of these words from the surrounding words in the passage. If you need further help, use your dictionary or the glossary in the back of this book.

Look up the medical terminology in your medical dictionary or the glossary. As you read the exercises in this chapter, write additional words you need to learn in the space provided.

MEDICAL TERMINOLOGY	GENERAL VOCABULARY
biomechanics	alignment
cervical	friction
disc	fulcrum
musculoskeletal	gravity
occipitoatlantal	holistic
pelvic	jargon
posture	leverage
psychosocial	momentum
symptoms	rapport
vertebrae	stability
__________	__________
__________	__________
__________	__________
__________	__________
__________	__________

• SURVEYING THE TEXTBOOK

Often the most difficult part of reading the textbook is getting started. Therefore, it's a good idea to buy your textbooks as soon as they are assigned. You can then become familiar with your textbook at the beginning of the semester. Don't procrastinate. Open your book and get started! Once you feel comfortable with a text, it will be easier for you to approach each reading assignment. You can learn to use the external structure of your textbook to acquaint yourself with the book and to help you become an active reader. Survey these seven parts of the text to help you read your nursing textbooks:

- Title page
- Preface
- Table of contents
- Glossary
- Bibliography
- Appendix
- Index

Title Page

The title page is the first printed page of the text and gives the following information:

- Title
- Author
- Edition
- Publisher
- City

EXERCISE 11–1

Directions. Look at the title page provided here, then answer the following questions:

1. The title of the book is ______________________________
2. The authors are ______________________________
3. The publisher is ______________________________
4. Is the copyright date (date of publication) given on this title page?

   Yes __________ No __________

Preface

The preface gives the author's objective in writing the text and explains the organization of the text. You can find the preface in the beginning of the book, following the title page.

EXERCISE 11–2

Directions. Read the preface from the Black and Matassarin-Jacobs book on the following page and answer the questions that follow.

Preface

Luckmann and Sorensen's Medical-Surgical Nursing: A Psychophysiologic Approach, 4th edition, presents up-to-date care of the adult client. On the "cutting edge" of current scientific, nursing, and medical knowledge, this new edition of the book retains the traditional strengths of previous editions: comprehensiveness, depth, authority, and strong pathophysiology. Improvements in the discussion of nursing management and the addition of special features designed to assist the nurse in the clinical setting allow a clear transition from the book to the bedside.

Philosophy and Approach

This book portrays the reality of nursing care, where often there is a clear differentiation between nursing management and medical management. The text represents our belief that although nurses and physicians do not compete with each other but collaborate for the benefit of the client, still, nursing and medicine are separate disciplines. In the text, Nursing Management and Medical Management are separate headings and are not intermingled with general management of clients. Because nursing and medicine are collaborative efforts, however, it is often difficult for nursing students to understand one without the other.

We used the nursing process to illuminate nursing care, but did not apply the nursing process to every disorder, electing instead to use the nursing process for prototypical disorders. Within the nursing process for a disorder, we developed nursing diagnoses and, as appropriate, collaborative problems, each with its own expected outcomes and implementation. Expected outcomes and implementation have been written for each nursing diagnosis because we have found, from our teaching experience, that lists of diagnoses followed by

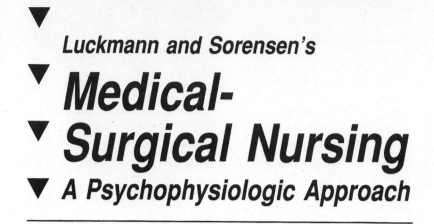

Luckmann and Sorensen's

Medical-Surgical Nursing

A Psychophysiologic Approach

Fourth Edition

JOYCE M. BLACK, M.S.N., R.N.,C.
Assistant Professor
College of Nursing
University of Nebraska Medical Center
Omaha, Nebraska

ESTHER MATASSARIN-JACOBS, Ph.D., R.N., O.C.N.
Associate Professor
Niehoff School of Nursing
Loyola University of Chicago
Chicago, Illinois

W.B. SAUNDERS COMPANY
A Division of Harcourt Brace & Company
Philadelphia London Toronto Montreal Sydney Tokyo

lists of expected outcomes and implementations cannot easily be teased apart and rebuilt into a care plan by the student. Collaborative problems define those areas of nursing practice that are not resolvable through independent nursing actions. Collaborative problems are potential complications that a client may develop due to the disorder, surgery, or other treatments. They complete the picture of nursing care and eliminate the need of force-fitting the various nursing diagnoses to each client problem that may be encountered.

A head-to-toe body systems approach is used in this edition. This is more easily adapted to a variety of conceptual frameworks than the use of a conceptual framework of our own. Concepts prevalent in medical-surgical practice, such as pain, perioperative care, shock, and chronic conditions, are found in the first quarter of the book.

Because a significant portion of medical-surgical disorders occur in the elderly, we added content on normal aging of individual body systems. Then, to help the student to modify care accordingly, there is a section at the end of each processed disorder called "Modification of Plan of Care for the Elderly."

The strong psychosocial underpinning of past editions of *Luckmann and Sorensen's Medical-Surgical Nursing: A Psychophysiologic Approach* has been reinforced by doubling the number of chapters on psychosocial content. There are chapters on ethics, cross-cultural nursing, spiritual needs, human sexuality, the family, and chronic conditions. This text focuses on not only the client's individual response to illness but also the effect of illness on a client's family. With shortened hospital stays, the family has become an extension of the medical-surgical nurse, who often works in tandem with the family to prepare them for their part in continued assessment and provision of care. This planning for home care is highlighted in the text in a section called "Discharge Teaching."

Special Features

Bridging the distance from the theoretical to the practical, and from the medical-surgical setting to the home, is essential in nursing. To that end, we have included several such "bridges" to clinical care.

In addition to a separate chapter on "Ethics" (Chap. 4), a feature called "Ethical Issues in Nursing" was written by a nurse ethicist and appears frequently throughout the book. An ethical dilemma is presented, not necessarily for resolution but for reflection.

The "Bridge to Home Health Care" feature also appears throughout the text, and gives practical suggestions on how to help clients in the home setting. These bridges were written by practicing home health care nurses.

Another feature, the "Bridge to Critical Care," highlights common modalities of treatment or assessment in critical care. Although there is no attempt to discuss all of critical care nursing, we present a basic understanding of hospital-based critical care treatments as they are used in post-hospital care. Some examples are pulmonary pressure monitors, ventilators, and arterial lines.

"Nursing Research" boxes provide illustrative examples to show students how nursing research may be used in client care.

Finally, in recognition of the need to make the client a collaborator in the care plan, we include "Client Education Guides." (Black and Matassarin-Jacobs, 4th ed., pp. xix–xx)

1. What is the purpose of the added special features in this fourth edition?

____

____

____

2. List the four concepts prevalent in medical-surgical practice found in the first quarter of the book:

____

____

____

____

Table of Contents

The table of contents, found in the front of the book after the preface, is the most important part of your survey of your nursing textbook. The table of contents provides you with the author's outline of the entire text. The format of the table of contents usually consists of sections divided into units and units divided into chapters. You will see at a glance how the text is organized.

EXERCISE 11–3

Directions. Survey the table of contents from the Luckmann and Sorensen book (Black and Matassarin-Jacobs, 4th ed., pp. xxv–xxx), then answer the questions that follow.

1. How many chapters are in Unit II?______________________________
2. What is the title of Unit IX?______________________________
3. Which unit deals with neurologic disorders?______________________________
4. What page gives you information about nursing care of people with thyroid and parathyroid disorders?______________________________

Glossary

A glossary, located in the back of the textbook, gives you an alphabetical listing of the vocabulary that is important for understanding the ideas in the text.

EXERCISE 11–4

Directions. Answer the following questions:

1. Write the definition of deciduous teeth. ______________________________

____

____

Text continued on page 144

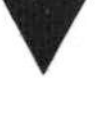 Contents in Brief

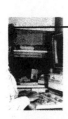

xxvi Contents in Brief

xxviii Contents in Brief

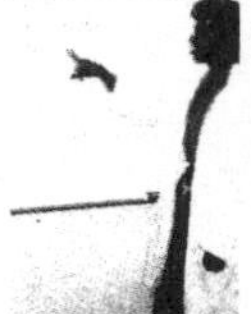

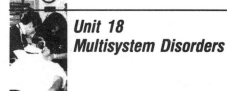

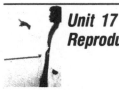

body in the thoracic and abdominal cavities and in the central nervous system. (31)

Cost containment: A variety of measures designed to reduce health care costs. (5)

Counterirritants: Agents that are applied locally to produce inflammatory reaction for the purpose of affecting some other body part, usually adjacent to or underlying the surface irritated. (48)

Countertraction: A force that pulls in the opposite direction from the force exerted by traction. (37)

CPU: Central processing unit—the main part of the computer, the part that performs calculations. (27)

Crackles (formerly known as rales): Noises created when air is traveling through vessels containing abnormal moisture. They are more pronounced on inspiration. (33)

Creams: Oils dispersed in 60 to 80 per cent water to form a thick liquid or soft solid. (46)

Criminal law: A type of law that punishes behavior that threatens the integrity of society and that may warrant the deprivation of personal liberty. (3)

Crisis: A disequilibrium in a steady state, occurring when usual problem-solving strategies are ineffective. (16)

Cross-contamination: The transmission of infectious agents from one person to another. (28)

CRT: Another name for a computer monitor. The letters stand for cathode ray tube. (27)

Cues: Subjective or objective pieces of information obtained through assessment. See Diagnostic cues. (8)

Cultural adaptation: Adjustment of an individual's behavior to the concepts, ideas, traditions, and institutions of a culture. (16)

Cultural competence: Being knowledgeable about health practices, beliefs, values, culture, and ethnicity within and between different groups and being able to provide health services that are acceptable to these groups. (19)

Cultural diversity: A term used to convey that there are differences among cultures as well as between subcultures and the dominant culture. (19)

Cultural sensitivity: Awareness of cultural generalizations and intragroup differences, as well as the avoidance of stereotypes. (19)

Culture: The accumulation of human experiences that evolve into a way of life for a group of people. (19)

Cursor: A symbol visible on a computer screen, the symbol that indicates the currently active portion of the screen (often a blinking line). (27)

Cutdown: Surgical incision made through the skin to expose a vein for venipuncture. (47)

Cyanosis: A bluish, mottled discoloration of the skin, nail beds, and mucous membranes caused by decreased oxygenation of the blood. (33)

Cystitis: Inflammation of the bladder. (44)

Cystoscopy: Endoscopic examination of the urinary bladder. (34)

Dandruff: Dry, white flakes that occur normally with scalp exfoliation. (38)

Dangling: Assisting the client to a position sitting on the side of the bed. Contrary to its name, the position assumed does not allow the client's legs and feet to hang loosely over the side of the bed. (35)

Data base: A series of pieces of information about an individual and significant others that is used to identify strengths and unmet needs and to establish the plan of care. (7); a program that organizes a collection of information so that it can be easily accessed or utilized for reports. (27)

Data gathering: Gathering of information about a person; includes information from nursing interview, medical history, health care documents, physical and psychosocial assessment, other health care professionals, and review of the literature. (7)

Dead space: Space where fluids may collect within an anatomic cavity, abscess cavity, or wound. (48)

Debridement: The removal of foreign material or dead or damaged tissue from a wound. This may be done surgically, enzymatically, or with certain types of wound dressings. (48)

Deciduous teeth: Temporary teeth that are shed in childhood. (38)

Decoder (receiver): The person to whom a message is aimed. This person must be able to decode the message sent so it is a clearly understood thought. (24)

Defamation: Intentional use of the spoken or written word to injure the reputation of another. (3)

Defense mechanisms: Unconscious psychologic and behavioral strategies that help protect a person from anxiety. (16)

Defensiveness: Argumentative behavior to justify beliefs, thoughts, or actions. (32)

Defervescence: The period in which a fever abates and the temperature returns to normal. (31)

Defining characteristics: Clinical cues that cluster as manifestations of a nursing diagnosis. (8)

Dehiscence: A breaking open of a surgical incision without organ protrusion. (48)

Delusional thinking: An intellectual mechanism that helps a person maintain a sense of power and control when security is threatened. (51)

Delusions: False beliefs that are firmly maintained in spite of obvious evidence to the contrary and lack of support from others. (32)

Democratic leadership: A leadership style in which the leader assumes a collaborative role with other members of the group and serves as a guide while other members take steps toward accomplishing group goals. (25)

Dental plaque: Soft, thin, film of food debris, mucin, and dead epithelial cells that is deposited on the teeth and provides a medium for the growth of bacteria. (38)

Dependent edema: The buildup of interstitial fluid in areas that normally rely on muscular contraction to help move the blood back to the heart against the force of gravity; edema in areas below heart level, e.g., in the distal portions of the arms and legs of standing or sitting individuals and in the sacral area and heels of persons lying on their backs. (35)

Depressed fracture: A fracture in which fragments of

2. How many of your other nursing textbooks contain glossaries?

____

____

____

____

Bibliography

The bibliography is found in the back of the text or at the end of each chapter. A bibliography lists the sources used by the author when compiling your textbook.

EXERCISE 11–5

Directions. Look at the bibliography from the Luckmann and Sorensen nursing textbook (Black and Matassarin-Jacobs, 4th ed., p. 372). Notice that the items are listed alphabetically by the last names of the authors. Then answer the following questions.

1. What is the title of the book written by Hickey, J.?______________________________

2. Write the name of the journal in which the article by M. S. Aldrich is found.

____

Appendix

The appendix, also found in the back of the book, lists supplemental material that may be useful when you are reading and studying from your textbook.

EXERCISE 11–6

Directions. Survey the appendix example from the Luckmann and Sorensen nursing textbook (Black and Matassarin-Jacobs, 4th ed., p. 2262), then answer the following questions.

1. What is the subject matter of the appendix?______________________________

2. How many items are listed under the heading "Antibiotics"?

____

Index

The index is found in the back of your textbook. The index is an alphabetical listing of important terms in a text with page references. These terms can be the headings of more client teaching to minimize the impact of sleep and sensory disturbances.

Bibliography

1. Aldrich, M. S. (1990). Narcolepsy. *The New England Journal of Medicine, 323*(6), 389-394.
2. Alexandre, A., Colombo, F., Nertempi, P., & Benedetti, A. (1983). Cognitive outcome and early indices of severity of head injury. *Journal of Neurosurgery, 59,* 751-761.
3. Anthonisen, N. R., & Kryger, M. (1986). Sleep and breathing in patients with lung disease. In N. Edelman & T. Santiago (Eds.), *Breathing disorders of sleep* (pp. 205-224). New York: Churchill-Livingstone.
4. Aurell, J., & Elmquist, D. (1985). Sleep in the surgical intensive care unit: Continuous polygraphic recording of sleep in nine patients receiving postoperative care. *British Medical Journal, 290,* 1029-1032.
5. Closs, J. (1988). Patients' sleep-wake rhythms in hospital: Part 2. *Nursing Times, 84*(2), 54-55.
6. Cohen-Mansfield, J., & Marx, M. S. (1990). The relationship between sleep disturbances and agitation in a nursing home. *Journal of Aging Health, 2*(1), 42-57.
7. Cox, H. C., Hinz, M. D., Lubno, M. A., Newfield, S. A., Ridenour, N. A., & Sridaromont, K. L. (1989). *Clinical applications of nursing diagnosis.* Baltimore: Williams & Wilkins.
8. Czeisler, C. A., & Allan, J. S. (1988). Pathologies of the sleep-wake cycle. In R. L. Williams, I. Karacan, & C. A. Moore (Eds.), *Sleep disorders: Diagnosis and treatment* (2nd ed., pp. 109-129). New York: John Wiley & Sons.
9. Diagnostic Classification Steering Committee, Thorpy MJ, Chairman (1990). *International classification of sleep disorders: Diagnostic and coding manual.* Rochester, MN: American Sleep Disorders Association.
10. Dinges, D. F., & Broughton, R. J. (1989). *Sleep and alertness: Chronobiological, behavioral and medical aspects of napping.* New York: Raven Press.
11. Feldman, R. (1983). Management of underlying causes and precipitating factors in epilepsy. In T. Browne, & R. Feldman (Eds.), *Epilepsy: Diagnosis and management* (pp. 129-138). Toronto: Little Brown & Co.
12. Fredrickson, P. A., Richardson, J. W., Esther, M. S., & Lin, S. (1990). Sleep disorders in psychiatric practice. *Mayo Clinic Proceedings, 65,* 861-868.
13. Hanly, P. J., Willar, T. W., Steljes, D. G., Baert, R., Frais, M. A., & Kryger, M. H. (1989). Respiration and abnormal sleep in patients with congestive heart failure. *Chest, 96*(3), 480-488.
14. Hauri, P. J. (1982). *The sleep disorders: Current concepts.* Kalamazoo, MI: Upjohn.
15. Hauri, P. J., & Exther, M. S. (1990). Insomnia. *Mayo Clinic Proceedings, 65,* 869-882.
16. Hickey, J. (1986). *Neurological and neurosurgical nursing* (2nd ed.). Philadelphia: J. B. Lippincott.
17. Hobson, J. A. (1988). Homeostasis and heteroplasticity: Functional significance of behavioral state sequences. In R. Lydic & J. F. Biebuyck (Eds.), *Clinical physiology of sleep* (pp. 199-220). Bethesda, Maryland: American Physiological Society.
18. Hoch, C. C., Reynolds III, C. F., & Houck, P. R. (1987). Sleep apnea in Alzheimer's patients and the healthy elderly. *Scholarly Inquiry for Nursing Practice, 1*(3), 221-235.
19. Hoch, C. C., Reynolds III, C. F., & Houck, P. R. (1988). Sleep patterns in Alzheimer, depressed and healthy elderly. *Western Journal of Nursing Research, 10*(3), 239-256.
20. Johnson, M. W., & Jemmers, J. E. (1984). Accessory muscle activity during sleep in chronic obstructive pulmonary disease. *Journal of Applied Physiology, 57*(4), 1011-1017.
21. Kaplan, J., & Staats, B. A. (1990). Obstructive sleep apnea syndrome. *Mayo Clinic Proceedings, 65,* 1087-1094.
22. Karacan, I., & Howell, J. W. (1988). Narcolepsy. In R. L. Williams, I. Karacan, C. A. Moore (Eds.), *Sleep disorders: Diagnosis and treatment* (pp. 85-105). New York: John Wiley & Sons.
23. Krueger, B. R. (1990). Restless legs syndrome and periodic movements of sleep. *Mayo Clinic Proceedings, 65,* 999-1006.
24. Lahaie, U. (1991). Shift-workers and seasonal affective disorder. *Canadian Nurse, 87*(5), 33-34.
25. Lavie, P. (1983). Incidence of sleep apnea in a presumably healthy working population: A significant relationship with excessive daytime sleepiness. *Sleep, 6*(4), 312-318.
26. Lee, K. A., Shaver, J. F. A., Giblin, E. C., & Woods, N. F. (1990). Sleep patterns related to menstrual cycle phase and premenstrual affective symptoms. *Sleep, 13*(5), 403-409.
27. Littrell, K. D., & Schumann, L. L. (1989). Promoting sleep for the patient with a myocardial infarction. *Critical Care Nurse, 9*(3), 44, 46-49.
28. Lipowski, Z. J. (1983). Transient cognitive disorders (delirium, acute confusional states) in the elderly. *American Journal of Psychiatry, 140*(11), 1426-1436.
29. Lipowski, Z. J. (1975). Sensory and information inputs overload: Behavioral effects. *Comprehensive Psychiatry, 16*(3), 199-221.
30. Lugaresi, E., Cirignotta, F., Mondini, S., Montagna, P., & Zucconi, M. (1988). Sleep in clinical neurology. In R. L. Williams, I. Karacan, C. A. Moore, (Eds.), *Sleep disorders: Diagnosis and treatment* (2nd ed., pp. 245-263). New York: John Wiley & Sons.
31. McCance, K. L., & Huether, S. E. (1990). *Pathophysiology: The biologic basis for disease in adults and children.* St. Louis: C. V. Mosby.
32. Mitchell, P. H. (1988). Consciousness: An overview. In P. H. Mitchell, L. C. Hodges, M. Muwaswes, & C. A. Walleck (Eds.), *AANN's neuroscience nursing* (pp. 57-66). Norwalk, CT: Appleton & Lange.
33. Orr, W. C. (1985). Sleep pathophysiology in medicine and surgery. In T. Riley (Ed.), *Clinical aspects of sleep and sleep disturbance* (pp. 159-180). Toronto: Butterworth Publishers.
34. Parkosewich, J. A. Sleep-disordered breathing: A common problem in chronic obstructive pulmonary disease. *Critical Care Nurse 6*(6), 60-64.
35. Parsons, L. C., & Ver Beek, D. (1982). Sleep-awake patterns following cerebral concussion. *Nursing Research 31*(5), 260-264.
36. Rasin, J. H. (1990). Confusion. *Nursing Clinics of North America, 25*(4), 909-918.
37. Ray, W., Griffen, M., & Downey, W. (1989). Benzodiazepines of long and short elimination half-life and the risk of hip fracture. *JAMA, 262*(23), 3303-3307.
38. Reimer, M. (1989). Sleep pattern disturbances related to neurological dysfunction. *Axon, 10*(3), 65-68.
39. Remmers, J. E. (1990). Sleeping and breathing. *Chest 97,* 77S-80S.
40. Reynolds III, C. F., & Kuppfer, D. J. (1987). Sleep research in affective illness: State of the art circa 1987. *Sleep 10*(3), 199-215.
41. Richardson, J. W., Fredrickson, P. A., Siong-Chi, L. (1990). Narcolepsy update. *Mayo Clinic Proceedings,* 65, 991-998.
42. Robinson, C. (1986). Impaired sleep. In V. K. Carrieri, A. M. Lindsey, & C. M. West (Eds.), *Pathophysiological phenomena in nursing* (pp. 390-417). Philadelphia: W. B. Saunders.
43. Shaver, J. L., & Giblin, E. C. (1989). Sleep. *Annual Review of Nursing Research, 7,* 71-93d.
44. Shepard, J. W., & Olsen, K. D. (1990). Uvulopalatopharyngoplasty for treatment of obstructive sleep apnea. *Mayo Clinic Proceedings, 65,* 1260-1267.
45. Sloane, P. D., & Mathew, L. J. (1990). The therapeutic environment screening scale. *The American Journal of Alzheimer's Care and Related Disorders & Research,* 22-26.
46. Suedfeld, P. (1985). Stressful levels of environmental stimulation. *Issues in Mental Health Nursing, 7,* 83-104.
47. Thorpy, M. (1988). Diagnosis, evaluation, and classification of sleep disorders. In R. L. Williams, I. Karacan, & C. A. Moor (Eds.), *Sleep disorders: Diagnosis and treatment* (2nd ed.; pp. 9-25). New York: John Wiley & Sons.
48. Welstein, L., Dement, W. C., Redington, D., Guilleminault, C., & Mitler, M. M. (1983). Insomnia in the San Francisco Bay Area: A telephone survey. In C. Guilleminault & E. Lugaresi, (Eds.), *Sleep/wake disorders: Natural history, epidemiology, and long-term evaluation* (pp. 73-85). New York: Raven Press, 1983.
49. Williams, R. L. (1988). Sleep disturbances in various medical and surgical conditions. In R. L. Williams, I. Karacan, & C. A. Moore, Sleep disorders: Diagnosis and treatment (2nd ed.). New York: John Wiley & Sons.

Reference Values for Therapeutic Drug Monitoring

	Therapeutic Range	Toxic Levels	Proprietary Names
Antibiotics			
Amikacin, serum	25 to 30 μg/ml	Peak >35 μg/ml Trough >5 to 7 μg/ml	Amikin
Chloramphenicol, serum	10 to 20 μg/ml	>25 μg/ml	Chloromycetin
Gentamicin, serum	5 to 10 μg/ml	Peak >12 μg/ml Trough >2 μg/ml	Garamycin
Tobramycin, serum	5 to 10 μg/ml	Peak >12 μg/ml Trough >2 μg/ml	Nebcin
Anticonvulsants			
Carbamazepine, serum	5 to 12 μg/ml	>12 μg/ml	Tegretol
Ethosuximide, serum	40 to 100 μg/ml	>100 μg/ml	Zarontin
Phenobarbital, serum	10 to 30 μg/ml	Vary widely because of developed tolerance	Luminal
Phenytoin, serum	10 to 20 μg/ml	>20 μg/ml	Dilantin
Primidone, serum	5 to 20 μg/ml	>15 μg/ml	Mysoline
Valproic acid, serum	50 to 100 μg/ml	>100 μg/ml	Depakene
Analgesics			
Acetaminophen, serum	10 to 20 μg/ml	>250 μg/ml	Tylenol Datril
Salicylate, serum	100 to 250 μg/ml	>300 μg/ml	
Bronchodilator			
Theophylline, serum (aminophylline)	10 to 20 μg/ml	>20 μg/ml	Theo-Dur
Cardiovascular Drugs			
Digitoxin, serum (specimen must be obtained 12 to 24 hours after last dose)	15 to 25 ng/ml	>25 ng/ml	Crystodigin
Digoxin, serum (specimen must be obtained 12 to 24 hours after last dose)	0.8 to 2.0 ng/ml	>2.4 ng/ml	Lanoxin
Disopyramide, serum	2 to 5 μg/ml	>5 μg/ml	Norpace
Lidocaine, serum	1.5 to 5.0 μg/ml	>6 to 8 μg/ml	Xylocaine
Procainamide, serum	4 to 10 μg/ml	>16 μg/ ml	Pronestyl
Measured as procainamide + *N*-acetyl procainamide	10 to 30 μg/ml	>30 μg/ml	
Propranolol, serum	50 to 100 ng/ml	Variable	Inderal
Quinidine, serum	2 to 5 μg/ml	>10 μg/ml	Cardioquin Quinaglute Quinidex Quinora
Psychopharmacologic Drugs			
Amitriptyline, serum (measured as amitriptyline + nortriptyline)	120 to 150 ng/ml	>500 ng/ml	Amitril Elavil Endep Entrafon Limbitrol Triavil
Desipramine, serum (measured as desipramine + imipramine)	150 to 300 ng/ml	>500 ng/ml	Norpramin Petrofrane
Imipramine, serum (measured as imipramine + desipramine)	150 to 300 ng/ml	>500 ng/ml	Antipress Janimine Presamine Tofranil
Lithium, serum (obtain specimen 12 hours after last dose)	0.8 to 1.2 mEq/L	>2.0 mEq/L	Lithobid
Nortriptyline, serum	50 to 150 ng/ml	>500 ng/ml	Aventyl Pamelor

specific concepts. The index helps you to quickly locate specific information within your text.

EXERCISE 11–7

Directions. Survey the page from the index from the Luckmann and Sorensen nursing textbook (Black and Matassarin-Jacobs, 4th ed., p. I-24), then answer the questions that follow.

1. Write the page number on which you would find information about a cough reflex. ______________________

2. Write the page on which you would find information about corneal abrasion.

____

Comprehending? Yes ___ No ___

EXERCISE 11–8

Directions. You have learned how to survey a textbook. Choose any nursing textbook and answer the following questions.

1. Write the following information from the title page.

a. Title: ______________________

b. Author(s): ______________________

c. Publisher: ______________________

2. Is there a preface? Yes __________ No __________. If yes, what is the author's objective in writing this text? ______________________

____

3. Survey the table of contents:

a. How many sections are in this text? ______________________

b. How many chapters are in Section 1? ______________________

4. Look in the back of the text:

a. Is there a bibliography? Yes __________ No __________

b. Is there a glossary? Yes __________ No __________

c. Is there an index? Yes __________ No __________

d. If yes, write the page number of each. ______________________

Now that you have had practice surveying a textbook as a whole, you are ready to concentrate on an essential strategy in reading the textbook—previewing the chapter.

• STRATEGIES FOR READING THE TEXTBOOK

Reading a textbook requires concentration strategies that are different from reading books for pleasure. You can learn these specific techniques, which will help you to concentrate on, comprehend, and retain textbook information. Reading concentration requires active reading. You must react to the material to stay focused on the subject.

The following strategies will help you concentrate on textbook information:

- Previewing
- Questioning
- Summarizing

Before Reading

PREVIEWING

Before reading the assigned textbook material, preview the reading assignment. As you recall from Chapter 2, previewing involves surveying the chapter. Read the *chapter title, introduction*, and *summary*. Notice *typographical* clues such as **boldface type** and *italics*, which are used to emphasize important ideas in the chapter. *Headings* and *key words* will also direct you to the main points discussed in the selection.

QUESTIONING

After previewing the reading assignment, try to anticipate the main ideas that will be discussed in the selection. Formulate questions to help you locate main ideas as you read. When you ask questions, you are reading with a purpose. Searching for the answers to your questions results in active reading. Questioning helps you to concentrate on textbook information.

An effective method for formulating questions is to turn boldface headings into questions. Look at the following example of creating questions from a boldface heading taken from a nursing textbook.

EXAMPLE 11–1

COMPONENTS OF PSYCHOSOCIAL HEALTH ASSESSMENT

The two components of the psychosocial health assessment are the history and the Mental Status Examination (MSE). Both components focus specifically on the psychologic, social, cultural, and spiritual dimensions of a person, with the physical dimension included only as a brief summary of the problems that were identified during the physical assessment. The psychosocial assessment allows you to collect data from each dimension of the client's experience and combine it with the physical dimension to form a holistic view of the person. (Bolander, 3rd ed., p. 630)

1. What are the components of psychosocial assessment?____________________

2. How does psychosocial assessment help the patient?____________________

____

Looking for the answers to these questions will help you concentrate while you read the text.

While Reading

THE 5 W'S

A strategy for helping you stay actively involved while reading your textbook is to use the 5 W's to lead you to the main idea and major details of a reading selection. The 5-W questions are:

- *Who* or what is the assigned reading about? (The answer to this question leads you to the topic, or subject.)
- *What* is the main point being made about the subject? (The answer to this question leads you to the main idea.)
- *When*?
- *Where*?
- *Why* or how?

} Provide the major details

As you read your assignments, thinking about the 5-W questions will help you to concentrate on the author's main ideas and major details. Read the chapter section by section. Ask the 5-W questions. You may want to write the answers to your questions or other comments concerning the text in the margins. Writing notes while you read helps you stay actively involved with the text.

EXERCISE 11–9

Directions. Read the following selection and formulate questions using the 5 W's.

Formulate your questions: ______________________________

____

____

COMPONENTS OF PSYCHOSOCIAL HEALTH ASSESSMENT

The two components of the psychosocial health assessment are the history and the Mental Status Examination (MSE). Both components focus specifically on the psychologic, social, cultural, and spiritual dimensions of a person, with the physical dimension included only as a brief summary of the problems that were identified during the physical assessment. The psychosocial assessment allows you to collect data from each dimension of the client's experience and combine it with the physical dimension to form a holistic view of the person. (Bolander, 3rd ed., p. 630)

Comprehending? Yes ___ No ___

SUMMARIZING

Monitor your comprehension by answering your questions. Your answers to the 5-W questions will give you a summary of each topic. Restate the author's information in your own words. This paraphrasing helps you to comprehend the text selection. Be certain that you understand the information before you proceed to the next boldface heading.

After Reading

UNDERLINING

Highlight the main ideas and details that you want to remember.

WRITING

Prepare a study guide. Write a summary or outline as a review of the chapter as a whole. Work from the general (main ideas) to the specific (details). This written summary or outline will later serve as a study guide.

STUDYING

Use your aids for retention. Review all underlined text material, summaries, and outlines.

Answer the review questions at the end of each chapter. Design a practice test based on your assigned reading. Answer the practice questions and correct your answers. Taking these practice tests is an invaluable method for reinforcing your knowledge of the material. Your improved comprehension and retention of textbook information will result in better test grades.

EXERCISE 11–10

Directions. Use all the reading comprehension strategies you learned in this chapter to concentrate on, comprehend, and retain textbook information. The questions and directions in this exercise will help guide your reading of the following selection from a nursing text. (Bolander, 3rd ed., pp. 629–630)

A psychosocial health assessment begins with an interview process that addresses all of the dimensions of an individual. It differs from the traditional medical-surgical history in which you collect only concrete, factual information relevant to the development of symptoms and past medical-surgical conditions. In a psychosocial assessment you also strive to form a picture of the person's unique personality characteristics, including strengths and weaknesses. This picture is subjective and therefore less tangible than assessment of purely physiologic data. A **psychosocial history** is the person's own story told in the person's own words from a personal point of view. The person being interviewed is considered the primary source of data. Valuable information and insight can also be obtained from secondary data sources such as family, friends, previous records, laboratory findings, and other diagnostic tests.

The purpose of the psychosocial health assessment is to establish a data base from which you can identify specific human responses and problems, make a nursing diagnosis, and develop an appropriate nursing care plan. Much of the completeness and accuracy of the information collected depends on your ability to communicate effectively.

OBTAINING A PSYCHOSOCIAL HEALTH ASSESSMENT

The Interview Process

Because good communication skills are crucial to conducting a psychosocial history, the communication techniques discussed in Chapter 25 are important in psychosocial assessment. As in all nurse-client communications, rapport is essential. **Rapport** implies that there is a sense of understanding and trust between you and your client and that both of you have a vested interest in the client's well-being. This rapport helps the client feel more comfortable in revealing personal facts. Your ability to establish good rapport affects the quality of the psychosocial health assessment and the information that you will get throughout the interview.

In preparing for a psychosocial interview, you must consider not only the person being interviewed but also yourself and the setting in which the interview will take place. Your initial contact with a person is extremely important because it sets the tone for the development of a therapeutic relationship in all subsequent interactions. One of the goals of the psychosocial health assessment is to elicit the person's feelings, thoughts, and values in order to identify individual needs. Meeting this goal depends on your approach.

The way in which you approach a client has a direct bearing on how that person will respond to you. You give messages verbally through what you say and nonverbally through your actions and behavior. You should be aware that your appearance, the way you ask questions, and nonverbal forms of communication all contribute to the way in which another person views you. Tone of voice; choice of words; facial expression; body language, such as degree of eye contact, crossed arms, a hurried manner; and whether you stand or sit all give direct messages.

The primary goal when initiating an interview is to establish trust. Your ability to be genuine, honest, and open fosters trust. Warm human interest enhances the interview process. Without this element the interview can become a monotonous, mechanical task of little value. For many clients, talking with another person who listens with nonjudgmental understanding rather than criticizing and admonishing is a unique experience. When you focus interest and concern entirely on the client without imposing advice or control, the psychosocial health assessment can be a very positive experience.

The ideal setting for the psychosocial interview is a private office free of interruptions. This, however, is not always feasible. The interview may be conducted in a home, in a clinic examination room, at the hospital bedside, in a vehicle, or in a variety of other settings. No matter where the interview takes place, the process should have a basic structure and a quality of formality and professionalism.

You should make an effort to provide as much privacy as possible. For example, if an individual is interviewed at the bedside in a multiple-patient room, you should draw the curtains. Affording some measure of privacy indicates respect for the person being interviewed. Even this small amount of privacy may influence the person's response to your questions.

Begin the interview by introducing yourself and identifying your position. In some cases it is helpful to obtain permission for the interview from the person being interviewed. If the person is reluctant to give a history, help the person explain the reason for this reluctance. Let the person know that one of your responsibilities as a nurse is to understand how an individual feels about and reacts to illness.

You may want to assure the person that the information collected during a psychosocial health assessment is confidential within the health care team and will be used to provide more thorough and individualized care. You should explain that a client does not have to talk about anything that the person does not want to discuss. This helps decrease anxiety and gives the person a greater sense of control. If possible, it is best to sit during the interview to communicate that you are interested and have time to listen.

The person you are interviewing may reveal many aspects about lifestyle, behaviors, and attitudes during this interview process. The person also may disclose details of life that you find distressing or objectionable.

It is imperative that you maintain a nonjudgmental attitude. The purpose of the psychosocial health assessment is to obtain a data base for making judgments about health, not judgments about the lifestyles, behaviors, or attitudes of another person.

If a family or significant others are present, you may ask them to step outside or wait elsewhere. If the client clearly prefers them to stay, however, respect the person's wish. Family and friends can be excellent sources of information. When others are present during the interview, you should also allow time for the client to speak with you in private. A private conference will give clients an opportunity to discuss things that they may not have wanted to talk about in front of others. In talking with persons receiving health care, it is important to speak at a level that they can understand. Therefore, it may be more appropriate to use lay terms and familiar language rather than medical jargon. Complex medical terminology and jargon can be frightening and block effective communication. Throughout the interview, you should listen for conflicting or missing information. Sometimes, you may need to rephrase a question to help the person gain a better understanding of the information you are seeking.

At the conclusion of the interview, it is always helpful if you briefly summarize or restate any major concerns. It is important to give the client a chance to ask questions, add information, and give other feedback. To make sure that the person agrees with your conclusion or understanding of the situation, it is also important for you to verify what you think you heard. At the end of the interview, you should thank the person for the time and cooperation provided. You may shake hands with the person if this step is appropriate.

Initially, you may find that conducting a psychosocial health assessment makes you uncomfortable. It takes time to develop good interviewing skills. With practice, you will become familiar with the interview process and begin to develop your own style.

BEFORE READING

Previewing

1. Identify the topic. Use heading and subheadings.
2. Read the first and last paragraph.
3. Pay attention to key vocabulary words, which are in italics.
4. After following these preview steps, choose one of the following as the best title for this selection.
   a. Social Networks
   b. Behavior and Sociologic Assessment
   c. The Psychosocial Health Interview
   d. The Role of the Nurse as a Primary Figure in a Patient's Social Network

Questioning

5. Based on your preview, formulate questions from the heading of the reading selection. Examples of questions:

   What is the goal of a psychosocial interview? ______________________

   How can a nurse conduct a psychosocial health assessment. Now formulate

   your questions: ______________________

   ____

WHILE READING

6. Ask the 5-W questions. Read the selection with the purpose of answering your questions. Remember to stop at each boldface heading to monitor your comprehension.

Summarizing

Answer your 5-W questions. Remember to monitor your comprehension as you complete each topic. Restate the author's information in your own words. This paraphrasing improves comprehension.

AFTER READING

Underlining

7. Highlight the main ideas and details that you will want to remember. Underline the main ideas and circle the details.

Writing

8. Write a summary or outline of the selection.

Studying

9. Review all underlined material and the written summary or outline. Design a practice test. Correct your answers.

Comprehending? Yes ___ No ___

EXERCISE 11–11

Directions. Read the following selection from Bolander (3rd ed., pp. 540–542, 544–545, and 554). Use the strategies for textbook reading discussed in this chapter. These strategies will help you to concentrate on, comprehend, and retain textbook information. Remember to *preview, question, read, underline, summarize, paraphrase, write,* and *study* the information in this excerpt from a nursing textbook.

Nurses frequently do lifting as part of their job activities. Lifting subjects the body to physical stresses that can result in musculoskeletal injury. Nurses are particularly at risk when the objects lifted are heavy, as when nurses lift clients who weigh as much as, or more than, they do. However, nurses need not lift heavy loads to injure themselves. Temporarily or permanently disabling injuries, particularly back injuries, can occur when nurses lift even small objects, if the lifting is done incorrectly.

Because musculoskeletal injuries are so common, most hospitals insist that nurses be trained in good body mechanics as a condition of employment. Good **body mechanics (biomechanics)** are the coordinated and efficient ways in which the body is used while moving from one position to another. Nurses are expected to come to their jobs in the hospital knowing and habitually using good body mechanics. Still, most hospitals provide a review of safe body mechanics as part of their employee orientation programs. In addition, most hospitals and nursing homes provide mechanical devices and may even provide teams of specially trained staff members to do the lifting or to assist in lifting and moving heavy loads. Employers are generally doing whatever they can to prevent musculoskeletal injuries on the job. They know that such injuries are significantly costly to their employees, to themselves, and to the clients they serve.

Try to imagine how you would feel if you were attempting to help a sick, weak person get out of bed and you hurt your back in the process. What if you could no longer hold the person up and caused a fall? How would you feel if the person broke a bone, received bruises, or suffered a head injury during the fall? Aside from your feelings, could you afford to be out of work with your back injury? Could you afford a legal defense if an injured person sued you? Would you have the means to pay if you lost a lawsuit? How would your employers feel about you dropping one of their patients? How would they feel about you causing them to be sued? Would your insurance rates go up because of such an incident? The implications of such a back injury can be enormous, particularly because musculoskeletal injuries are often preventable. And, because they are preventable, you may bear the responsibility for their occurrence.

For your own protection, as well as for the good of your clients and your employers, you must learn proper body mechanics and use them consistently in all of the work that you do. Consistently using good body mechanics will be difficult as you are learning new nursing skills.

As you learn and practice new skills, you will have to think consciously about everything you do and how you are holding your body as you do it. You will be tempted to think only of the steps of each new skill you need to master and to forget about your body. Forgetting can be a costly mistake.

This chapter will provide you with some basic principles that will help you to learn body mechanics. In addition to attending to your health and safety, these principles can be applied to help ensure the safest and easiest completion of certain tasks. In fact, these are principles you should be using, often without thinking about them, every day for the rest of your professional life. Your instructors will do their part in insisting that you follow through with good body mechanics as they observe all that you do throughout your nursing education. However, in the final analysis, it will be your own attention to forming new, and correct, habits that determines how successful you will be at preventing your own injury.

In this chapter, we focus on scientific principles that will help you to protect yourself from back injury. In subsequent chapters, these principles will be integrated into procedures you will use as you provide client care.

SELECTED PHYSICS PRINCIPLES

As a nurse, you will frequently be called on to apply principles from the sciences to your work in providing client care. In particular, three sets of scientific principles from physics will be of assistance to you in preventing musculoskeletal injuries. These include principles relating to stability, leverage, and motion.

Stability of Objects

Stability is steadiness of position. Three important principles concerning the stability of an object relate to the **base of support** (foundation on which an object rests), the **center of gravity** (center, or heaviest part, of an object), and the **line of gravity** (imaginary line going straight down through an object's center of gravity). Figure 11–1 shows these areas on a human male in correct body alignment, and the three principles concerning stability are illustrated in Figure 11–2. The three principles are as follows:

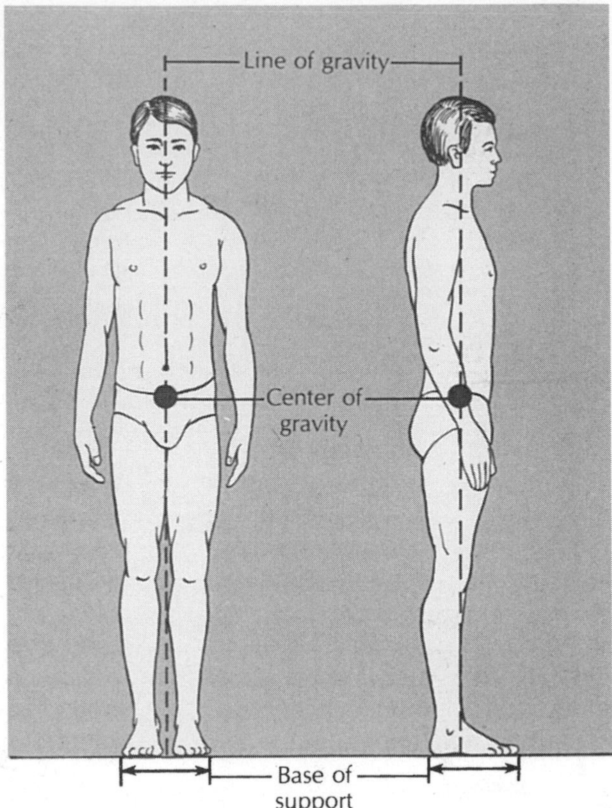

Figure 11–1 The base of support, center of gravity, and line of gravity in a man who is in correct body alignment. The center of gravity would be slightly lower in a woman. Note how the line of gravity passes through the center of the base of support.

- The wider the base of support, the more stable the object. For example, the pyramids of Egypt are very stable. A tall lamp with a small base is less stable. A typewriter is stable. A dime balanced on its edge is not. A briefcase that is standing with its handle up is less stable than when placed on its side, ready to be opened. A nurse with feet spread so as to provide a wider base of support is more stable than a nurse with feet held together.
- The lower the center of gravity, the more stable an object. For example, when lying flat, a brick is very stable. A long pole, if placed on one end, lacks stability and can easily topple. A merry-go-round is stable. A Ferris wheel is much less stable. A heavy book is less stable when placed upright on its bottom edge than when placed flat on its side. A nurse who needs to reach down (to pick up an object, for example) is more stable if the center of gravity is lowered in a squat than if the body is bent at the hips and the center of gravity remains high.
- The closer the line of gravity is to the center of the base of support the more stable is the object. For example, the Eiffel Tower is stable. The Leaning Tower of Pisa is far less stable. In fact, the Leaning Tower of Pisa leans just a bit more each year, and if its line of gravity is allowed to fall too far outside of its base of support, it will surely topple. A nurse who leans too far from the base of support is much less stable than when standing upright.

Use of Leverage

The wise nurse uses principles of leverage to assist in lifting and moving objects. **Leverage** is the use of a **lever** (a rigid or firm structure) supported on a **fulcrum**, or **axis** (fixed

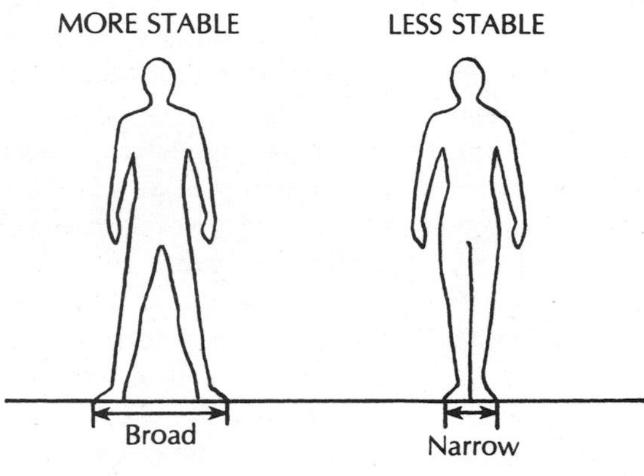

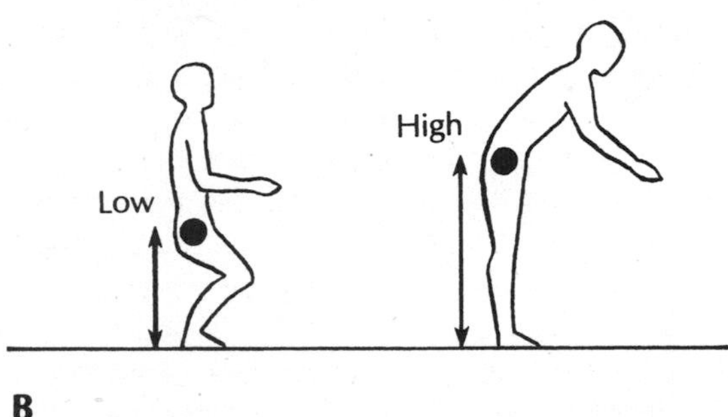

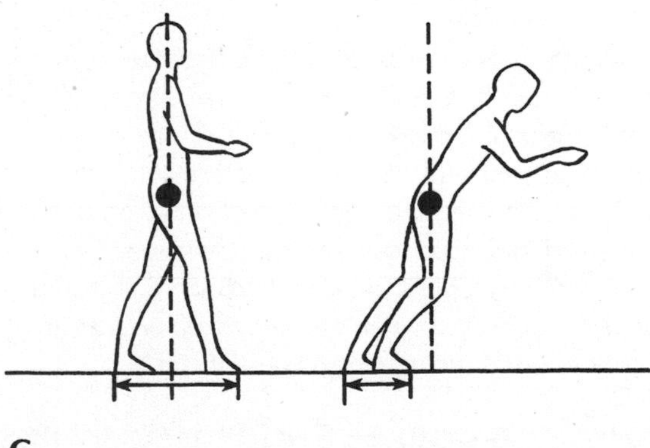

Figure 11–2 Factors affecting stability. *A,* The wider the base of support, the more stable the object. *B,* The lower the center of gravity, the more stable the object. *C,* The closer the line of gravity to the center of the base of support, the more stable the object.

point on which a lever moves), to move a **load** (weight of an object or person, often referred to as resistance) more easily by the application of **force** (effort exerted). There are three classes of levers:

- Class I levers consist of a load on one end, a fulcrum in the middle, and downward force exerted on the opposite end of the lever. The force can be a pushing downward from above or a pulling downward from below. For example, a person pushes downward (applies force) on one end of a crowbar (lever) over a log (fulcrum) to move a heavy rock (resistance) more easily.
- Class II levers consist of a fulcrum at one end, an upward effort at the other end, and the load in between. The upward effort can be a pushing upward from below or a pulling upward from above. For example, a wheelbarrow's wheel serves as a fulcrum, and the load in the middle is lifted by applying an upward force on the handles at the opposite end.
- Class III levers consist of a fulcrum at one end, a load at the opposite end, and an upward (pushing or pulling) force in the middle. For example, a fishing rod is held in one hand (the fulcrum) as the other hand applies an upward force further up the pole to help lift a heavy fish on the opposite end of the pole.

The human musculoskeletal system is a series of leverage systems that help us move with minimal effort. The bones serve as levers; the joints serve as fulcrums; and the muscles and tendons work to apply force as needed to move the body parts and to move loads added to the body. For example, the occipitoatlantal joint serves as a fulcrum as the longissimus capitis muscles in the posterior cervical area contract and apply a downward force at the back of the neck that moves the posterior portion of the head downward and the anterior portion of the head (the load) upward. This movement is an example of a Class I lever.

A nurse might exemplify the use of a Class II lever in lifting a client. You would begin to lift the client by putting your arms under the person's body so that your radius and ulna bones served as levers, your wrists rested on the bed to serve as fulcrums, and you applied an upward force with your entire upper body to pull your forearms (and the added weight on them) upward. As you shifted the person's weight in your arms to continue with the lift, you would use your elbows as fulcrums and your forearms as levers. You also would contract your biceps muscles to apply a lifting force between elbow and wrists. This lifting force, which would lift your wrists and the person upward, would be an example of a Class III lever.

Motion

Nurses frequently make use of Newton's first law of motion. This law pertains to inertia. **Inertia** is the property of matter that causes it to tend to remain at rest (if it is at rest) or to remain in motion (if it is in motion). The law of inertia states that objects at rest will tend to remain at rest and objects in motion will tend to remain in motion at a constant speed and along a straight line unless acted on by an outside force. Two such outside forces are gravity and friction. Because you must work against the force of gravity, more effort is needed to lift a heavy object than to push or pull it along a horizontal plane. **Friction** is the resistance encountered when two irregular surfaces are moved across each other. Friction makes even horizontal movement more difficult.

GUIDELINES FOR CORRECT BODY MECHANICS

As a nurse, you must apply your knowledge of stability, leverage, and motion so that you use the correct body alignment and effective body movements that will help you to prevent back injuries. Scientific principles related to these three areas are summed up in Table 11–1.

Correct Body Alignment

Body alignment, or **posture**, is the proper relationship of body parts to one another. Correct body alignment is important for proper body functioning, reduces strain, and helps

TABLE 11–1 Selected Scientific Principles and Related Nursing Interventions for Body Mechanics

Principle	Nursing Interventions
The wider the base of support, the more stable the object.	When lifting clients or heavy objects, stand with your feet apart.
The lower the center of gravity, the more stable the object.	When picking up an object from the floor, squat rather than bend from the waist.
The closer the line of gravity to the center of the base of support, the more stable the object.	When reaching for something a short distance from you, do not let your line of gravity fall outside of your base of support
Leverage is the use of a lever supported on a fulcrum to move a load more easily by the application of force.	Use leverage whenever possible to reduce strain and prevent injury to yourself and others.
An object at rest tends to stay at rest, and an object in motion tends to stay in motion at a constant speed and along a straight line unless acted on by an outside force such as:	To turn heavy clients more easily, change the center of gravity and begin the turn that will tend to continue.
Gravity	To help overcome gravity, lower the head of clients' beds before attempting to slide them upward on the mattress.
Friction	To move a client more easily, decrease friction by applying powder to lubricate the skin, using a lift sheet to move the client, or rolling rather than pushing or pulling the client.

maintain balance. When standing in correct alignment, as Figure 11–1 illustrates, the body is held in the following ways:

- back is straight
- head is erect, not leaning forward, backward, or sideways
- chin is tucked in, not jutting forward
- arms are at sides with elbows slightly flexed
- the lower abdominal area is pulled up and in
- buttocks are tucked under to prevent excessive curvature of the lumbar spine
- knees are slightly flexed
- toes are pointed forward

It is important to practice proper body alignment yourself and to demonstrate it to others. Also it is essential to position those people in your care in proper body alignment.

Effective Body Movement

Good body mechanics begins with proper body alignment and continues with adherence to several guidelines. These guidelines can be used in many of the tasks you will have to perform in nursing. If you are able to understand the underlying principles and apply them appropriately as new situations arise, your work will be a good deal easier and safer.

Come to work dressed appropriately for lifting and moving. For example, you should wear clothing that will allow you to maintain a broad base of support and to squat to keep your center of gravity (your pelvis) low and over your base of support as necessary. Do not wear clothing that will subject you to embarrassment if you assume certain positions. You should wear comfortable clothing that is loose enough to allow freedom of movement and that will not cause you to be self-conscious about what you are wearing.

Plan your movements. Before beginning, assess the situation and determine the best (e.g., the safest, most efficient, and least difficult) method of movement. Be aware of the space allowed for the movement. The space available for the move can vary depending on the amount of equipment and other furniture in the room. Adequate space is important to move a person safely and effectively. Rearrange the room, if necessary. When moving a client to or from a bed, the height of the bed can make a considerable difference in the amount of effort you will have to make. Adjust the bed to the best height for the work you are going to do (a working height). Do not begin the move until you have planned adequately. Do not hurry unless you face an emergency.

Be realistic about your ability to lift the weight involved. Be aware of your personal abilities, muscle strength, and limitations.

Generally, nurses should not lift more than 35 per cent of their body weight without assistance. For example, a 60-kg (132-lb) nurse should not lift a load greater than 21 kg (46 lbs).

Obtain help if at all in doubt about whether or not you can manage the move. If you know that help will be needed, determine the number of persons required to complete the move safely and correctly.

If you are moving a client, assess the amount of assistance the person can provide. Assess the person's strengths, limitations, and ability to move. Why does this person require help? What is the goal of the move? People vary in their weights (load), abilities, and willingness to assist with moves. Does the person want to move and to help with the move? Is the person able to understand and follow directions?

Let people move themselves as much as possible and allowed. They know what hurts; you do not. They can protect themselves from pain better than you can.

If clients are unable to move independently, it is usually safer for all concerned if they can participate in the move. To prepare clients for participation, carefully describe the planned moves to them. Discuss exactly how they can participate. Consider the clients' suggestions and preferences concerning the move and integrate them into your plans whenever possible.

Coordinate your movements. When working with others to move an object or person, identify one person to be the "leader." Movements are more coordinated when directed by one person. The leader clarifies what each person will do (e.g., "Debbie, you take his feet" or "I'll count '1-2-3-lift' and we'll all lift on the word 'lift' "). Following a leader's directions helps to ensure that the move is coordinated, with everyone beginning and moving at the same time, and that the move is safer for all concerned.

Maintain a broad base of support. Keep your feet apart to increase your stability. This stance also allows you to shift your weight readily from one foot to the other.

Keep your center of gravity low. Bending your knees while your feet are spread apart not only lowers your center of gravity but also widens your base of support to provide for extra stability and balance.

Be sure your line of gravity passes through the center of your base of support. You ensure the correct position by moving your center of gravity (pelvic area) directly over the space between your two feet. Alternatively, you can position your feet so as to widen your base of support, helping to ensure that it remains under your center of gravity. If you are shifting your weight (and center of gravity with it) as you move, you may move your line of gravity outside of your base of support unless you have planned correctly and widened your base of support before the move.

Use leverage to increase the efficiency of the energy you use. Levers help move heavy objects by decreasing the amount of force required to complete a lift and move. Nurses frequently use their elbows as fulcrums and their hands and arms as levers. To help lift a sick child and place a pad or bedpan under the child, for example, you might place your hands and forearms under the child's back and contract your biceps to lift the weight. These maneuvers use your body's natural levers.

Bring the load to be lifted or moved as close as possible to your center of gravity. Notice what happens to your body as you take a heavy bowling ball in one hand and hold it down by your side. Your head and shoulders shift and flex your spine in the opposite direction because the weight added to one side of your body by the ball has moved your center of gravity toward the ball, and you must move your body in the opposite direction to reestablish the center of gravity over your base of support. Failure to make such a compensating move would make you unstable, and you would topple over unless you compensated in some other way.

One way to compensate is to use your muscles to hold the ball in place at your side. This method, however, would cause a strain on your back muscles and on your leg muscles on the side holding the ball. A better way to compensate for the additional load on your body, without flexing your spine in the opposite direction, is to bring the ball as near as possible to your center of gravity by holding the ball in both hands in front of your body just below waist level. This position reestablishes your center of gravity over the center of your base of support and provides stability. However, what do you do if you cannot bring the object you want to move close to your center of gravity? For example, suppose the object to be moved is a stuck window you want to raise. In such a case, you should bring your center of gravity as close as possible to the windowsill. Even if the load to be lifted is not particularly heavy, bringing it closer to your center of gravity lessens the amount of work your muscles have to do to lift it. If you doubt this statement, try holding this textbook out at arm's length for awhile and then try holding it in, near your center of gravity. Compare for yourself which position is easier to maintain.

Move in a straight line and avoid twisting. When pushing or pulling an object or person, face the direction in which the movement will be made. Point your toes in that direction, placing one foot in front of the other to widen the base of support. Place the object in motion by exerting pressure on it as you move your body forward. For example, if you stand at the side of a person's bed and try to pull the person more toward the head of the bed, you should face the head of the bed and move toward the head of the bed. If you were to face the side of the bed and attempt to move the person toward the head of the bed, you might have to twist your back to complete the movement. Twisting movements can cause strains that can be severely painful and disabling.

Move heavy loads forward while maintaining a wide base of support. Once you have a good hold on a heavy object, it is close to your base of support, you are facing in the direction you wish to move, and your feet are apart with one leg in front of the other providing a wide base of support, you are ready to move. How do you move without lifting one foot to take a step (i.e., how do you lift one foot without causing the other foot to become the sole base of support)? When you do not have to move very far, you can simply shift your weight (and the weight of the load) from one foot (the one behind) closer to the other (forward) foot rather than taking a step to effect movement. Shifting your weight in such a manner avoids strain on muscles.

Use smooth, continuous, rhythmic movements. More energy is required to make many short movements than to make one continuous movement. Smooth rhythmic movements permit the efficient use of muscles by allowing more time for muscle contraction.

Use larger muscle groups, such as those in the legs and thighs, for heavier work. These muscles fatigue less quickly than smaller muscles, such as those of the arms and back. The use of long, strong muscles of the legs and thighs also helps to protect the back and prevent damage to the intervertebral disks (cushionlike structures between the vertebrae of the spinal column). These disks can be damaged when sudden or extreme force is exerted on them (e.g., by incorrectly lifting or trying to lift too heavy a weight).

Use your entire hand rather than your fingers. The hand has a broader area than individual fingers do, and hand muscles are stronger than finger muscles.

For longer tasks, change positions and alternate the larger muscle groups being used. Changing the muscles being used lessens the chance of fatigue in the muscles (e.g., bear weight more on your right leg for awhile and then shift to your left leg).

Put on your "internal girdle" before lifting and moving heavy objects. To put on your internal girdle, contract your abdominal muscles, so that you feel them move in and up, and contract your gluteal (buttocks) muscles in a firm movement, drawing them upward. The internal girdle helps protect the intervertebral disks of the lower back. For additional methods to protect the lower back, see Box 29–1.

When attempting to lift a heavy object, apply the lifting force at the area of the object's greatest weight. This procedure will help to overcome the object's inertial mass. If you apply the lifting force at any other point, the greatest weight will most likely be farther from your base of support and will cause you unnecessary strain. For example, you might easily lift a small table by grasping both sides of its top, but you would probably find it difficult or impossible to lift the same table by grasping only one of the table legs.

To roll heavy, helpless persons, change the center of gravity more toward the direction you wish it to go. For example, before attempting to roll a completely helpless man to his left side, cross his right arm over his body toward the left side and cross his right leg over his left leg. The rest of his body will be easier to roll as it follows the limbs that have led the way.

To move a heavy object, rock it back and forth several times to help it gain <u>momentum</u> *before providing the full effort necessary to move it when you want it to go.* This maneuver shows that you can apply Newton's first law and start an object in motion with the understanding that it will tend to stay in motion.

Use pulling or pushing rather than lifting movements whenever possible. Pulling or pushing an object or person across a level surface uses less effort than lifting because lifting requires overcoming the effects of gravity, whereas pulling or pushing requires only overcoming the effects of friction.

When moving an object or person up an incline, change the degree of incline, if possible, to best take advantage of gravity. Pushing a person or object up an incline is more difficult than moving the same person or object across a level surface. Moving a person or object across a level surface is more difficult than sliding the person or object down an incline. For example, helpless clients frequently keep the heads of their beds in an elevated position, causing them to slide downward in their beds and be in abnormal body positions. Nurses then have to move them back toward the head of their bed. This maneuver is much easier to do if the head of the bed in lowered to a flat position before attempting such moves.

When moving an object across a horizontal surface, use a pulling motion rather than pushing. Pushing an object along a horizontal plane creates more friction than does pulling it. It is therefore easier to pull than to push.

When necessary, decrease friction before pushing or pulling an object across a surface. Decreasing friction can reduce your workload. Friction may be decreased by measures to smooth the two surfaces that will come into contact. Sometimes, cleaning, drying, or lubricating one or both surfaces reduces friction. Sometimes, covering one surface with something that will cause less resistance during the movement reduces friction. For example, you may place a lift sheet (a flat bed sheet that has been folded in quarters) under your client and pull on the lift sheet to slide the client over the surface of the bed. In this case, sheeting comes into contact with sheeting, and both are smooth enough to reduce friction.

If possible, when moving an object over a horizontal surface, roll it rather than pull it. Rolling an object creates less friction than pulling does. If it is feasible, rolling may be easier. Some objects (e.g., square boxes) do not roll well. In such cases, it may be possible to place one or more sets of rollers under the object to ease movement.

Maintain consistency of method when moving a client. Evaluate the success of your method of movement, and write the method on the client's care plan so the same method will be used consistently.

Comprehending? Yes ___ No ___

• VOCABULARY CHECK

Directions. Below are 10 words taken from the key words section of this chapter. Circle the letter of the best definition from the four choices.

1. Biomechanics

a the study of biology as applied to the laws of nature
b the application of mechanical laws to living structures
c mechanical plants or animals, robotics
d the study of machines and mechanical laws governing them

2. Gravity

a weight
b weightlessness
c imaginary force
d a sinking object

3. Disk

a the backbone
b a rupture
c cushion-like structures
d the spine

4. Stability

a changing conditions
b the strength to endure
c the inability to endure
d a plan of action

5. Posture

a a mental attitude
b an attitude of the body
c problems with the back
d deviation of the spine

6. Jargon

a slang
b foreign language
c specialized vocabulary
d medical terminology

7. Psychosocial

a pertaining to the inability to socialize
b pertaining to psychic and social elements
c pertaining to pathologic social behavior
d pertaining to attempts of the mentally ill to seek peers

8. Friction
   - **a** a head-on collision of two vehicles
   - **b** an argument that is easily resolved
   - **c** the rubbing of one body against another
   - **d** a pressure point painful to the touch

9. Vertebrae
   - **a** segments of the spine
   - **b** injuries to the spine
   - **c** segments of the body
   - **d** broken bones

10. Fulcrum
   - **a** support to the spine
   - **b** support to a lever
   - **c** emotional support
   - **d** a psychological crutch

• CRITICAL THINKING LOG

List the strategies you learned in this chapter.	Select the strategy that is most useful for your school success.	How can you apply this strategy to your nursing studies?

• SUMMARY

Reading a textbook is different from reading books for pleasure. Learn to survey your textbooks. Survey the title page, preface, table of contents, glossary, appendix, and index. Becoming familiar with your text as a whole helps you to get ready to learn the information in each chapter. You can learn the specific strategies that will help you to concentrate on, comprehend, and retain textbook information. These strategies are:

- Previewing
- Questioning
- Summarizing

After reading, underline the main ideas and details you want to remember. Write a summary or outline to use as a study guide. Study all underlined text material, summaries, outlines, and end-of-chapter review questions. Design and take your own practice test.

These active reading strategies will ensure your success in reading nursing textbooks.

CHAPTER 12

Graphic Aids

• OBJECTIVE

To develop techniques for reading and studying graphs, pictures, tables, and diagrams.

• KEY WORDS

Pay attention to the following key words, which are underscored the first time they appear in this chapter. Try to determine the meaning of these words in the passage. If you need further help, use your dictionary or the glossary in the back of this book.

Look up the medical terminology in your medical dictionary or the glossary. As you read the exercises in this chapter, write additional words you need to learn in the space provided.

MEDICAL TERMINOLOGY

congestive
diuretics
gout
immobility
postoperative
pulse
receptive
tachycardia

GENERAL VOCABULARY

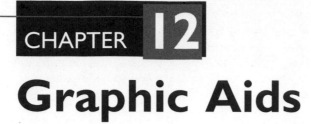

caption
collaborate
concise
enhances
expedient
footnotes
graphic
legend

thrombus

vital signs

statistics

systematic

____

____

____

____

____

____

• WHY READ GRAPHIC AIDS?

Many students skip over visual materials such as graphs, pictures, tables, and diagrams. It is tempting to look for ways to shorten textbook assignments, but ignoring the visual materials in your nursing textbooks will undermine your efforts to succeed in your studies.

Nursing textbooks are filled with visual materials. These graphs, pictures, tables, and diagrams contain visual information that is pertinent to your understanding the main ideas in a chapter. Furthermore, when you interpret this visual information and paraphrase the ideas in language you understand, you will remember this material. Therefore, visual aids serve to improve your:

- Concentration, by visually attracting your attention.
- Comprehension, by your interpreting the visual information into verbal language.
- Retention, by reinforcing your memory when you learn information visually and verbally.

Graphic materials are designed to be clear and accurate so they will help you learn unfamiliar concepts.

Be aware of the help you receive from graphic aids and focus on these materials to help you learn the information in your nursing textbooks.

• HOW GRAPHIC AIDS RELATE TO THE WRITTEN TEXT

Graphic aids make it easier to understand and read the written text. Below are pages copied from a nursing book (Arnold and Boggs, pp. 515–516). Carefully read the text describing the four steps in the advocacy process. Then study Table 12–1. Note especially how the table summarizes, in an easy-to-read format, the main points of the written text.

EXAMPLE 12–1

STEPS IN THE ADVOCACY PROCESS

The nurse, as the client's advocate, uses a four-step informational process, as presented in Table 12–1. The nurse's power base in advocacy is relevant knowledge and information. Basically, the nurse needs to be aware of personal and professional ethics, values, and prejudices. "One needs to have a good knowledge and understanding of personal views on how human beings relate to each other in a framework or philosophy of fairness" (Kohnke, 1982). For example, if the nurse thinks of elderly clients as helpless and equates aging with being taken care of, then the nurse will be likely to "take charge" of all client health activities, even those the client is still capable of performing with little or no assistance. In this situation, personal values have gotten in the way of individualized professional nursing values associated with client advocacy.

TABLE 12–1 Informational Steps in Client Advocacy

Knowledge of the personally held values of nurse and client.
Awareness of treatment and of professional and personal goals.
Information about professional nursing, environmental, and interpersonal protocols and of the bureaucratic structure of the organizational work system.
Knowledge of potential power or recognition needs that could compromise the integrity of the client advocacy process.

From Arnold and Boggs, p. 516.

Self-awareness is important. Nurses should have a firm understanding of their personal as well as their professional goals in nursing situations. Frequently both goals are unstated and remain a part of the blind self until they are called into conscious awareness by circumstance. For example, the nurse may have an unstated personal goal of wanting to be liked by every client or an unspoken professional goal of never making a mistake in the delivery of clinical nursing care. Each implied goal will have as much effect on the nurse's interpersonal behaviors with clients and coworkers as a stated professional goal of wanting to learn the latest tracheal suctioning technique.

Understanding the System

To be successful as client advocates, nurses also need to know the environmental, interpersonal, and bureaucratic system within which they work. For example, how do all the units—nursing and hospital administration, the medical staff, and other health system disciplines—relate to one another, and how does the system relate to the community at large? It is important to understand how the communication flow filters through the different systems. Usually a combination of formal and informal communication with other staff is necessary for complete understanding.

The professional nurse can gain some of this knowledge by observing how communication is passed from person to person and by asking many questions. Knowing how the various units are influenced by outside pressures such as politics, financial constraints, consumer groups, and regulatory agencies is as important as knowing who is in charge and who is influential in facilitating change. All of these understandings add to the nurse's power base in effecting change on the client's behalf. With this knowledge base, the nurse is in a position to inform and assist the client in making the most of health care choices with the least amount of effort.

Finally, the nurse needs to recognize personal power needs that stem from his or her personal insecurities and to analyze how those needs affect professional relationships with clients. To a greater or lesser extent, everyone has power needs and insecurities. The important thing is to recognize their presence.

Comprehending? Yes ___ No ___

Thus, one major way graphic aids relate to the written text is by summarizing concisely the major points of the selection. Graphic aids make the textbook more comprehensible.

Graphic aids actually save you time in reading. Instead of writing a lengthy description of a concept, the author may choose to use a graphic aid.

Following is a page taken from a nursing book (Arnold and Boggs, p. 532). Pay attention to how the writer introduces an important idea with a graphic aid rather than writing about it at length.

EXAMPLE 12–2

UNDERSTANDING THE ORGANIZATIONAL SYSTEM

Whenever one works in an organization, either as a student or professional, one automatically becomes a part of an organizational system with established political norms of acceptable behavior. Each organizational system defines its own chain of command and rules about social processes in professional communication. Even though your idea may be excellent, failure to understand the chain of command or an unwillingness to form the positive alliances needed to accomplish your objective dilutes the impact. For example, if your instructor has been defined as your main contact, then it is not in your best interest to seek out staff personnel or other students without also checking with the instructor.

Although side-stepping the identified chain of command and going to a higher or more tangential resource in the hierarchy may appear less threatening initially, the benefits of such action may not resolve the difficulty. Furthermore, the trust needed for serious discussion becomes limited. Some of the reasons for avoiding positive interactions stem from an internal circular process of faulty thinking. Because communication is viewed as part of a process, the sender and receiver act on the information received, which may or may not represent the reality of the situation. Examples of the circular processes that block the development of cooperative and receptive influencing skills in organizational settings are presented in Table 12–2.

TABLE 12–2 Examples of Unclear Communication Processes That Block the Development of Cooperative and Receptive Influencing Skills

Low Self-Disclosure

Consequently
No one knows my real thoughts, feelings, and needs.
Consequently
I think no one cares about me or recognizes my needs.
Others see me as self-sufficient and are unaware that I have a problem.
Consequently
Others are unable to respond to my needs.

Reluctance to Delegate Tasks

Consequently
Other people think I don't believe that others can do the job as well as I can.
Consequently
The others work at a minimum level.
I don't expect or ask others to be involved.
Consequently
Other people don't volunteer to help me.
Consequently
I feel resentful and others feel undervalued and dispensable.

Making Unnecessary Demands

I expect more from others than they think is reasonable.
Consequently
I feel the others are lazy and uncommitted, and I must push harder.
Others see me as manipulative and dehumanizing.
Consequently
Others assume a low profile and don't contribute their ideas.
Consequently
Work production is mediocre.
Morale is low.
Everyone, including me, feels disempowered.

From Arnold and Boggs, p. 532.

Often a person is not directly aware of personal communication blocks in professional relationships. Asking for feedback and engaging in self-reflection give the nurse an honest appraisal of personal communication strategies in professional situations.

As you can see, it is much more expedient (that is, faster and easier) to look at Table 12–2, "Examples of Unclear Communication Processes That Block the Development of Cooperative and Receptive Influencing Skills," than to read the many lines it would take to describe the same information. Graphic aids make the textbook easier to read. Rather than ignoring graphic aids when you read your chapters, you should get in the habit of consulting them to make your reading clearer and ultimately faster.

Comprehending? Yes ___ No ___

• TYPES OF GRAPHIC AIDS

When looking through your nursing textbooks, you have probably noticed the many varieties of graphic aids. Indeed, it would be hard to find a page without at least one. However, a careful examination would show that they are primarily of four types: graphs, pictures, tables, and diagrams.

Graphs

Graphs readily show a comparison between two or more facts or items. Look at Figure 12–1 and notice how people in their sixties, seventies, and eighties are being compared to the mortality rate from hip fracture.

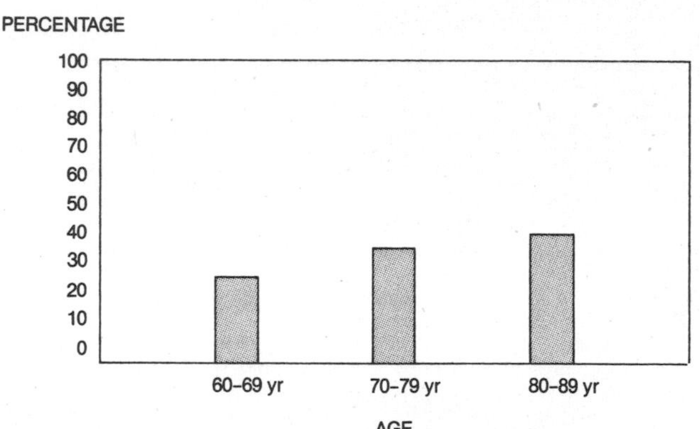

Figure 12–1 Mortality rates associated with hip fractures by age. (From Matteson et al., p. 177)

Pictures

The purpose of pictures is to help you visualize what is being described in the written text. They are included not only to illustrate a major point, but also to add interest to what you are reading. Consider the following example (Matteson and McConnell, pp. 186–187). Note how the picture of acute gouty arthritis enhances the written words (Fig. 12–2).

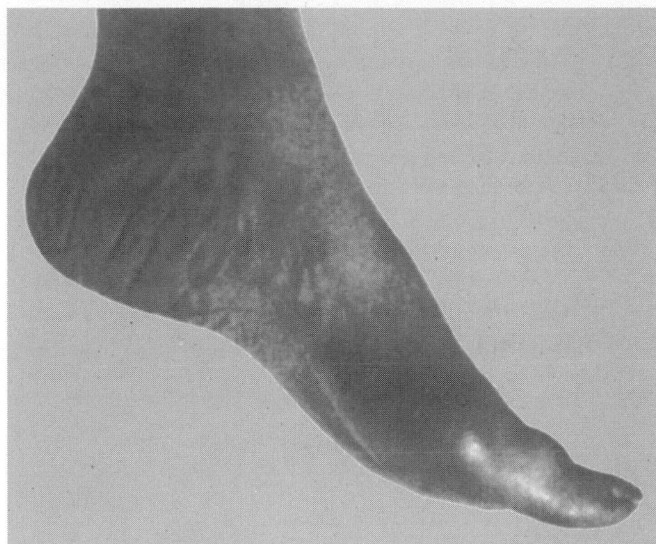

Figure 12–2 Acute gouty arthritis involving the first metatarsophalangeal joint (great toe) (podagra). (From Wyngaarden, J.B., and Smith, L.H. [eds.]: Cecil textbook of medicine, ed. 17, Philadelphia, 1985, W.B. Saunders, p. 1137.)

EXAMPLE 12–3

GOUTY ARTHRITIS

Gout is characterized by episodes of acute arthritis, followed by chronic damage to joints and other structures. The disease tends to run in families and is seen primarily in middle-aged men. It is rarely seen before the age of 30, and studies have shown that the highest incidence occurs in the thirties, forties, and fifties.

Hyperuricemia, an excess of uric acid in the blood and tissues, is the major cause of gout. Increased serum uric acid levels are related either to increased formation of uric acid or decreased excretion of uric acid. Other related factors include sex, age, genetic factors, obesity, higher social class and intelligence, indulgence in alcohol, and high plasma lipid levels. When hyperuricemia is due principally to an inherited metabolic abnormality, the condition is called *primary gout*; when it is due to acquired disease or some environmental factor, it is known as *secondary gout*. Primary gout is seen primarily in men; however, men and women are equally affected by secondary gout.

An acute attack of gouty arthritis is an inflammatory reaction resulting from the presence of sodium urate crystals within a joint. It most often occurs in the great toe, which is affected in 50 percent of the cases. Acute gout also may appear in other joints, mainly in the periphery, such as the feet and ankles, hands, knees, and elbows. Precipitating factors are loss of body weight, high-fat diet, ingestion of certain drugs (penicillin, thiamine chloride, vitamin B_{12}, insulin, folic acid, sulfa, ergotamine tartrate, and mercurial and thiazide diuretics), joint trauma, emotional turmoil, surgery, or overindulgence in food or alcohol.

Each acute episode lasts for a short period of time and is followed by intervals during which there is freedom from symptoms. Some people have only one or two attacks during their lifetime, while others may have repeated occurrences of increasing duration, severity, and frequency with multiple joint involvement. The affected joint becomes reddened, tender, swollen, and hot [see Fig. 12–2]. Individuals may have a sensation of discomfort that, over a period of hours, develops into excruciating pain. Larger joints, such as the knee, may have accumulations of inflammatory effusion. Chalky deposits of urate (tophi) form around joints and areas associated with cartilage, such as the ear: in the elderly, tophi are prone to infection.

Diagnosis is made by means of clinical presentation, serum uric acid levels, identification of uric acid crystals in aspirated synovial fluid, examination of tophi, and radiographs. Serum uric acid levels are elevated to 8 to 10 mg per 100 ml in gouty arthritis as opposed to normal levels of 7 mg per 100 ml. Treatment for an initial acute attack is with colchicine, which is 95 percent effective in providing symptomatic relief. This drug also can provide diagnostic confirmation of the disease. Prophylactic management usually consists of colchicine 0.5 mg and Benemid (probenecid) 0.5 mg every day, weight loss, restriction of foods high in purines (liver, kidney, sweetbreads), and a high fluid intake; however, treatment of asymptomatic hyperuricemia with uric acid–lowering agents is rarely necessary. The drugs must be used judiciously in the elderly because they tend to experience toxicity and adverse reactions.

Tables

The function of tables is to present data (statistics, facts, or numbers) in a systematic way for efficient reading and studying. In Table 12–3, see how the table is organized into columns and headings. Make sure you read all title and column headings. Try to see the relationships among the data given.

Diagrams

Diagrams summarize information that, if written in words, would be lengthy and complicated. From Figure 12–3, try to imagine what it would be like to have to read the same information presented in text form.

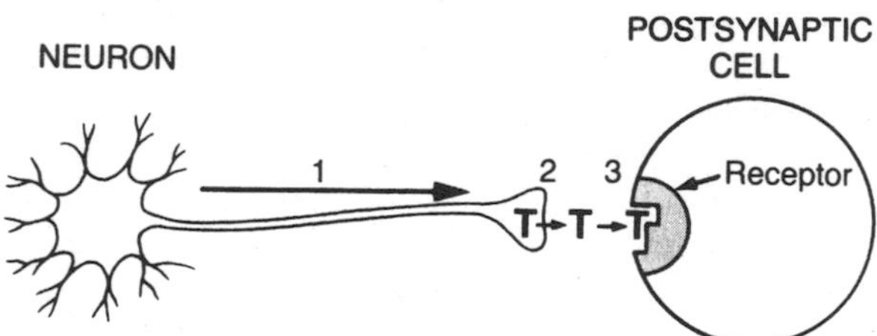

Figure 12–3 How neurons regulate other cells.
1. Action potential
2. Release of neurotransmitter (T)
3. Interaction of T with receptor
} Synaptic transmission
(From Lehne, p. 102)

Regardless of the different types of graphic aids you may encounter in your nursing textbooks, they all serve a similar purpose—to present, in an interesting, concise, and visual way, information that would otherwise be given in long and complicated written text.

Comprehending? Yes ___ No ___

TABLE 12–3 Food and Nutrition Board, National Academy of Sciences—National Research Council Recommended Dietary Allowances,[a] Revised 1989[74]

		Weight[b]		Height[b]		Energy		Fat-Soluble Vitamins				Water-Soluble Vitamins							Minerals					
	Age (years) or Condition	(kg)	(lb)	(cm)	(in)	(kcal)	Protein (g)	Vitamin A (μgRE)[c]	Vitamin D (μg)[d]	Vitamin E (mg α-TE)[e]	Vitamin K (μg)	Vitamin C (mg)	Thiamine (mg)	Riboflavin (mg)	Niacin (mg NE)[f]	Vitamin B_6 (mg)	Folate (μg)	Vitamin B_{12} (μg)	Calcium (mg)	Phosphorus (mg)	Magnesium (mg)	Iron (mg)	Zinc (mg)	Iodine (μg)
Infants	0.0–0.5	6	13	60	24	650	13	375	7.5	3	5	30	0.3	0.4	5	0.3	25	0.3	400	300	40	6	5	40
	0.5–1.0	9	20	71	28	850	14	375	10	4	10	35	0.4	0.5	6	0.6	35	0.5	600	500	60	10	5	50
Children	1–3	13	29	90	35	1300	16	400	10	6	15	40	0.7	0.8	9	1.0	50	0.7	800	800	80	10	10	70
	4–6	20	44	112	44	1800	24	500	10	7	20	45	0.9	1.1	12	1.1	75	1.0	800	800	120	10	10	90
	7–10	28	62	132	52	2000	28	700	10	7	30	45	1.0	1.2	13	1.4	100	1.4	800	800	170	10	10	120
Males	11–14	45	99	157	62	2500	45	1000	10	10	45	50	1.3	1.5	17	1.7	150	2.0	1200	1200	270	12	15	150
	15–18	66	145	176	69	3000	59	1000	10	10	65	60	1.5	1.8	20	2.0	200	2.0	1200	1200	400	12	15	150
	19–24	72	160	177	70	2900	58	1000	10	10	70	60	1.5	1.7	19	2.0	200	2.0	1200	1200	350	10	15	150
	25–50	79	174	176	70	2900	63	1000	5	10	80	60	1.5	1.7	19	2.0	200	2.0	800	800	350	10	15	150
	51+	77	170	173	68	2300	63	1000	5	10	80	60	1.2	1.4	15	2.0	200	2.0	800	800	350	10	15	150
Females	11–14	46	101	157	62	2200	46	800	10	8	45	50	1.1	1.3	15	1.4	150	2.0	1200	1200	280	15	12	150
	15–18	55	120	163	64	2200	44	800	10	8	55	60	1.1	1.3	15	1.5	180	2.0	1200	1200	300	15	12	150
	19–24	58	128	164	65	2200	46	800	10	8	60	60	1.1	1.3	15	1.6	180	2.0	1200	1200	280	15	12	150
	25–50	63	138	163	64	2200	50	800	5	8	65	60	1.1	1.3	16	1.6	180	2.0	800	800	280	15	12	150
	51+	65	143	160	63	1900	50	800	5	8	65	60	1.0	1.2	13	1.6	180	2.0	800	800	280	10	12	150
Pregnant	2nd and 3rd trimester					+300	60	800	10	10	65	70	1.5	1.6	17	2.2	400	2.2	1200	1200	320	30	15	175
Lactating	1st 6 months					+500	65	1300	10	12	65	95	1.6	1.8	20	2.1	280	2.6	1200	1200	355	15	19	200
	2nd 6 months					+500	62	1200	10	11	65	90	1.6	1.7	20	2.1	260	2.6	1200	1200	340	15	16	200

[a]The allowances, expressed as average daily intakes over time, are intended to provide for individual variations among most normal persons as they live in the United States under usual environmental stresses. Diets should be based on a variety of common foods in order to provide other nutrients for which human requirements have been less well defined.

[b]Weights and heights of Reference Adults are actual medians for the U.S. population of the designated age, as reported by National Health and Nutrition Examination Survey II (NHANES II). The use of these figures does not imply that the height-to-weight ratios are ideal.

[c]Retinol equivalents. 1 retinol equivalent = 1 μg retinol or 6 μg β-carotene.

[d]As cholecalciferol. 10 μg cholecalciferol = 400 IU of vitamin D.

[e]α-Tocopherol equivalents. 1 mg *d*-α-tocopherol = 1 α-TE.

[f]1 NE (niacin equivalent) is equal to 1 mg of niacin or 60 mg of dietary tryptophan.

From Bolander, 3rd ed.

• HOW TO READ GRAPHIC AIDS

1. Look over the graphic aid to get a general impression of the visual material.
2. Read the title carefully to determine the subject of the graphic aid.
3. Pay close attention to:
   Headings—titles found above a graphic aid.
   Legends—symbols that explain a graphic aid.
   Captions—an explanation accompanying a graphic aid.
   Footnotes—an explanatory note found below a graphic aid.
   Keys—information used to interpret a graphic aid.
4. Determine the purpose of the graphic aid. For example, ask yourself, "What is being compared?"
5. Examine the units of measurement.
6. Ask:
   a. What information is given in this graphic aid?
   b. How does this information relate to the ideas discussed in the chapter?
   c. How does this graphic aid add to or clarify the ideas discussed in the chapter?
7. Try to make a general statement that relates the graphic aid to the ideas covered in the text.

Figure 12–4 is an example that shows you how to read and interpret a graphic aid.

EXAMPLE 12–4

1. What is the subject of the graph in Figure 12–4? __________
   (vital signs graphic sheet)

2. What is being compared? __________
   (vital signs and time)

3. How is the temperature listed? __________
   (°F and °C)

4. List the vital signs that are being examined. __________
   (body temperature, pulse, blood pressure, respiration)

5. What is the person's body temperature (°F) on the second postoperative day? __________
   (102.2°)

6. Why is this graph included in a chapter titled, "Assessing Pulse, Respiration and Blood Pressure"? __________
   (to give a visual representation of the concepts in the chapter)

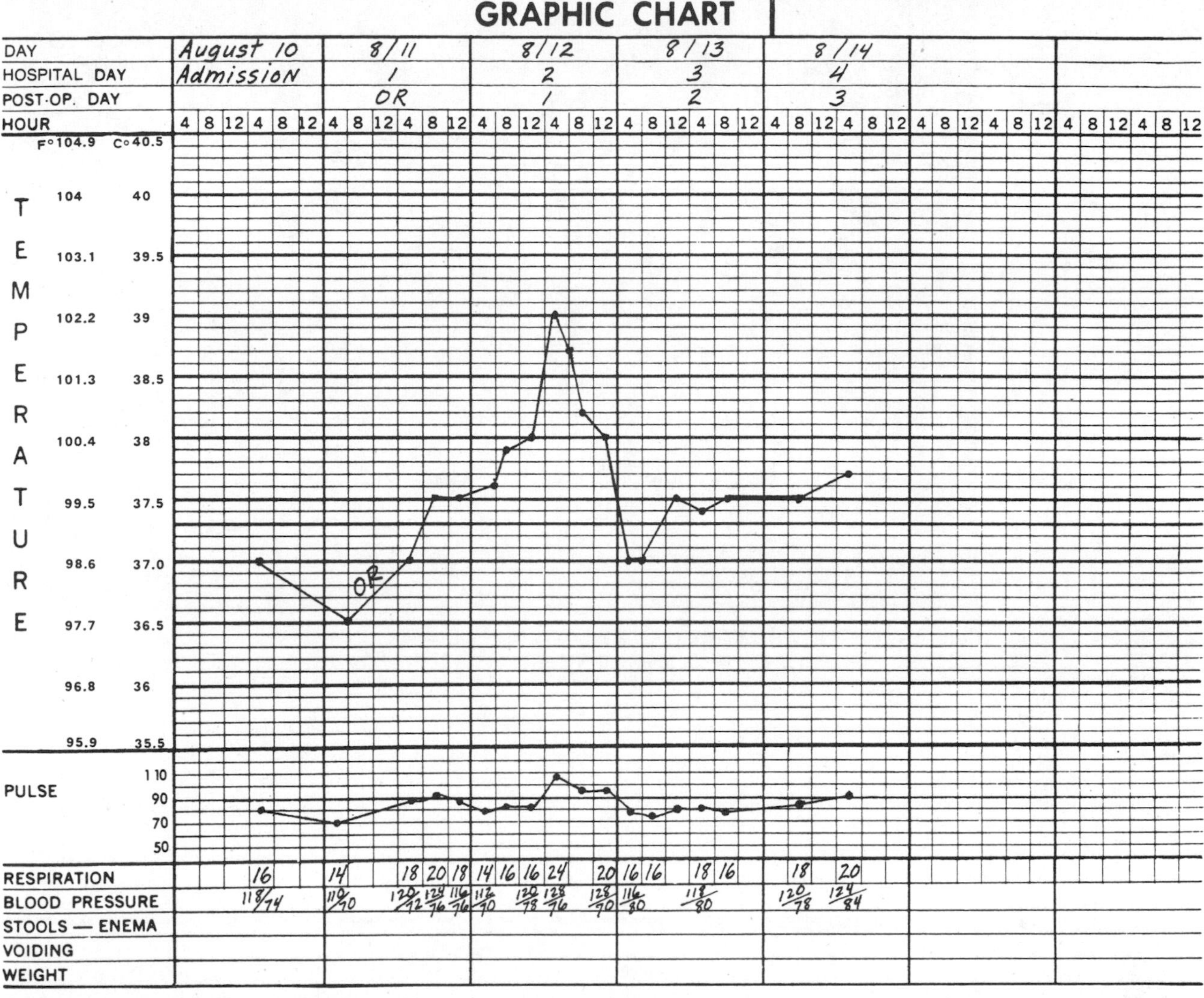

Figure 12–4 Sample of a vital signs graphic sheet. Note vital signs when this person has a fever on first postoperative day. Also note increased frequency of measurement as nurse suspects a developing trend. (From Sorensen, K.C., and Luckmann, J.: Basic nursing: a psychophysiological approach, ed. 2, Philadelphia, 1986, W.B. Saunders, p. 547.)

EXERCISE 12–1

Directions. Read and study the following graphic aid (Fig. 12–5). Answer the questions and write your answers in the space provided.

1. What is the subject of this picture? ______
2. How would you describe the person's problem? ______
3. Who is the person? ______
4. What does the equipment suggest? ______
5. What impact does this picture have? ______

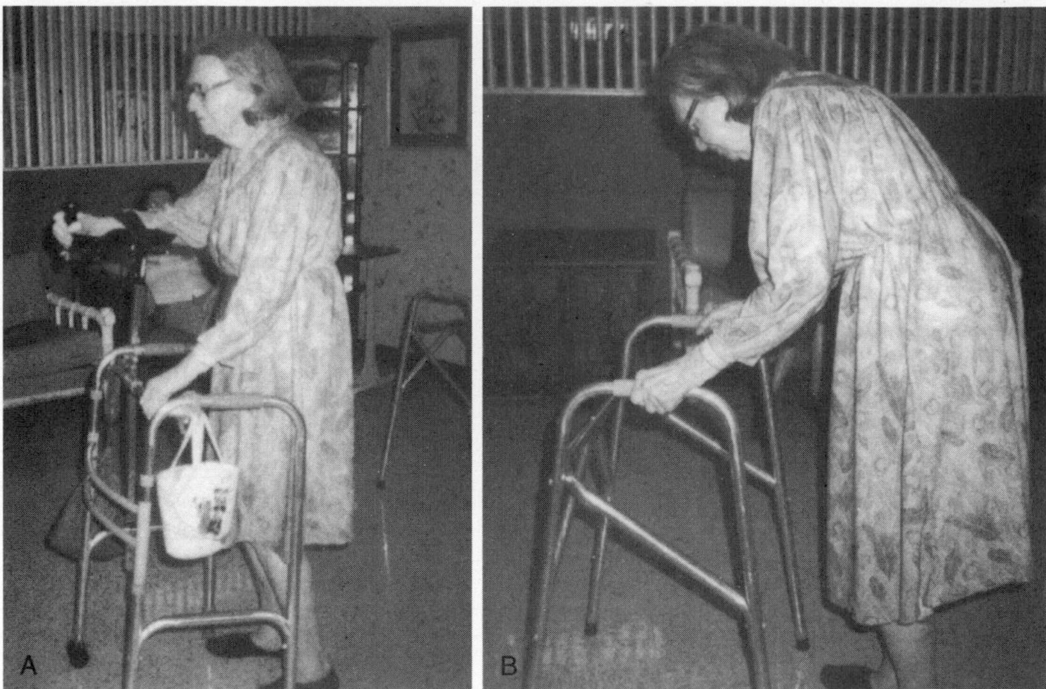

Figure 12–5 Note the difference in a person's body alignment when a walker is properly fitted *(A)*, compared with posture when an improperly fitted walker is used *(B)*. (From Matteson et al., p. 372)

EXERCISE 12–2

Directions. Read and study the following graphic aid (Table 12–4). Answer the questions and write your answers in the space provided.

1. What is the title of this table? ______
2. What are the heading names of the three columns? ______
______
3. Why should ACE inhibitors not be used for pre-eclampsia? ______
______
4. What drugs should be avoided for gout? ______
5. What is the overall purpose of this table? ______

TABLE 12–4 Pathophysiologic Conditions that Require Cautious Use or Complete Avoidance of Certain Antihypertensive Drugs

Pathophysiologic Condition	Drugs to Be Avoided or Used with Caution	Reason for Concern
Cardiovascular		
Congestive heart failure	Beta blockers Labetalol Verapamil Diltiazem	These drugs act on the heart to decrease myocardial contractility and can thereby further reduce cardiac output.
A-V heart block	Beta blockers Labetalol Verapamil Diltiazem	These drugs act on the heart to suppress A-V conduction and can thereby intensify A-V block.
Coronary artery disease	Guanethidine Hydralazine	Reflex tachycardia induced by these drugs can precipitate an anginal attack.
Post myocardial infarction	Guanethidine Hydralazine	Reflex tachycardia induced by these drugs can increase cardiac work and oxygen demand.
Other		
Renal insufficiency	K^+-sparing diuretics K^+ supplements	Use of these agents can lead to dangerous accumulations of potassium.
Asthma	Beta blockers Labetalol	$Beta_2$ blockade promotes bronchoconstriction.
Depression	Reserpine	Reserpine causes depression.
Diabetes mellitus	Thiazides Furosemide Beta blockers	Thiazides and furosemide promote hyperglycemia; beta blockers suppress glycogenolysis and can mask signs of hypoglycemia.
Gout	Thiazides Furosemide	These diuretics promote hyperuricemia.
Hyperkalemia	K^+-sparing diuretics ACE inhibitors	These drugs cause potassium accumulation.
Hypokalemia	Thiazides Furosemide	These diuretics promote potassium loss.
Collagen diseases	Hydralazine	Hydralazine can precipitate a lupus erythematosus–like syndrome.
Liver disease	Methyldopa	Methyldopa is hepatotoxic.
Pre-eclampsia	ACE inhibitors	These drugs can injure the fetus.

From Lehne, p. 494.

EXERCISE 12–3

Directions. Read and study the graphic aid (Table 12–5). Answer the questions and write your answers in the space provided.

1. What is the title of this table? ____________________

2. How many tricyclic antidepressants are listed? ____________________

3. What is the tradename for phenelzine? ____________________

4. What is the initial dose for Paxil? ____________________

5. What type of antidepressant is Prozac?

____

TABLE 12–5 Adult Dosages for Antidepressants

Generic Name	Trade Name	Initial Dose*† (mg/day)	Dose After 4–8 weeks* (mg/day)	Maximum Dose‡ (mg/day)
Tricyclic Antidepressants				
Amitriptyline	Elavil, Endep	50–150	100–200	300
Desipramine	Norpramin, Pertofrane	50–150	75–200	300
Doxepin	Adapin, Sinequan	50–150	100–200	300
Imipramine	Tofranil	50–150	100–200	300
Nortriptyline	Aventyl, Pamelor	25–100	75–150	150
Protriptyline	Vivactil	10–40	15–40	60
Trimipramine	Surmontil	50–150	75–250	250
Monoamine Oxidase Inhibitors				
Isocarboxazid	Marplan	20–30	20–30	30
Phenelzine	Nardil	45–75	45–75	75
Tranylcypromine	Parnate	20–30	20–30	30
Selective Serotonin Reuptake Blockers				
Fluoxetine	Prozac	20	20–40	80
Fluvoxamine§	Floxyfral	50–100	50–300	300
Paroxetine	Paxil	20	20–50	50
Sertaline§	Zoloft	50	50–200	200
Trazodone	Desyrel	150	150–200	400
Miscellaneous Antidepressants				
Amoxapine	Asendin	50–150	200–300	400
Bupropion	Wellbutrin	200	300	450
Maprotiline	Ludiomil	50–100	100–150	225

*Doses listed are *total daily doses.* Depending on the drug and the patient, the total dose may be given in a single dose or in divided doses.
†Initial doses are employed for 4–8 weeks, the time required for most symptoms to respond. The smaller dose within the range listed is used initially. Dosage is gradually increased as required.
‡Doses higher than these may be needed for some patients with severe depression.
§Investigational agent. (From Lehne, p. 279.)

EXERCISE 12–4

Directions. Read and study the following graphic aid (Fig. 12–6). Answer the questions and write your answers in the space provided.

1. What is the subject of the diagram? ______________________________

2. List three physical complications of immobility. ______________________________

____

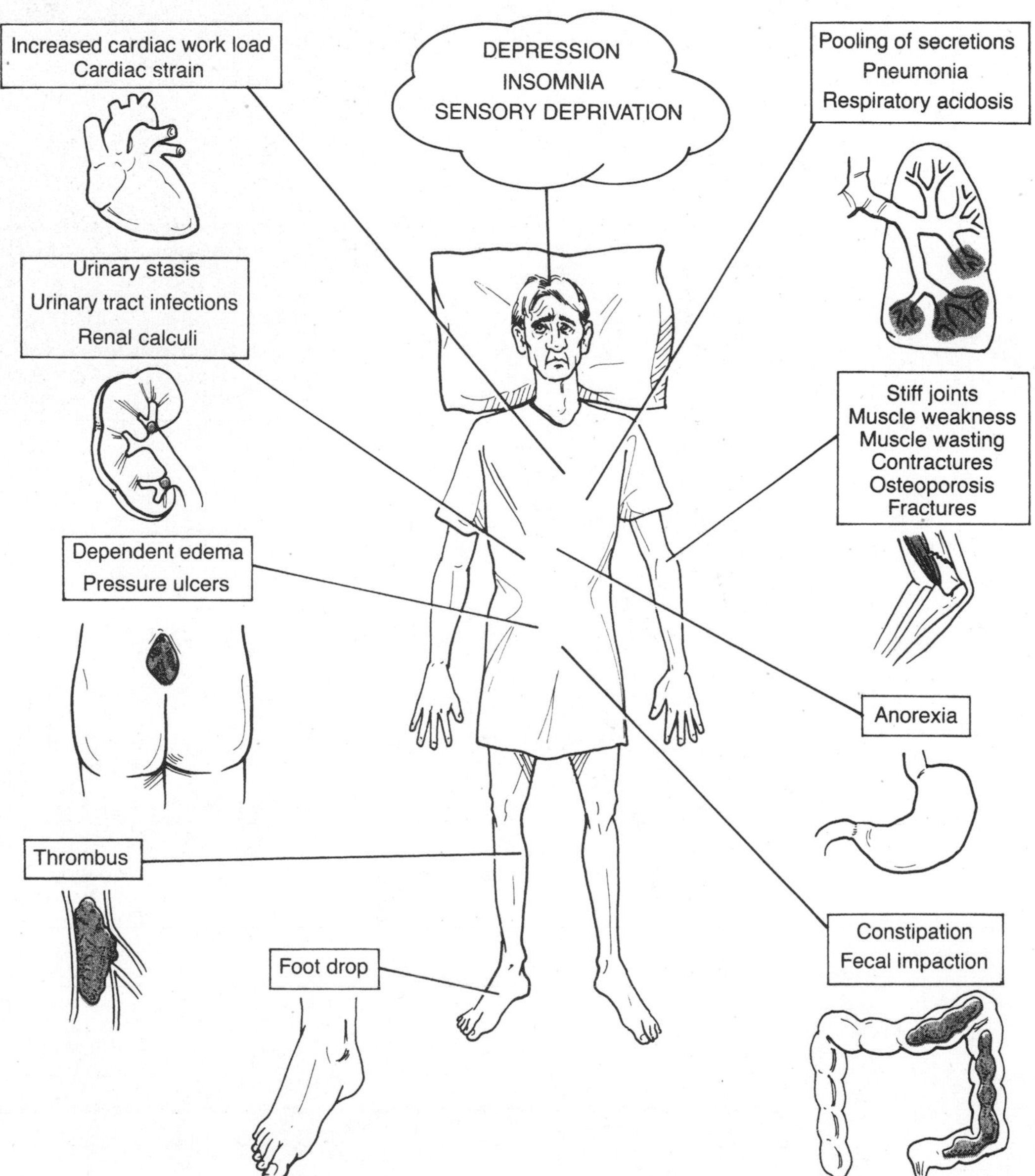

Figure 12–6 Some major complications of immobility. (From Sorensen, K.C., and Luckmann, J.: Basic nursing: a psychophysiological approach, ed. 2, Philadelphia, 1986, W.B. Saunders, p. 591.)

3. List three psychological complications of immobility. ______________________

____

4. Thrombus is pointing to what part of the body? ______________________

5. What general feeling about this patient do you get from this diagram? ______________________

6. List the facts that lead you to this general feeling. ______________________

____

EXERCISE 12–5

Directions. Read and study the following graphic aid (Fig. 12–7). Answer the questions and write your answers in the space provided.

1. What is this graphic aid about? ______________________

2. List the five basic steps depicted in Figure 12–7. ______________________

3. What do the arrows indicate? ______________________

____

4. Which step is concerned with reviewing the planned intervention?

____

5. In which step do you review the literature and do consultations?

____

Comprehending? Yes ___ No ___

EXERCISE 12–6

Directions. Using your own nursing textbook and a separate sheet of paper, copy the format of one graphic aid. Read and study the written text that accompanies this graphic aid. Then fill in as much of the graph, picture, table, or diagram as you remember. When you are finished, check your version with the original. Correct and make changes, if necessary.

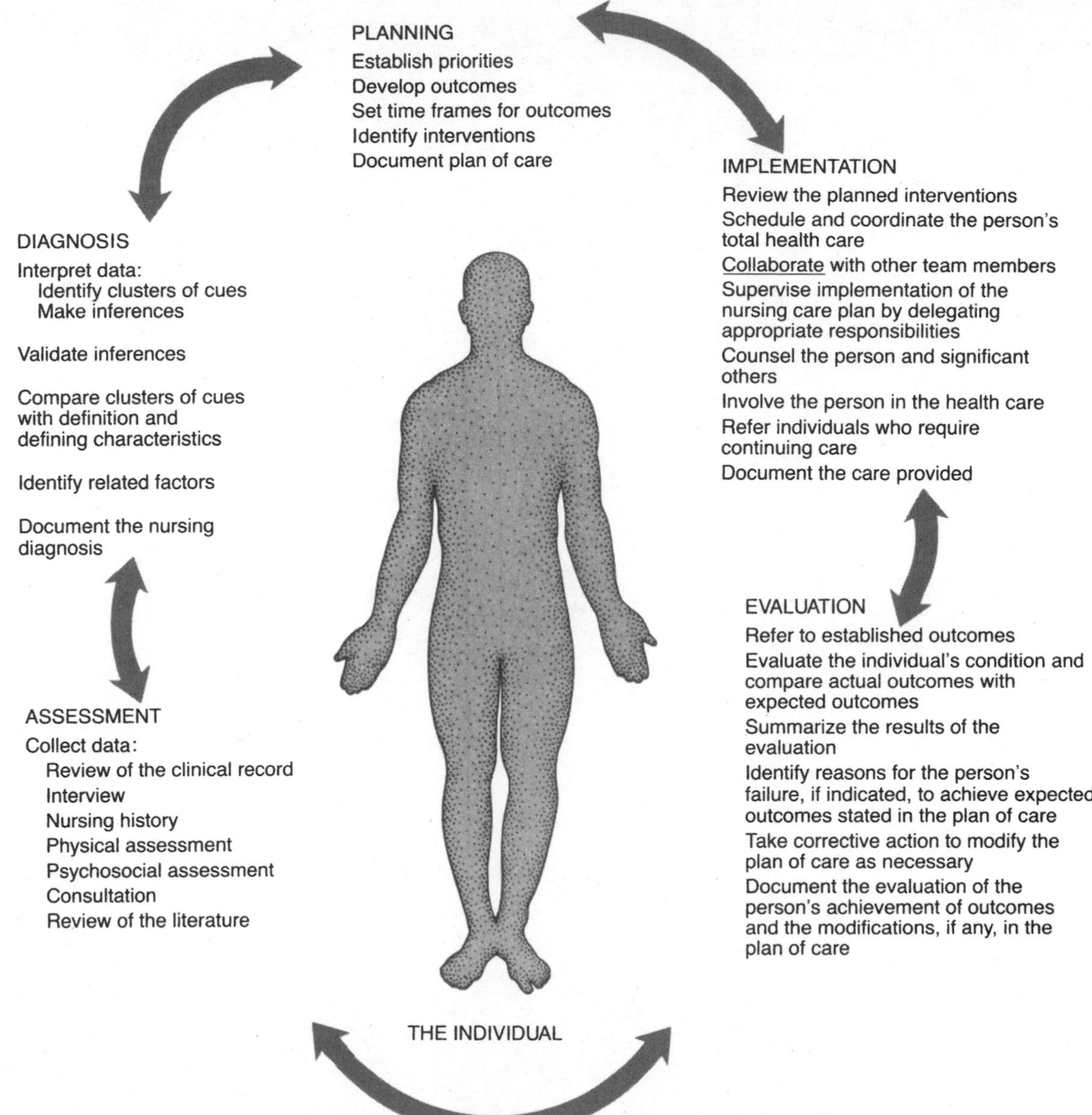
PLANNING
Establish priorities
Develop outcomes
Set time frames for outcomes
Identify interventions
Document plan of care
IMPLEMENTATION
Review the planned interventions
Schedule and coordinate the person's total health care
Collaborate with other team members
Supervise implementation of the nursing care plan by delegating appropriate responsibilities
Counsel the person and significant others
Involve the person in the health care
Refer individuals who require continuing care
Document the care provided
DIAGNOSIS
Interpret data:
Identify clusters of cues
Make inferences
Validate inferences
Compare clusters of cues with definition and defining characteristics
Identify related factors
Document the nursing diagnosis
EVALUATION
Refer to established outcomes
Evaluate the individual's condition and compare actual outcomes with expected outcomes
Summarize the results of the evaluation
Identify reasons for the person's failure, if indicated, to achieve expected outcomes stated in the plan of care
Take corrective action to modify the plan of care as necessary
Document the evaluation of the person's achievement of outcomes and the modifications, if any, in the plan of care
ASSESSMENT
Collect data:
Review of the clinical record
Interview
Nursing history
Physical assessment
Psychosocial assessment
Consultation
Review of the literature
THE INDIVIDUAL

Figure 12–7 Diagram of the nursing process. The nursing process consists of five steps: assessment, diagnosis, planning, implementation, and evaluation. The purposes are to maintain health, prevent illness, promote recovery, restore wellness and maximal function, and provide support in peaceful death. Note that the nursing process is a cyclical, problem-solving method that allows for change. When the evaluation step indicates that some problems are unresolved or are unidentified, the process continues with data gathering, problem identification, and so forth. (From Sorensen & Luckmann, p. 111)

• VOCABULARY CHECK

Directions. Below are 10 words taken from the key words section of this chapter. Circle the letter of the best definition from the four choices.

1. Pulse

a the arteries in which blood flows from the lungs
b a method of treating heart problems without invading the body
c damage to the heart because of arterial blockage
d the beat of the heart as felt through the wall of the arteries

2. Footnotes
a alphabetized listing of subjects at the back of the text
b introductory comment or preface
c the appendix located at the end of the text
d explanatory notes found at the bottom of the page

3. Postoperative
a before surgery
b after surgery
c during surgery
d an operation

4. Caption
a an illustration in a text
b a design in a journal
c an addition to a text
d an explanation accompanying a picture

5. Immobility
a movement
b incapacity to be moved
c a sudden movement
d ability to move with ease

6. Legend
a an explanatory list of symbols on a graphic aid
b the title or heading of a graphic aid
c a map or chart that acts as a graphic aid
d the outline or structure of graphic aids

7. Vital signs
a signs of distress
b signs of life
c high temperature
d respiratory illness

8. Graphic
a pertaining to a lead substance
b pertaining to a grape
c pertaining to a visual representation
d pertaining to trauma

9. Gout
a a clotting disease that affects only males
b urinary infections brought on by pregnancy
c a form of arthritis in which uric acid appears in excessive quantities in the blood
d protein found in the blood

10. Concise
- **a** brevity of expression
- **b** expandable
- **c** elaborately detailed
- **d** speechless

• CRITICAL THINKING LOG

List the strategies you learned in this chapter.	Select the strategy that is most useful for your school success.	How can you apply this strategy to your nursing studies?

• SUMMARY

Graphic materials are an important part of your textbook and should not be skipped over. They give you information in a visual form that attracts your attention and holds your concentration. Understanding the visual material and paraphrasing the information into language you comprehend help you to remember the ideas. Graphic aids are easy to read because they are designed to be clear and accurate. When you read graphic aids, focus on the title, all other headings, and descriptions and determine the purpose of the visual aid. Make a general statement that relates the information of the graphic aid to the ideas covered in the chapter. Graphic aids improve your reading concentration, comprehension, and retention. Paying close attention to graphic aids will help you to read your nursing textbooks.

CHAPTER 13

Active Listening and Successful Note-Taking

• OBJECTIVE

To learn procedures for active listening and the organizing, taking, and studying of notes from nursing school lectures.

• KEY WORDS

Pay attention to the following key words, which are underscored the first time they appear in this chapter. Try to determine the meanings of these words from the surrounding words in the passage. If you need further help, use your dictionary or the glossary in the back of this book.

Look up the medical terminology in your medical dictionary or the glossary. As you read the exercises in this chapter, write additional words you need to learn in the space provided.

MEDICAL TERMINOLOGY	GENERAL VOCABULARY
ambulatory care	abbreviations
anatomy	chronological order
care plans	concepts
charting	conversely
clotting	dilemma
coagulation	former
physiology	regardless
psychotherapy	sabotage
pulmonary	streamlined
self-concept	supplemented
______________	______________
______________	______________
______________	______________

• CHECKLIST

Directions. Evaluate your listening skills and note-taking system. Check yes or no.

1. Do you daydream during class lectures? Yes ________ No ________
2. Do you sometimes pretend to pay attention during class? Yes ________ No ________
3. Do you attempt to write every word instead of listening for your instructor's main points? Yes ________ No ________
4. Do you turn off subjects or speakers without giving them a chance? Yes ________ No ________
5. Are you easily distracted? Yes ________ No ________
6. Do you skip some lectures? Yes ________ No ________
7. Is your notebook disorganized? Yes ________ No ________
8. Are your notebook papers messy and in disorder? Yes ________ No ________

9. Do you fail to know how much information to write? Yes ________ No ________

10. In a lecture, do you not know how to tell the important facts from the unimportant facts? Yes ________ No ________

11. Do you take notes slowly? Yes ________ No ________

12. Are your notes incomplete? Yes ________ No ________

13. Do you quit taking notes before the end of the session? Yes ________ No ________

14. Do you not have a method for studying from your notes? Yes ________ No ________

If you answered yes to most of these questions, you need help in taking classroom notes. This chapter will teach you techniques for active listening and organizing, taking, and studying your lecture notes.

• IMPORTANCE OF GOOD LECTURE NOTES

A good portion of your time in nursing school will be spent listening to lectures on various nursing topics. While these lectures will be supplemented by reading assignments in your textbooks, it is important to listen and take accurate and complete classroom notes for the following reasons:

- Your instructor may want you to learn additional concepts not covered in your nursing book.
- Your instructor may restate facts you have already encountered in your reading, thereby reinforcing learning.
- Your instructor may indicate what information will appear on tests.

Thus listening well and taking good lecture notes have many advantages.

• NEED FOR ACTIVE LISTENING

Many people think that listening is synonymous with hearing, but there is an important difference. Listening involves comprehension. An active listener concentrates on and reacts to a speaker's message. Hearing, on the other hand, is passive. The sounds are heard, but they are not deciphered into information that is understood.

When you are listening to an instructor's information during your nursing class lectures, you need to be an active listener. You must pay attention during class lectures because you will be responsible for knowing these facts when you take your exams.

• LISTENING PROBLEMS

Unfortunately, many students have listening problems that interfere with their ability to get the most out of their classroom lectures. Do you have any of the following listening problems?

- *Daydreaming*. Your mind wanders during the lecture. You then try to jump back in. You've probably missed several important facts. Daydreaming is the most common listening problem. You daydream because your mind works faster than the speaker can talk. In this chapter you will learn strategies to use this extra mental time to focus on a person's ideas, rather than letting your mind wander.
- *Pretending attention*. You are pretending to pay attention in class, but you are really mentally asleep behind open eyes. This is even worse than daydreaming because you are missing all the information, and you are not fooling your instructor. Your instructor knows from your blank expression that you are not concentrating. An active listener reacts to a speaker's ideas. The facial muscles move.
- *Rote note-taking*. You can think faster than a speaker can talk, but you can't write as fast as the speaker can talk. If you try to write every word, without thinking about what is being said, you will end up with unfinished sentences. This is a listening problem because you are not focusing on the most important information. Concentrate on writing the most important main ideas and details.
- *Closing off the subject or speaker*. We are all subjective. However, if you make up your mind before your class begins that you find the information too controversial or difficult or the subject or speaker boring, you may tune out. If you refuse to listen during class, you are preventing yourself from learning. Your task, as a nursing student, is to concentrate on and comprehend your instructor's information. Learn to put your initial impression aside. Be open to receiving your instructor's message, and you will be successful when you take your exams.
- *Giving in to distractions*. All students have a tendency to let external noises and events distract them during class lectures. However, it is up to you, the listener, to block out these distractions and concentrate on your instructor's main ideas. Using external distractions as an excuse for losing attention will only result in a loss of information.

EXERCISE 13–1

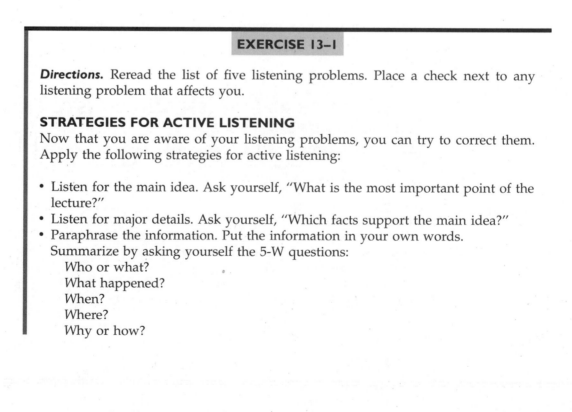

Directions. Reread the list of five listening problems. Place a check next to any listening problem that affects you.

STRATEGIES FOR ACTIVE LISTENING

Now that you are aware of your listening problems, you can try to correct them. Apply the following strategies for active listening:

- Listen for the main idea. Ask yourself, "What is the most important point of the lecture?"
- Listen for major details. Ask yourself, "Which facts support the main idea?"
- Paraphrase the information. Put the information in your own words. Summarize by asking yourself the 5-W questions:
  - Who or what?
  - What happened?
  - When?
  - Where?
  - Why or how?

EXERCISE 13–2

Directions. Practice applying the strategies for active listening by keeping a listening journal for one week of classes. Fill in the following listening journal. Each day, evaluate your listening habits.

Class	*Type of Listening Problem*	*What Listening Strategy Would Be Helpful?*
Monday		
Tuesday		
Wednesday		
Thursday		
Friday		

• HINTS ON IMPROVING YOUR LISTENING

You can be actively involved in improving your listening skills. Focus attention on the speaker by looking directly at your instructor. Ask questions and listen for the answers. Sit in front of the room if you have trouble seeing, hearing, or concentrating. Be aware of your body language. Sit up straight. Slouching in your chair makes it easier for you to fall mentally asleep. Evaluate the instructor's information. Do you agree? Disagree? *React*! Focus on the subject.

• RELATIONSHIP BETWEEN ACTIVE LISTENING AND NOTE-TAKING

Study skills research indicates that successful students take good notes. It is imperative to be an active listener to take effective notes. Applying active listening strategies will help you to take good notes.

- Listen for your instructor's main ideas.
- Pay attention to key words that signal important ideas.
- Mentally summarize the information, then write an outline or summary that includes all main ideas and major details.
- Pay extra attention to the beginning and end of your classroom lectures; that's when important points are introduced and summarized.

• BENEFITS OF ACTIVE LISTENING

Use your active listening strategies to help you concentrate on and comprehend the main points discussed in your nursing class lectures. Active listening will help you to improve your grades in nursing school. You will:

- Get more out of class lectures.
- Take better notes.
- Be an active participant in your nursing studies.
- Be actively involved in your success in nursing school.

• BE PREPARED

Before attending any lecture, read all the textbook assignments that pertain to the lecture topic. By reading beforehand, you will have a foundation of knowledge on which to add the new information you will be getting in lectures. In other words, you will have background knowledge or a framework to which you can relate new facts and ideas. After the lecture, you should reread these same textbook assignments. Not only will you gain a stronger understanding of what you have previously read, but you may also interpret the concepts differently after hearing the lecture. Reading your assignments before and after the lecture will greatly improve your success on exams.

• ATTENDANCE

To take the best possible notes and to get the greatest benefit from lectures, attend all your classes. At times all students are tempted to skip a class. Staying home or studying in the library seems easier, but once you have missed a lecture, you must rely on some secondhand method for obtaining the information you have missed. You may also have lost the chance to gain invaluable information and ask questions. So make it a point to attend all lectures, regardless of the weather, headaches, or the argument you had with your friend. Eventually, you will be glad you were there to record the information yourself.

Plan your schedule so you can arrive on time. Many instructors introduce the main points in the beginning of their lectures. This introduction, of course, is something you would not want to miss.

• ORGANIZED NOTEBOOK

A reliable pen and a well-organized notebook are essential for taking good classroom notes. You should invest in the following:

- A different 8-1/2 × 11 inch spiral-bound notebook for each class, *or*
- An 8-1/2 × 11 inch spiral-bound notebook divided into different sections, *or*
- An 8-1/2 × 11 inch loose-leaf notebook with dividers that separate one subject from another

You do not want to mix your anatomy and physiology notes with your nursing notes. So make sure you have organized your notebook so that one subject is distinct from another.

• ORGANIZED NOTE PAPER

In the minutes while you are waiting for your instructor to begin, you should be organizing the sheets of paper on which you will be taking your notes. At the top of the first sheet, on the right-hand side, write the date of the lecture. All lecture notes must begin with the date so you can keep them in sequential order. If you are using an individual spiral-bound notebook or one divided into sections, the earlier lectures will be in the front of the notebook and the later lecture notes will be in the back. If you prefer a loose-leaf notebook, you should place the beginning lecture notes in the back with the more current ones in front. Keeping your lecture notes dated and in chronological order is important when it comes time to study for exams.

In addition to dating your sheet of paper while you are waiting for the lecture to begin, you should draw a second left-hand margin line, about 1-1/2 to 2 inches to the right of the first, on all the sheets of paper to be used (Fig. 13–1).

During the lecture you will write only on the portion of the paper marked "B" in Figure 13–1. The area you have created by drawing a second margin line ("A") should remain blank. The purpose of area "A," as shown in the figure, is to provide a space for later adding information you have missed, such as summaries, headings, and comments. With this method of organizing your paper, you not only have room to jot down additional information after the lecture but also have space to write in when you study or review your notes for a test. Your paper is now ready for the actual lecture notes.

• HOW MUCH INFORMATION TO WRITE

When attending a lecture class, you are faced with a dilemma—how much information should you be writing? Should you try to write down "everything," or will focusing on the main ideas and major details be sufficient? Time, experience, and a little knowledge will help you to judge the situation.

When you get the results of your first exam, you will be able to assess whether your note-taking was adequate. If possible, compare the items on your exam to the topics you covered in your notes. If you see that your notes contain the majority of items asked about on your exam, you know your notes are sufficient. If you see many omissions, however, you know you need to write more to be prepared for the next exam. Conversely, if your notes contain many items that were not mentioned on your test, you may want to write more succinctly next time.

Once you are experienced and familiar with your instructor's lecture style, you may have a greater sense of how much to write down in your notes. In fact, your instructor may let you know during the course of her talk just what she feels you should be

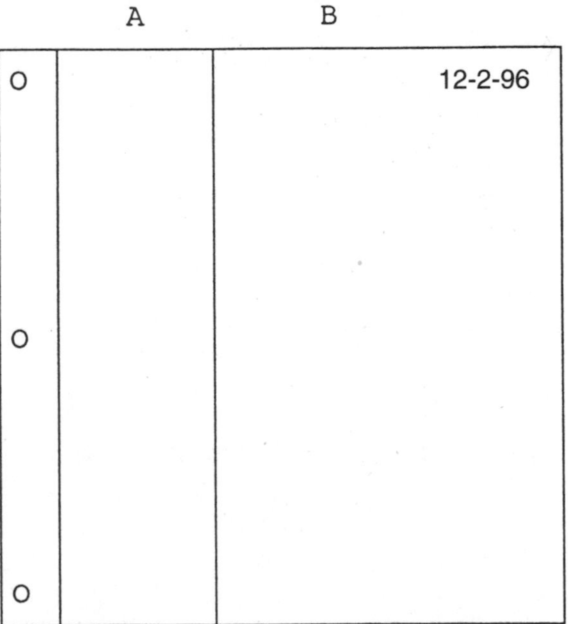

Figure 13–1 Hand-drawn second left-hand margin.

writing down. So stay alert and listen for an instructor's cues that let you know when and what to write.

Knowing something in advance about the course you are taking will also dictate how detailed your notes should be. If, for example, you are in a nursing lecture and you have heard that the exams are multiple-choice focusing on the application of terms and concepts to clinical situations, you will need to write down all definitions and examples given during the lecture. If you have heard that the psychology instructor gives essay tests on major concepts only, it may be necessary only to write down the main points and actively listen to the rest of the lecture.

Reliable ways of finding out about your course are:

- Asking the instructor or your advisor
- Checking with former students who did well in the class
- Reading the course description in the nursing school catalogue.

Once you know something about your course requirements, you will be in a better position to judge how much information you should be writing.

• LESS DETAILED NOTE-TAKING

When the situation in your lecture class requires that you familiarize yourself with just the broader concepts of the course, the best approach to note-taking is to summarize the material. To summarize, you must first listen to what your instructor is saying. Write, *in your own words*, the main points of what was just said. Summarizing consists in a large part of listening and reflecting and, in smaller part, of writing. When you listen, pay attention to the most important concepts and examples the instructor is presenting. You do not have to concern yourself with minor details or incidental facts and examples (see Chapters 8 and 9). When you reflect, you want to quickly translate the instructor's most important points into your own words. You do this by first listening and then silently in your mind phrasing in your own words what you just heard. You capture this paraphrasing by writing it in your notebook.

EXERCISE 13–3

Directions. Below is an excerpt from a nursing textbook (Matteson and McConnell, p. 144). Read it silently, reflect on the content, and in the space provided summarize the main points of the selection.

FREE RADICAL THEORY

Free radicals [consist of] the separated electrons [that] have a large amount of free energy and oxidatively attack adjacent molecules. The O_2 molecule most commonly generates free radicals, and the most vulnerable sites are the mitochondrial and microsomal membranes rich in unsaturated lipids. Lipid molecules are especially vulnerable to attack by free radicals, resulting in structural changes and malfunctions. Chemical and structural changes are progressive with a potential for a chain reaction in which free radicals generate other free radicals. Free radicals do not contain useful biological information and replace genetic order with randomness; thus faulty molecules and cellular debris accumulate in the nucleus and cytoplasm over a lifetime.

Lipofuscin is a pigmented material rich in lipids and proteins that accumulates in many organs with aging. The pigments originate from a peroxidation of components of polyunsaturated acids located in mitochondrial membranes. Lipofuscin appears to have some relationship to free radicals and the process of aging because the substance is associated with oxidation of unsaturated lipids. The accumulation of lipofuscin interferes with the diffusion and transport of essential metabolites and information-bearing molecules in the cells and may play an important part in the aging process.

Comprehending? **Yes** ___ **No** ___

• MORE DETAILED NOTE-TAKING

When you are in a course that requires you to know a lot of factual information, your notes will necessarily be more detailed. When taking detailed notes, you listen and write to a large extent and reflect to a lesser extent. You write as quickly as possible to catch as many of the instructor's ideas as possible. This does not mean that you try to copy verbatim what the instructor is saying. That would be impossible, since we can talk much faster than we can write. It does mean, however, that you try to write as much as you can of what is being said in the most concise way. Following are four suggestions for taking notes efficiently.

Streamlined Handwriting

Eliminating all extraneous, or extra, strokes in your handwriting will make note-taking a quicker process. Use script, or cursive, rather than printing, or manuscript. Since you pick up the pen less often when writing script than when printing, your writing speed is naturally increased. Eliminate all fancy loops in your handwriting. A streamlined writing style is more conducive to speed than an ornate one. See the example below.

Nursing is a great profession

Nursing is a great profession

EXERCISE 13–4

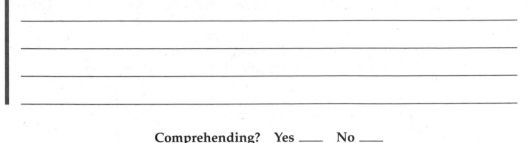

Directions. In the space provided, copy the following short selection. Make sure your handwriting is streamlined—no extra strokes or loops.

Once the plan is formulated, the nurse should share care plans with the rest of the staff. This is critical to success. Though the nurse may have consulted the staff about different aspects of the plan, it is useful to summarize initial plans with other staff members. This simple strategy accomplishes two purposes: Staff will support the nurse's efforts, and often staff have additional input that can prove useful. Failure to involve staff in the initial planning stages can sabotage the most careful and creative plan (Arnold and Boggs, p. 88).

Comprehending? Yes ___ No ___

Abbreviations

When it is necessary to take many pages of notes as quickly as possible, you should not write out every word in its entirety. Instead, you will want to abbreviate as many of these words as possible. This does not mean that you have to know and use the standard medical abbreviations. Instead, you can make up your own system of abbreviations; just be sure that days or weeks later you will know what the abbreviations stand for. Below are suggestions for abbreviating some common nursing terms.

EXAMPLE 13–1

TERM	ABBREVIATION
Nurse	Nrs.
Nursing	nrsg.
Care plan	C.P.
Ambulatory care	Amb. c.
Cardiac	Card.
Pulmonary	Pulm.
Diagnosis	Diag.
Inflammation	Inflam.

EXERCISE 13–5

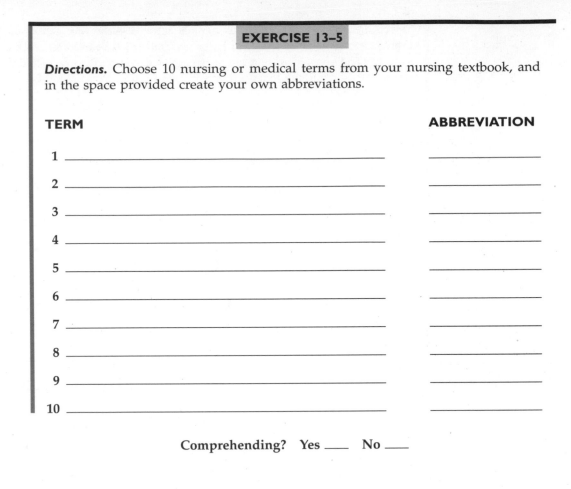

Directions. Choose 10 nursing or medical terms from your nursing textbook, and in the space provided create your own abbreviations.

TERM	ABBREVIATION
1 ______________________	____________
2 ______________________	____________
3 ______________________	____________
4 ______________________	____________
5 ______________________	____________
6 ______________________	____________
7 ______________________	____________
8 ______________________	____________
9 ______________________	____________
10 ______________________	____________

Comprehending? Yes ___ No ___

Shorthand System

Another suggestion to help you take more rapid notes is to create your own shorthand system. To do this most simply, eliminate some vowels from key words. See the example below.

EXAMPLE 13–2

Longhand: You must learn to write careful and complete care plans.
Shorthand: You mst lrn to writ carfl and complt cps.

Remember that you must be able to understand your shorthand style days or weeks later.

EXERCISE 13–6

Directions. Below is a short excerpt from a nursing textbook. Practice using the shorthand system above by rewriting the passage in the space provided, leaving out some vowels from key words.

Some dietary habits can enhance blood clotting. Diets high in vitamin K may increase the rate of blood coagulation. (Ignatavicius and Bayne, p. 1032)

____

____

____

____

Comprehending? Yes ___ No ___

Symbols

The last suggestion for writing more rapidly is to use symbols instead of words. Some symbols that you might already be familiar with are:

&	for "and"
w/	for "with"
w/out	for "without"
#	for "number"
=	for "equals"
≠	for "not equal to"

EXERCISE 13–7

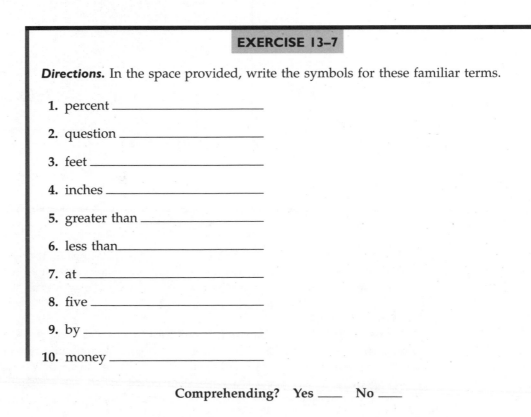

Directions. In the space provided, write the symbols for these familiar terms.

1. percent ______________
2. question ______________
3. feet ______________
4. inches ______________
5. greater than ______________
6. less than ______________
7. at ______________
8. five ______________
9. by ______________
10. money ______________

Comprehending? Yes ___ No ___

Using streamlined handwriting, abbreviations, a shorthand system, and symbols will help you to take more pages of detailed notes quickly. You can decide through practice which of these hints for increasing note-taking speed will benefit you.

• INDICATING MAJOR AND MINOR POINTS

While you are taking your lecture notes, you need to make a distinction between the major and minor points being presented. One way to do this is by using an indentation method. Starting at your hand-drawn left margin, write down the main ideas. If the next idea presented is a major detail supporting this main idea, indent a bit to the right as you write it down. If you need to write a minor detail, indent this even more to the right (Fig. 13–2).

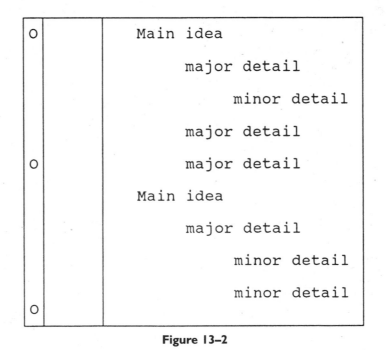

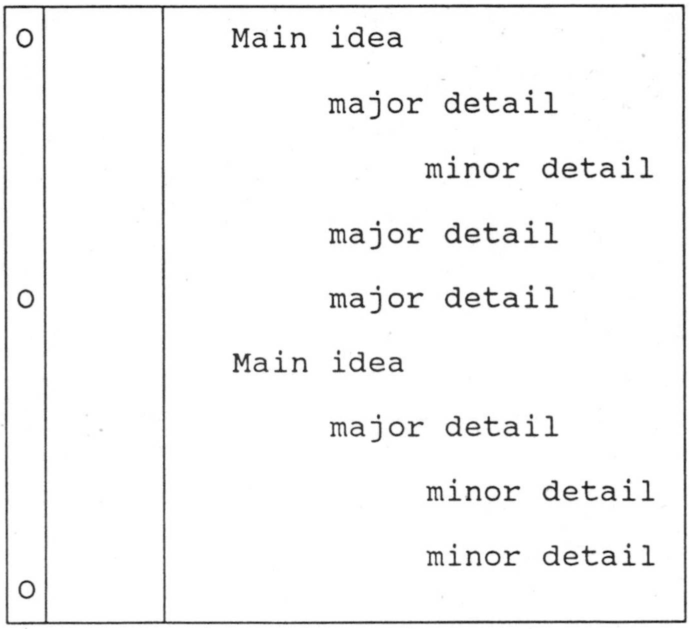

```
o          Main idea
                major detail
                     minor detail
                major detail
o               major detail
           Main idea
                major detail
                     minor detail
                     minor detail
o
```

Figure 13–2

EXERCISE 13–8

Directions. Read the selection below from a nursing textbook (Matteson and McConnell, p. 155). Following the indentation system described above, take notes in the space provided, indicating the main ideas and major and minor details.

SKIN GLANDS

The two major types of skin glands are *sebaceous glands* and *sweat glands*. Sebaceous glands originate in the dermis and secrete *sebum*, an oily, colorless, odorless fluid, through hair follicles. Sweat glands originate in the subcutaneous tissue and are of two major types: *eccrine* and *apocrine*. Eccrine sweat glands are unbranched, coiled, tubular glands that are widely distributed and open directly onto the skin surface. They promote body cooling by allowing the sweat secretions to evaporate from the skin surface. The apocrine sweat glands are large, branched, specialized glands located chiefly in the axillary and genital regions that empty into hair follicles. They are responsible for body odor through bacterial decomposition of the sweat secretions.

Sebaceous glands show little atrophy or histological change with age; however, their function tends to diminish as seen by a decrease in sebum secretion. In men the decrease is minimal, but in women there is a gradual diminution in sebum secretion after menopause with no significant changes after the seventh decade. There are fewer sebaceous glands in older people, which appears related to the loss of hair follicles. The decrease in sebum secretion and in the number of sebaceous glands results in the dryer, coarser skin associated with aging.

Sweat glands generally decrease in size, number, and function with age. In the eccrine glands, the secretory epithelial cells become uneven in size, ranging from normal to small, and there is a progressive accumulation of lipofuscin in the cytoplasm. In the very old, the secretory coils of many eccrine glands are replaced by fibrous tissue, which drastically diminishes their capacity to produce sweat. The thermal threshold for sweating is raised, so that the amount of sweat output at a body temperature of 38 degrees centigrade decreases. This may be due to the fact that there are fewer blood vessels and nerve cells around the glands that enable the body to respond to temperature changes. Apocrine glands do not decrease in number or size, but they do decrease in function. An accumulation of lipofuscin has also been noted in apocrine glands. The diminished functioning of sweat glands in the elderly greatly impairs the ability to maintain body temperature homeostasis.

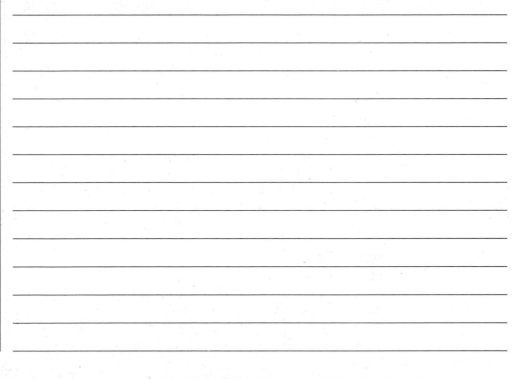

Comprehending? Yes ___ No ___

• CUES FOR DETERMINING WHAT IS IMPORTANT

During the course of the lecture, your instructor will directly and indirectly give you cues that indicate what is important to write down. Being able to recognize these cues is critical to taking good notes. Below are some cues you should watch for in the lecture.

Ideas Written on the Board

Whatever information your instructor writes on the board, make sure you copy it accurately in your notes. Most instructors take the time and make the effort to write on the board only those facts they feel are most important. After you have copied what was on the board, write a "B" for board in your handwritten margin by these notes.

Verbal Tips

Sometimes your instructors will tell you what is important. They may use such words as "important," "chief," "significant," "essential," or "key." Make sure you have written in your notes any facts that follow these or similar cues.

Your instructors may say that the information they are presenting will appear on a test. Make sure these concepts are written accurately in your notes and indicate that you must know this for the test. The easiest way to do this is by writing "T" for test in the handwritten margin by these notes.

Reading from a Text

At some point in the lecture your instructor may read aloud from a text or other sources. This added reference is a cue that your instructor believes that the information is important. Copy as much information as you believe significant and write an "R" for "read aloud" in the handwritten margin by these notes.

Enumerations and Terminology

Any ideas that are presented in numerical order should be considered important. For example, if your instructor presents information saying "first," "second," "third," and so on, make sure you have written down all these components. Also, include in your notes any new terms presented orally or written on the board.

Subtle Cues

Watch your instructor carefully to catch any indirect cues that indicate important information. A louder voice emphasizing a point, repeating an idea, pausing for you to write, and overt hand gesturing are all indications that what is being said is significant. Sit close to your instructor and pay attention to these indirect cues.

End of Lecture

As the class comes to an end, you may be tempted to stop listening and taking notes and to start packing up books. This may not be wise, since many instructors take these final moments to summarize their main points. You should be listening and taking notes right up to the last word. Don't cheat yourself out of critical information just to get a jump start in leaving the classroom.

EXERCISE 13–9

Directions. In your next nursing lecture, practice taking notes using the suggestions described above. Pay attention to the direct and indirect cues given by your instructor. Make sure you annotate the relevant information in the handwritten margin with a "B" for facts copied from the board, "T" for items that will appear on tests, and "R" for what the instructor read aloud. Write down all enumerations and terms. Keep taking notes until your instructor is finished.

• REVIEWING YOUR NOTES

Soon after the lecture, review your notes for completeness. If you feel that you have left out something important, you may have to ask to see another student's notes. Make sure that person is available to explain the notes because one person's note-taking style may not be clear to someone else. It makes no sense to copy something you do not understand.

• TAPING THE LECTURE

A way to verify the completeness of your lecture notes is to tape the lecture. This method has many advantages. First, you will have the opportunity on your own, during your study period, to replay and hear the entire lecture again. This is wonderful reinforcement. Second, you can review your notes and fill in any blanks without having to rely on anyone else. Third, you can prepare for your exam by listening to the tape of the lecture when you are at home, driving, or commuting to school.

Before you tape, make sure you get permission from your instructor. Use a portable battery-operated recorder. Make sure the casettes are long-playing and that you have extra batteries in case the power begins to run out. Sit as close to the lecturer as possible, so the recording will be clear and the speaker's words distinct.

• STUDYING YOUR NOTES

The purpose of note-taking is to have a permanent record of the information you will need to learn in order to pass exams in nursing school. The note-taking is just the first part of the procedure. You also need a good system for studying your notes.

• HEADINGS IN NOTES

Just as sections in your nursing textbooks are divided by headings, so should your notes be divided by headings. Read over your notes and decide where one topic ends and a new one begins. This is the most natural place for a heading. Ask yourself, "What is the section mostly about?" The answer will be the topic, and this should be used as the heading. Write the heading in a different color ink than you used for note-taking. See the example below, in which an excerpt from a nursing book is used to represent your lecture notes.

EXAMPLE 13–3

Short-term dynamic psychotherapy is usually indicated when a person has a specific symptom or interpersonal problem he or she wants to work on. The therapist participates actively and influences the direction of the content more than in either of the models discussed previously.

Although many of the tools employed in traditional psychotherapy are used, such as uncovering unconscious processes through transference and dream interpretations, other methods such as free association are discouraged. Sessions are held weekly, and the total number of sessions to be held (anywhere from 12 to 30) is determined at the onset of therapy. This type of intervention is successful for highly motivated individuals who have insight and who indicate a positive relationship with the therapist from the beginning. (Varcarolis, p. 33)

What is this passage mostly about?
(Short-term dynamic psychotherapy = topic = heading.)

EXERCISE 13–10

Directions. Take a page from your nursing lecture notes. Decide on the appropriate places for headings. Ask, "What is this section mostly about?" (The brief answer will be the topic, which can be used for the heading.) Write these headings where you think they belong.

Comprehending? Yes ___ No ___

• QUESTIONS

Once you have written headings for the different topics in your lecture notes, turn these headings into questions. Use the 5-W questions (who, what, when, where, and why or how). Referring back to Example 13–3, you see the heading is "short-term dynamic psychotherapy." You can turn this into a question by asking, "What is short-term dynamic psychotherapy?" Once you have turned all the headings in your notes into questions, you will read and remember the facts in your notes that answer the questions. This will keep you focused on your studying and help you distinguish the more important information from the less important. Underline or highlight all facts in your notes that answer the heading question.

EXERCISE 13–11

Directions. Below are headings. In the space provided, turn these headings into questions.

HEADING	QUESTION
Perceptual processes related to	____________________
self-concept	____________________
Engagement phase	____________________
Using physical and nonverbal	____________________
behavioral cues	____________________
Creating personal space in	____________________
hospital situations	____________________
Computer-assisted charting	____________________

Comprehending? Yes ___ No ___

EXERCISE 13–12

Directions. Using your notes from Exercise 13–10, turn all the headings you have made into questions. Then underline all the information that directly answers these questions.

• OTHER WAYS OF STUDYING FROM YOUR NOTES

When studying from your notes, be creative. Don't just read over the same words with the hope of memorizing them. In addition to the heading and questions method of studying from notes, other activities can keep you actively involved in the studying task:

- Write out quizzes based on your notes.
- Take these quizzes at the beginning of each of your study sessions.
- Make a chart covering the main points from your notes. Then fill in the details without looking at your notes.
- Dictate into your cassette recorder the main points from your lecture notes and listen to it at some later time.
- Create flashcards of the important terms from your notes and practice learning these words with them.
- Create your own ideas for making studying your notes exciting.

You have learned new techniques for organizing, taking, and studying lecture notes. Use these methods conscientiously in your upcoming lectures. Eventually you will see rewards for your efforts—improved grades.

EXERCISE 13–13

Directions. After a few weeks of practicing your new note-taking system, reread the checklist at the beginning of this chapter. See if your responses have improved.

• VOCABULARY CHECK

Directions. Below are 10 words taken from the key words section of this chapter. Circle the letter of the best definition from the four choices.

1. Concepts
- **a** thoughts
- **b** feelings
- **c** suspicions
- **d** fears

2. Anatomy
- **a** science dealing with fetal development
- **b** science dealing with organ structures
- **c** science dealing with physical processes
- **d** science dealing with the form and structure of living organisms

3. Streamlined
- **a** a rough finish
- **b** functioning at top speed
- **c** stripped of nonessentials
- **d** gauge of water depth

4. Pulmonary
- **a** pertaining to the brain
- **b** pertaining to the lungs
- **c** pertaining to the kidney
- **d** pertaining to the spinal cord

5. Dilemma
- **a** a heated discussion
- **b** an abrasive response
- **c** an unattainable goal
- **d** difficult or persistent problem

6. Coagulation
- **a** to fend off microorganisms
- **b** to form clots
- **c** to conceal
- **d** to bond

7. Conversely
- **a** reacting in a negative way
- **b** acting in anger
- **c** reversed in order, action
- **d** responding in like manner

8. Ambulatory care
  a care of patient in the ambulance
  b care of patient outdoors
  c care of patient confined to bed or chair
  d care of patient who is not confined to bed

9. Regardless
  a despite everything
  b not noticing
  c not caring
  d not usual

10. Self-concept
  a one's own fears
  b one's reaction to other people
  c when someone perceives another to be similar to herself or himself
  d the way someone views himself or herself

• CRITICAL THINKING LOG

List the strategies you learned in this chapter.	Select the strategy that is most useful for your school success.	How can you apply this strategy to your nursing studies?

• SUMMARY

In this chapter you learned techniques for becoming an active listener. You also learned a new system for organizing, taking, and studying lecture notes. You were shown the value of reading before the lecture and being organized. You were taught not only how to assess how much information to write, but also how to determine which ideas are important. Suggestions were given on how to take notes more efficiently and how to differentiate major concepts from minor ones. You were then given suggestions for studying your notes.

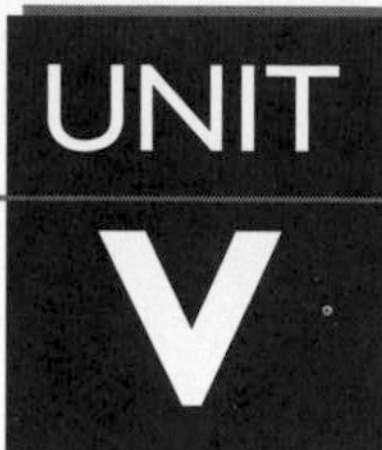

TAKING TESTS

Test-taking strategies will help you improve your grades on exams in nursing school. These strategies will work together with your knowledge of the content so you understand what is being asked in a test item. You will then be able to respond more often with the correct answer. Chapter 14, "Improving Your Strategies for Test Preparation," will help you learn how to prepare for tests more successfully. Chapter 15, "Preparing for and Taking Tests," will help you learn how to improve your scores on both objective and essay examinations. Successful students know how to prepare carefully for their tests, and how to take them in a pressure situation. Their high scores reflect their mastery of these skills.

CHAPTER 14

Improving Your Strategies for Test Preparation

• OBJECTIVE

To learn the strategies to help you prepare for tests more successfully.

• KEY WORDS

Pay attention to the key words, which are listed below. They are underscored the first time they appear in this chapter. Try to determine the meanings of these words from the surrounding words in the passage. If you need further help, use your dictionary or the glossary in the back of this book.

Look up the medical terminology in your medical dictionary or the glossary. As you read the exercises in this chapter, write additional words you need to learn in the space provided.

MEDICAL TERMINOLOGY	GENERAL VOCABULARY
ataxia	acronyms
diphtheria	aggravates

epistaxis	alleviates
hepatitis	analogy
hyperventilation	assessment
melena	components
myalgia	dysfunction
seizures	haphazard
syncope	interaction
wheezing	mnemonics
______________	______________
______________	______________
______________	______________

• PREPARING FOR EXAMINATIONS

You have learned the strategies for reading the textbook, active listening, and note-taking in the preceding chapters of this textbook. These study skills will help you to learn the material in your liberal arts and nursing textbooks and nursing lectures as you keep up with your weekly assignments. To do well on tests, however, you must do more than keep up with your assignments. You have to prepare for doing well on your exams. Test preparation is a planned series of steps. It is not haphazard. If you want to be successful, you should develop a plan that works for you and then follow it.

Successful students use their calendars to plan ahead for study time. Even if you feel you already know the information that will be on the test, you will forget a certain amount of material by the time you have the exam. That is why a review is essential.

• PLAN AHEAD

Be sure that you know **what** to study. Do you know which information from your textbooks, class lectures, notes, or labs will be covered on the test? Then make sure that your outlines and notes are complete and accurate.

Decide **when** you will study for the test. Get organized for study. Budget enough study time into your schedule. Use your time management skills to help you plan ahead. Monthly, weekly, and daily calendars help you to schedule study hours. Follow your schedule. Avoid procrastination and cramming, studying at the last minute. Falling behind in your work or leaving your work until the last minute will increase your anxiety. You will have better test results if you are prepared, calm, and confident.

Ask your instructor whether the test will be essay or objective. This information will help you decide **what** to study, **how** to organize the material for effective comprehension and retention, and **which** questions you should include in your practice tests.

EXAMPLE 14–1

Jason's chemistry exam was scheduled for Friday afternoon. On Thursday evening, he was nervously reviewing his lecture notes and textbook summaries. He felt anxious and disorganized.

What did Jason do wrong?

Jason didn't plan ahead. He left his studying for the night before the exam. He forgot about using his time management strategies. Last-minute cramming increases anxiety. He didn't give himself time to organize his test preparation.

EXERCISE 14–1

Directions. Answer the following question.

How can you plan ahead for your next exam? Write the steps that you should follow.

____

____

____

____

____

Comprehending? Yes ___ No ___

• KEEP UP WITH ASSIGNMENTS

The most effective way to understand and remember information is to do your assignments on a regular basis. Follow your class syllabus carefully to keep up with all the assigned work. As you read your textbooks, remember to be an **active reader. Preview** the assigned reading. **Ask questions**. Write **summaries** and **outlines**. Pay attention to **key vocabulary** words and **illustrations, tables,** and **formulas** that help you understand the ideas in each reading assignment. **Monitor** your comprehension. When you complete each assignment, make sure that you understand the information before you move on to the next chapter.

Use **active listening** and **effective note-taking** strategies. Attend your classes regularly, and take organized, accurate notes so that you can later review the lecture information. Apply your active listening strategies so that you will grasp the main ideas and major details presented in your lectures and labs. Ask questions if you do not understand the information. You need precise and comprehensive notes as an effective study tool.

EXAMPLE 14–2

Talia was scheduled to take her nutrition exam on Wednesday morning. It was Tuesday evening, and she felt confident because she had kept up with all assignments and attended every lecture except the last class before the exam. She didn't think that the information from one class would be that important.

What is her error?

Talia is taking a chance to go into an exam with incomplete information. The instructor may have used the last class to review highlights or even to introduce new points. She should have called another classmate to find out what she missed.

EXERCISE 14–2

Directions. Examine the following checklist of steps to follow in keeping up with assignments. Check any strategy that you feel you could improve. In the space provided, write how you could do better when you prepare for your next test.

Strategy	***Needs Improvement***	***How to Improve***
Active reading		
Monitoring comprehension		
Active listening		
Effective note-taking		

Comprehending? Yes ___ No ___

• STUDY AND LEARN MATERIAL

Even if you have kept up with your assignments on a regular basis and attended every class lecture and lab, you still have to study before every test. Review all lecture and lab notes, summaries, outlines, and underlined material from your textbooks. Organize the information by outlining, listing, or mapping the main ideas and details. It is easier to remember organized information than random facts.

A precise knowledge of medical terminology is important in your nursing studies. Review key vocabulary because these definitions will help you to understand the information. Keep words and definitions in a file of 3×5 inch index cards. Use the illustrations, tables, and formulas to help you understand the text. These pictures and numbers often clarify information in the chapters. Monitor your comprehension. Don't give up if you have difficulty understanding the material. Look up difficult vocabulary words, or try to paraphrase complex passages. Ask your instructor or other students to explain complicated material before the exam.

Find a study technique that works best for you. Do you learn best by reading, listening, writing, or discussing information? Is using a combination of strategies most effective for you? Do you prefer studying individually, with a study partner, or in a group? Once you find and use a study method that works well for you, you will improve your test results.

Some students use mnemonics, a memory technique to learn formulas, definitions, or ideas from a text. These mnemonic devices are easily remembered words, sentences, or rhymes that help you to learn more difficult information. Mnemonic devices work by association. Some common mnemonic devices are rhymes ("Thirty days hath September, April, June, and November . . ."), and acronyms, e.g., **RACE** for procedures to remember in case of fire:

R = **R**escue
A = **A**larm
C = **C**onfine the area
E = **E**xtinguish

EXAMPLE 14–3

Irina went into her biology test feeling prepared. She knew every definition and every detail. When she looked at the test, she was surprised to find that the format was mainly essay questions. She needed to organize the details under generalizations. She had just learned random facts.

What did Irina do wrong?

She should have tried to find out if the test was essay or objective. Irina also should have tried to organize the details under headings so that the facts would relate to main ideas. She should have tried to outline, map, or list the information.

EXERCISE 14–3

Read the following selection. Organize the main ideas and major details by outlining, mapping, or listing the information.

MAJOR COMPONENTS OF A HEALTH HISTORY

Chief Complaint

The **chief complaint** is a person's description of the major problem he or she is experiencing. It is written in the person's own words and is contained within direct quotes. Help the person be specific. A person's main concerns are often a change in usual condition or the presence of pain or dysfunction. The chief complaint provides a broad beginning for assessment. It usually consists of one statement, containing one to two symptoms and the duration. Examples of a chief complaint are "I've been having chest pain for the last 2 days" and "I've been short of breath for 3 to 4 weeks."

Present Illness

The present illness is derived from the chief complaint. It details the course of the illness or the sequence of events leading up to the present illness. The history of the present illness usually identifies major disease mechanisms and may even establish the diagnosis when symptoms are precise.

To reconstruct the events leading up to the present illness, you must acquaint yourself with the seven variables central to obtaining pertinent information from the person:

Body Location. Pinpoint the body system or organs involved. A question you may ask is "Where does it hurt?"

Quality. Usually a person will equate a symptom with an analogy, by stating it is "like" something. For example, "My chest pain feels like a knife is being thrust in my chest."

Quantity. You need to quantify the symptom according to the level of intensity, how it affects activities of daily living, frequency, volume, number, and size or extent of the symptom. For example, ask the person, "On a scale of one to ten with ten most severe, what is your level of pain?"

Chronology. You need to consider the symptom in relation to time. For example, when did the symptom first appear? Does the symptom begin gradually or suddenly? Does it stay the same in quality and intensity? How often does it occur? Does it wake the person from sleep?

Setting. Consider where and what the person was doing when the symptom occurred.

Aggravating or Alleviating Factors. Identify what worsens (aggravates) or relieves (alleviates) the symptom. For example, does the chest pain increase during physical activity? Does it require rest? Does emotional upset make the symptom worse?

Associated Factors. Assess the associated factors or symptoms. Some disorders produce symptoms in various body parts. For example, a person with congestive heart failure may have swollen ankles and abdomen and may experience shortness of breath. Exploration of associated factors may reveal useful information. For example, an acutely ill child may have eaten a poisonous substance, or a desperately ill adult might have been traveling recently and developed malaria or some other regional disorder.

Past Health History

The past health history reflects a chronologic review of previous disorders and contacts with health professionals. The first information you will need to obtain is a description of the person's general health immediately prior to the present illness. You may ask the person to describe health prior to this particular illness. The following are areas to be included in the past health history:

- Pediatric and adult illness: Inquire whether the person has ever had measles, mumps, chickenpox, hypertension, polio, hepatitis, pneumonia, diabetes, cancer, mental illness, scarlet fever, anemia, rheumatic fever, seizures, chronic bronchitis, heart disease, whooping cough, stroke, diphtheria, or malaria. If the person answers yes to any of these illnesses, question the person concerning the time frame and any complications resulting from the illness
- Previous hospitalizations: Obtain the date, physician, disorder, and hospital location
- Operations and injuries without hospitalization
- Immunizations
- Allergies or sensitivities, e.g., asthma, hayfever, food, skin, drugs (note drug allergies or sensitivities and manifestations)
- Transfusions
- Current medications: This should include medications prior to and during hospitalization. Remember to include prescription as well as over-the-counter medications
- Current treatments, e.g., physical or occupational therapy, respiratory therapy

Family Health History

The family health history is a past medical history of relatives. You will need to assess the person's family history with respect to the present illness and future health risks. The following are areas to be included in the family health history:

- Present status of parents and siblings: Question the person concerning the age and health status of the mother, father, and each of the siblings, or the age at death and cause.
- Medical problems: Question the person concerning the family history of disorders that may be influenced by heredity (familial disorders) or contact. Also ask about family allergies, deformities, or serious illnesses. Include the following: diabetes, hypertension, heart disease, renal disease, cancer, tuberculosis, stroke, deafness, anemia, gout, arthritis, mental illness, alcoholism, seizures, obesity.
- Similar illness or symptoms in family: Is anyone in the family experiencing an illness or symptoms resembling a person's present illness?

Personal and Social History

The personal and social history pertains to information concerning the person's personality and lifestyle. Some of the information may be emotionally charged and difficult for the person to describe. Question the person concerning the following areas (only information needed to care for the person should be obtained):

- Marital status
- Number of dependent children
- Other people in the household
- Religion
- Occupation
- Military service
- Daily routines, e.g., food intake, elimination, sleep pattern, exercise
- Habits, e.g., tobacco, caffeine, alcohol, drugs
- Pets
- Housing and living arrangements
- Family responsibilities
- Interests
- Daily activity, e.g., description of an average day
- Source of income
- Health insurance
- Travel
- Past development, e.g., childhood and adolescence, educational experiences, occupational experiences
- Patterns of interaction and communication, e.g., sexual relations, personality (mood, feelings, temperament, and general attitudes)

Systems Review

A review of systems is included in the client health history. You will be questioning the person about the structure and function of the body systems in order to identify symptoms that the person may not have previously reported. Some of the terms used will be new to you, but they are common medical terms you will have to know in your role as a nurse. You are urged to look them up and become familiar with them. The following systems should be addressed:

- Integument: color change, pruritus, nevi, infections, inflammations, rash, tumor, hair changes, nail changes, excessive bruising, cuts failing to heal
- Eyes: visual acuity, glasses/contact lenses, blurring, diplopia, pain, inflammation, excessive tearing, visual defects, date of last eye examination
- Ears: hearing loss, tinnitus, discharge, hearing aid, earache, vertigo, infection
- Nose and sinuses: frequent colds, sinusitis, epistaxis, discharge, obstruction, postnasal drip, pain

- Mouth and throat: gums, teeth, partial/full dentures, sore tongue, sore throat, difficulty swallowing, hoarseness, voice change, goiter, bleeding gums, date of last dental examination
- Neck: pain, thyroid or lymph node enlargement, limitation of motion
- Respiratory: cough, sputum, hemoptysis, wheezing, dyspnea, recurrent respiratory tract infections, night sweats, recent chest x-ray, pain, positive tuberculin test (date)
- Cardiovascular: chest pain, dyspnea, orthopnea, palpitations, murmur, hypertension, syncope, anemia, edema, varicosities, thrombophlebitis, claudication, pain
- Gastrointestinal: appetite changes, dysphagia, eructation, nausea, vomiting, hematemesis, pain, gas, indigestion, jaundice, change in bowel habits, food intolerance, constipation, diarrhea, stools (color, character), hemorrhoids, hernia, melena, use of laxatives, weight change, rectal itching
- Genitourinary/reproductive: frequency, nocturia, urgency, dysuria, incontinence, albuminuria, flank pain, venereal disease, discharge, lesions, contraception, hesitancy, hematuria, pyuria, infections, stones, glycosuria, infertility, libido, testicular mass or pain, impotence, menarche, LMP (last menstrual period), cycle, duration, regularity, dysmenorrhea, gravida, para, abortions, spotting, leukorrhea, pruritus, last pelvic examination, last Pap smear, menopause, complications
- Musculoskeletal: myalgia, weakness, pain, swelling, heat, limitation of motion, stiffness, redness
- Endocrine: sensitivity to environmental temperature, change in body configuration, changes in scalp or hair, body weight in relation to appetite, sweating, polyuria, postural hypotension, change in voice, polydipsia, polyphagia
- Neurologic: headache, syncope, convulsions, seizures, vertigo, diplopia, paralysis, paresis, spasm, muscle weakness, paresthesia, tremor, ataxia, memory change, unconsciousness, speech problems, coordination
- Psychologic: nervousness, insomnia, depression, nightmares, indecisiveness, hyperventilation, work difficulty, mood, emotional difficulty, sense of failure, social withdrawal, memory loss

A variety of printed forms are available for recording the client's health history. It is important to remember that a client health history is privileged information. Information should not be sought unless it will be used in a professional, confidential manner. (Bolander, 3rd ed., pp 651–653)

Comprehending? Yes ___ No ___

• TACKLING TEST-TAKING ANXIETY

Test-taking anxiety occurs because of worrying about not learning the information or worrying about time.

Research in study skills indicates that overpreparation is the best cure for test-taking anxiety. Keep up with your assignments. Take notes, underline, write summaries and outlines, and review, and you will go into a test feeling confident. This preparation can be done either alone or in study groups with other students.

• VALUE OF PRACTICE TESTS

Take timed practice tests when you have completed your review. Use the questions at the end of the chapter or create your own test questions. This type of rehearsal before the performance helps you go into your test feeling prepared and positive. Remember, nothing succeeds like success.

• VOCABULARY CHECK

Directions. Below are 10 words taken from the key words section of this chapter. Circle the letter of the best definition from the four choices.

1. Haphazard
- **a** backward
- **b** slanted
- **c** wrong direction
- **d** lack of a plan

2. Analogy
- **a** likeness
- **b** difference
- **c** antonym
- **d** error

3. Syncope
- **a** sneezing
- **b** fainting
- **c** headaches
- **d** steroids

4. Epistaxis
- **a** hemorrhage from the eyes
- **b** hemorrhage from the ears
- **c** hemorrhage from the nose
- **d** hemorrhage from the mouth

5. Assessment
- **a** problem
- **b** solution
- **c** appraisal
- **d** cost

6. Aggravates
- **a** worsens
- **b** relieves
- **c** cures
- **d** eases

7. Seizures
- **a** setbacks
- **b** fractures
- **c** dizzy spells
- **d** convulsions

8. Mnemonics
- **a** an essay test
- **b** an objective test
- **c** a memory technique
- **d** a survey

9. Myalgia
- **a** muscular pain
- **b** back pain
- **c** heartburn
- **d** inflammation

10. Alleviates
- **a** worsens
- **b** relieves
- **c** deteriorates
- **d** destroys

• CRITICAL THINKING LOG

List the strategies you learned in this chapter.	Select the strategy that is most useful for your school success.	How can you apply this strategy to your nursing studies?

• SUMMARY

Improving your strategies for test preparation will help you to get better grades on both objective and essay tests in nursing school. Plan ahead so that you can schedule your study time. Use active reading strategies as you keep up with weekly assignments. Review all your notes, underlined material, summaries, outlines, key words, and graphic information from texts.

Find out whether the test will be objective or essay. Take practice tests from end-of-chapter questions or create your own questions. A positive attitude, careful preparation, and practice will ensure your success.

CHAPTER 15

Preparing for and Taking Tests

• OBJECTIVE

To learn the strategies that will help you to improve your scores on both objective and essay examinations.

• KEY WORDS

Pay attention to the following key words, which are underscored the first time they appear in this chapter. Try to determine the meaning of these words from the surrounding words in the passage. If you need further help, use your dictionary or the glossary in the back of this book.

Look up the medical terminology in your medical dictionary or the glossary. As you read the exercises in this chapter, write additional words that you need to learn in the space provided.

MEDICAL TERMINOLOGY

anorexia
arthritis
hallucinations
malnutrition
mobility
obesity
paralysis
resuscitate
scoliosis
sensory

____

____

____

GENERAL VOCABULARY

construct
deficit
deviation
exotic
impairments
ingrained
myths
revisions
stringent
upheld

____

____

____

• TAKING THE TEST SUCCESSFULLY

Learning how to take tests successfully will improve your test scores. You can learn test-taking strategies that will help you improve your results in both essay and objective tests. Apply the following strategies to improve your grades on tests:

- Follow the test directions carefully. Read all directions before you answer any questions. Check the grading system, before you write your answers. You should spend extra time on questions that are worth more points.
- Monitor your test-taking time.
- Answer the questions that you are sure of first. Then go back to finish the more difficult questions.
- Read the question carefully. Be sure that you are providing information that is asked for.
- Save time at the end of the test to review your answers and make any correction or additions.
- Revise and edit your writing so that your answers are well organized.

• TAKING OBJECTIVE TESTS

Objective tests—those with multiple-choice, short-answer, matching, or true-false questions—require you to know both details and main ideas. You have to retain facts as well as understand general concepts. To study for objective tests:

- Review class notes carefully.
- Review all underlined material, outlines, and summaries from your text.
- Take practice tests.
- Go over any end-of-chapter questions.
- Try to predict the test questions. Then prepare answers to your own questions.

Learning How to Answer Multiple-Choice Questions

Practicing how to answer the specific types of questions on multiple-choice tests will help you improve your grades in your nursing and liberal arts courses. When answering multiple-choice questions, you select one answer from several choices. The following strategies will help you select the correct answer:

- If two choices are the same, they are both incorrect. Therefore, you eliminate both of these choices.
- When "all of the above" is given as a choice, it is usually correct unless you determine that one of the choices is obviously wrong.
- Be aware of directional words such as "but," "except," and "however," since they signal opposite meanings.
- Read all answer choices before making your decision.

To answer multiple-choice questions you need to know how to:

- Find main ideas.
- Locate and retain the details that support the main idea.
- Make inferences.
- Learn vocabulary meanings through context.

The following techniques will help you to answer questions on each of these skills.

Main-Idea Question

The answer to a main-idea question will be: (1) Who or what is the selection about? (2) What is the main point being made about the selection?

The following are examples of questions that require you to find the main idea:

The primary concern is:
The major purpose is:
The idea primarily discussed is:
The main point is:
What is the most important idea?

Eliminating Answers to the Main-Idea Question

Learning how to eliminate answers is an important test-taking strategy in multiple-choice tests. When answering main-idea questions, you should eliminate any answers that are:

- Too general. The answer covers more information than is discussed in the passage.
- Too specific. The answer covers just a detail from the selection, not the main idea.
- Not mentioned. The answer is an idea not discussed in the passage.

EXAMPLE 15–1

Directions. Read the following excerpt from a nursing textbook (Iyer et al., 3rd ed., p. 240) and the explanation of the answer to the main-idea question based on the selection.

Age also affects ability to learn. The very young child may have difficulty in grasping concepts unless they are presented in very concrete terms. Some elderly clients may have ingrained ideas or "myths" that affect their ability to accept new changes. Additionally, they may have physiological deficits that interfere with their ability to learn (e.g., vision or hearing problems).

The main point of this passage is:

a learning disabilities in children
b age affects learning
c physiological deficits interfere with learning
d ability to learn

The correct answer to this passage is (b), age affects learning. Choice (a) is not mentioned in the passage. Choice (c) is too specific; it is just a detail from the selection. Choice (d) is too general; the answer covers more information than is discussed in the passage.

EXERCISE 15–1

Directions. Read the following excerpt from a nursing textbook (Black and Matassarin-Jacobs, 4th ed., p. 692). Then answer the five multiple-choice main-idea questions based on this selection. Use the test-taking strategy of eliminating any answers that are too general, too specific, or not mentioned before you choose the correct answer.

CLINICAL MANIFESTATIONS

The earliest sign of a metabolic brain disorder is a disorder of attention. The client may report the loss of concentration or appear preoccupied. At the same time, restlessness, emotional lability, insomnia or drowsiness, and vivid nightmares may begin. Clients may appear anxious and fear that they are "going crazy." As the disorder progresses, stupor and coma develop. Data seen in the client are reflective not of personality but of the cause of the disorder. For example, barbiturate/alcohol abuse and withdrawal and liver disorders cause agitated delirium. In contrast, anoxia and kidney and lung disorders cause a more quiet response. Disorders that develop rapidly are more likely to cause an agitated response than are those that develop slowly.

Fluctuations in cognition (the ability to think and reason) are common in clients with metabolic brain disorders. Clients may be totally out of context one moment and lucid the next. Some of the fluctuations are due to the environment, and delirious clients become more disoriented at night, in unfamiliar surroundings, and in situations in which restraints are used, unfamiliar noises are heard, or unfamiliar people are seen. The lack of a window in the room has caused many clients to become disoriented.

The client will commonly have difficulty with immediate recall and ability to abstract. Loss of memory for recent events is a hallmark of metabolic brain disorders (sometimes called organic brain disease). Clients who are delirious quickly lose orientation to time. Normal subjects can readily recall six or seven digits forward and five or six backward and identify the commonalities between an orange and an apple or a tree and a bush. Delirious clients cannot do this. However, the client's general intelligence level can have an impact on the data seen. If possible, the level of education should be known before assessment.

Perceptual errors (e.g., mistaking the nurse for a daughter) as well as hallucinations, illusions, and delusions are common accompaniments of delirium.

Hallucinations are sensations occurring in the absence of external stimuli. A client may hear, see, feel, smell, or taste something that is not present. The client may or may not realize that the experience is "unreal."

Illusions differ from hallucinations in that illusions are the misinterpretation of something in the environment. For example, if a client sees a shadow on the drape and mistakes it for a real person, the client is experiencing an illusion.

Delusions are thoughts or beliefs that have no basis in fact. For example, a client may think that he has been robbed or poisoned, when there is no basis for this thought.

Diagnostic Assessment

There are no specific diagnostic tests for confusion. The client would have a CT or MRI scan for determining whether there is a structural cause of the confusion, such as a tumor. In addition, a series of laboratory studies would be performed to determine whether there is a metabolic cause. Common studies include a complete blood count, electrolyte determinations, vitamin B_{12} and folate levels, thyroid and liver function studies, drug toxicity screening tests, and an electroencephalogram. A lumbar puncture may be performed for the analysis of CSF.

MEDICAL MANAGEMENT

The medical management of the confused client begins by determining the cause of the confusion and correcting it if possible. When no specific cause is found, the medical management focuses on controlling symptoms. At times, haloperidol can be given to calm agitation. Nutritional needs must also be monitored.

SURGICAL MANAGEMENT

There are no operations for confusion, unless the confusion is due to a structural disorder such as a tumor or hematoma. For those clients, craniotomy may be performed to remove the growth or accumulation of blood.

1. Hallucinations, illusions, and delusional thinking are examples of:
   a. physical diseases of the elderly
   b. organized group behavior
   c. patterns of organized behavior
   d. disorganized thought and behavior patterns
2. Hallucinations are:
   a. always present in the physical world
   b. external stimuli found in the material world
   c. sensory impressions occurring in the absence of external stimuli
   d. created by the absence of taste or other sensory stimuli
3. The earliest sign of a metabolic brain disorder is:
   a. a disorder of attention
   b. increased concentration
   c. caused only by exotic drugs
   d. a brain tumor
4. Illusions are:
   a. the same as hallucinations
   b. correctly interpreted stimuli
   c. a misinterpretation of a real stimulus
   d. caused by reduction of environmental stimuli

5. Delusional thinking:
   a. is caused by persecution
   b. is the result of persecution
   c. is based on reality
   d. is false thoughts and beliefs

Detail Questions

When you are reading for details, concentrate on reading accurately. The most minor misinterpretation of a fact can cause you to choose an incorrect answer. When you study, try to retain facts. A helpful study strategy is to try to classify facts under main ideas. Retaining organized information is easier than remembering random facts. When answering detail questions: Read the question carefully. Are you asked to know when, why, or how? You must understand the question before you can choose an answer.

Be careful of such words as *all, only, always, every,* and *never.* These words are too general. Their presence in a multiple-choice response often means the response is incorrect.

EXAMPLE 15–2

Read the following excerpt from a nursing textbook (Sorensen and Luckmann, 3rd ed., p. 810) and the explanation of the answer to the detail question based on the selection.

The concept of *Impaired Physical Mobility* is difficult to grasp because mobility is such an important, basic need that virtually all other aspects of life relate to it in some manner or other. As a result, you will note that many nursing diagnoses include a mention of mobility (or activity) somewhere in their definition, defining characteristics, risk factors, or related factors.

Mobility:

a threatens our physical, psychological, emotional, and economic well-being
b prevents numerous bodily movements
c is an important basic need
d is underestimated by everyone

The correct answer is choice (c), which is stated in the first sentence of the passage. A careful reading of the passage will eliminate choices (a) and (b) because those statements are true of immobility, not mobility. Choice (d) is incorrect because the word "everyone" is too general.

EXERCISE 15–2

Directions. Read the following excerpt from a nursing textbook (Bolander, 3rd ed., p. 806). Then answer the five detail questions based on this selection. Concentrate on reading and understanding the questions before you choose your answers.

CAUSES OF IMMOBILITY

Clients should be assessed for impaired physical mobility when they have either a prescribed or an unavoidable decrease in musculoskeletal activity.

Unavoidable causes of immobility include

- pain severe enough to limit motion and curtail activity. For example, persons with diseases such as rheumatoid arthritis may be able to move joints, but severe pain causes them to limit movement. Chronic pain increases the risk of complications of immobility.
- impairments of motor nervous function that seriously and sometimes permanently decrease body movements. Examples of conditions in this category include progressive degenerative disorders such as muscular dystrophy, Parkinson's disease, and amyotrophic lateral sclerosis. Paralysis from a stroke and spinal cord injury are other examples.
- structural problems like scoliosis (lateral deviation of the spine), degenerative joint disease, joint contractures, or osteoporosis.
- generalized weakness from chronic illness (e.g., cancer, anorexia with resulting malnutrition, or profound obesity).
- psychologic problems such as severe depression, acute confusion, and certain other mental disorders. (See Applying Research to Nursing Practice.)

Prescribed causes of immobility include

- orthopedic (musculoskeletal) problems that require treatment by immobilization of the spine or one or more extremities (e.g., traction or the application of a cast). **Orthopedics** is the branch of medicine that specializes in the treatment of musculoskeletal disorders.
- other health problems that require restriction of mobility as a part of the treatment (e.g., the person who requires restraints or bed rest).

1. The risk of complications from immobility is increased by:
   a. severe pain
   b. chronic pain
   c. only arthritis
   d. the lack of pain
2. Impairments of motor nervous function:
   a. decrease pain
   b. decrease all body movements
   c. inhibit movements
   d. sometimes permanently decrease body movements
3. Scoliosis is a:
   a. joint contracture
   b. deviation of the spine
   c. cause of structural problems
   d. cause of paralysis
4. Immobility can be:
   a. caused only by a physical disease
   b. caused only by psychological problems
   c. caused by severe depression
   d. cured by improved nutrition
5. Immobility is the result of:
   a. bed rest
   b. removal of a cast
   c. new medical and nursing treatments
   d. all orthopedic problems

Inference Questions

An inference question requires you to understand unstated meanings. When you are answering inference questions, choose an answer that is based on information you have studied in your nursing and liberal arts courses. Do not choose an answer that is not related to ideas or facts in the material.

The following are examples of statements that require you to make inferences:

You can conclude . . .
It is implied that . . .
One can infer . . .
Which is most probably . . .

EXAMPLE 15–3

Directions. Read the following excerpt from a nursing textbook (Iyer et al., 3rd ed., p. 322) and the explanation of the answer to the inference question based on the selection.

During an attempt to resuscitate a woman in the intensive care unit the client opened her eyes. She said to the nurse, "Let me go. Leave me alone." The physician, who was standing by her side, verified that the client wanted no further treatment. The resuscitation effort ended and the client was allowed to die. You can conclude that the resuscitation effort ended because:

a the nurse had no hope for the patient's recovery
b the doctor failed to save the patient's life
c the patient has the right to refuse care
d the patient had only a few hours to live

Choice (a) is not based on any statement in the passage. The nurse's feelings about the patient's chances for recovery are not mentioned. Choice (b) is incorrect because the doctor was not involved in the resuscitation effort and merely was a witness to the patient's request to end treatment. Choice (c) is correct based on the third sentence, in which the physician verified that the client wanted no further treatment. Choice (d) is incorrect because the reader is not given any information on the life expectancy of the patient.

EXERCISE 15–3

Directions. Read the following excerpt from a nursing textbook (Iyer et al., 3rd ed., pp. 323–324). Then answer the five inference questions based on the selection. Remember to use the test-taking strategy of basing your answer on information stated in the selection.

NURSE'S RIGHTS

Under this principle of law you have rights and responsibilities as an employee and professional.

Right to a Safe Environment. You have a right to a safe working environment according to the Occupational Safety and Health Administration (OSHA) laws. The regulations permit you to refuse to work in proven unsafe conditions. Your employer is obligated to provide you with safety equipment and you have a responsibility to use the equipment. For example, you are expected to wear gloves when handling blood and body fluids. If you do not wear gloves when drawing blood and contract hepatitis, you would not be entitled to compensation from the employer.

Right to Be Free from Sexual Harassment. There is no precise definition of what constitutes sexual harassment. The courts have defined three situations that are unlawful:

- Submission to sexual harassment is either explicitly or implicitly a term or condition of an individual's employment.

Example. You are told that tolerating sexual harassment is required in order to keep your job.

- Submission to or rejection of such conduct is used as the basis for employment decisions affecting you.

Example. You are told that if you tolerate sexual harassment you will be promoted.

- Sexual harassment has the effect of substantially interfering with your work performance or creating an intimidating, hostile, or offensive working environment.

Example. Two male employees of an Ohio hospital "groped" a female unit clerk on a deserted elevator. Both lost their jobs following an investigation that they had violated the hospital's rules prohibiting sexual harassment (Tammelleo, 1993).

You have a right to expect your school and your employer to have policies for the reporting of sexual harassment. If you are ever the victim of sexual harassment, you have the responsibility to report it through the appropriate channels.

1. Occupational Safety and Health Administration laws are designed:
   a. to discharge nurses with AIDS
   b. to encourage litigation
   c. to protect only the patients
   d. to establish standards of hospital safety controls
2. One can infer that lack of safety equipment:
   a. creates security problems
   b. always prevents adequate care of patients
   c. may interfere with safe care
   d. injures all patients and nurses
3. A nurse can sue a hospital if an injury results:
   a. while refusing to use safety equipment
   b. while using safety equipment
   c. while drawing blood without gloves
   d. outside hospital grounds
4. It is implied that situations have been defined by the courts as sexual harassment because:
   a. no precise definition of sexual harassment exists
   b. nurses employed by hospitals always face sexual harassment
   c. trouble exists with the union
   d. improvement of hospital-patient relations is required

5. According to this article, the responsibility for reporting sexual harassment is:
   a. the nurse's responsibility
   b. the patient's responsibility
   c. the victim's responsibility
   d. the hospital administration's responsibility

Vocabulary in Context Questions

Follow these three steps when you are asked to define a word in context, that is, to define an unknown word by looking at surrounding words:

1. Decide on the part of speech of the unknown word.
2. Use clues in the surrounding words to find the meaning.
3. Check your answer choice by placing it in the original sentence and reading to see if it makes sense.

EXAMPLE 15–4

Note how the word "resuscitation" is used in the following sentence. "The **resuscitation** effort ended and the client was allowed to die" (Iyer et al., 3rd ed., p. 322). Resuscitation means:

a life-saving
b lifesaver
c failed
d resentful

Choice (a) is the correct answer. Since the effort ended, resuscitation had to have a meaning opposite of "to die." Choice (b) is incorrect because a lifesaver is a person and therefore a noun, while resuscitation is used as an adjective. Choice (c) is incorrect because the phrase "allowed to die" lets the reader know that the effort was stopped; it didn't fail. Choice (d) is incorrect because there is no basis in the sentence for the negative word "resentful."

EXERCISE 15–4

Directions. Read the following five sentences. Use the three-step plan learned in this chapter to define each boldface word.

1. "This **principle** of confidentiality applies to families who are seeking detailed information." (Iyer et al., 3rd ed., p. 322)
   a. administrator of a school
   b. to theorize
   c. pressure point
   d. question

2. "The client who decides to file a malpractice suit is called the **plaintiff**." (Iyer et al., 3rd ed., p. 329)
   a. lawyer
   b. person who is suing
   c. person who is being sued
   d. judge
3. "There are guidelines for a nurse's conduct and mechanisms for **enforcing** those rules." (Iyer et al., 3rd ed., p. 327)
   a. procedure
   b. putting into action
   c. arresting
   d. changing
4. "For instance, the board may be asked to rule on whether licensed practical nurses may **insert** intravenous needles." (Iyer et al., 3rd ed., p. 327)
   a. remove
   b. an order
   c. stick in
   d. request
5. "The board is expected to take disciplinary action when a nurse has a physical, mental, or substance abuse **impairment**." (Iyer et al., 3rd ed., p. 325)
   a. weakness
   b. disease
   c. habit
   d. license

Comprehending? Yes ___ No ___

Answering Other Types of Objective Test Questions

In your nursing classes most objective test questions will be multiple-choice. However, in your liberal arts classes some objective test questions will be in other forms. Therefore, you should learn how to answer the other types of objective test questions, such as:

- *Short answers.* Short-answer questions ask you to fill in the blank. Since you will be completing sentences, make sure that your answer choice fits grammatically and contextually.
- *Matching.* When matching items, keep track of the answers you've already used. In this way you monitor your progress.
- *True-false.* When answering true-false questions, focus on the part of the statement that makes it either true or false. Usually, close attention to detail is needed in reading true-false questions. The entire statement has to be correct for the answer choice to be true. If a part of the statement is incorrect, the answer is false.

EXERCISE 15–5

Directions. Read the following excerpts from a nursing textbook (Iyer et al., 3rd ed., pp. 327–328 and 324–326). Study the material, then answer the objective test questions based on the selection.

LAW IS BASED ON A CONCERN FOR FAIRNESS AND JUSTICE

The third principle of law seeks to protect a person's rights from infringement by the actions of another person. It defines appropriate conduct under the law and creates a mechanism to enforce this conduct. The laws are designed to achieve a fair outcome in legal disputes, and to provide structure for managing the complexities of the health care system.

There are guidelines for a nurse's conduct and mechanisms for enforcing those rules. The expectations of professional conduct are defined by the state board of nursing in the nurse practice act, the ANA and other specialty organizations, by standards published by the Joint Commission, and other accrediting bodies. The state board of nursing consists of a group of nurses and, in some states, non-nurses who are appointed by the governor. The board is charged with a number of responsibilities:

1. Approval of the curriculum of schools of nursing located in the state.
2. Inspection of employer records to be sure the nursing employees are credentialed and complying with professional standards (Markowitz, 1982).
3. Rulings on questions that are submitted to it. These questions clarify the scope of nursing practice. For instance, the board may be asked to rule on whether licensed practical nurses may insert intravenous needles.
4. Determining who is competent to be licensed as a nurse and the granting of licenses.
5. Disciplining of nurses who are found to be unfit or incompetent to practice nursing.

Nurse's Responsibilities

There are many nursing responsibilities. A few are highlighted below.

Safe Practice. You are expected to practice nursing in such a manner that you do not jeopardize the safety of the clients entrusted to your care. A nursing license is a legal document that permits the nurse to offer certain skills and knowledge to the public of the state, where such practice would otherwise be unlawful without a license (Creighton, 1986). Nurses are required to hold a current license issued by their state in order to practice. You must be in good health to apply for an initial license, to renew your license, or to receive a license in another state (licensure by endorsement). Schools of nursing are expected to screen out those individuals who have physical and mental disabilities that would prevent them from practicing safely. Those with physical or mental disabilities who are applying for a license renewal or obtaining a license by endorsement are required to present evidence that they are able to practice nursing in a safe and competent manner in spite of their disability (Champagne et al, 1987). The Americans with Disabilities Act provides new rights to individuals with handicaps. Physical disabilities that have led to concern about safe practice include legal blindness, severe hearing impairment, and the loss of motor skills and normal speech.

The Board of Nursing is the regulatory agency that is charged with the authority to discipline nurses who do not practice in a safe, professional manner. The Board is expected to take disciplinary action when a nurse has a physical, mental, or substance abuse impairment. Through surveys of state boards of nursing, Champagne et al (1987) and Swenson et al (1987a, 1987b, 1989), found that:

- 99 percent of the boards had dealt with cases of illegal substance abuse.
- 76 percent with alcohol abuse.
- 70 percent with legal substance abuse that impaired practice.
- 20 percent with cases of mental impairment.
- 5 percent with cases of physical impairment.

Murphy and Connell (1987) studied 100 records of Arizona nurses who had violated the state's nurse practice act and discovered that 60 percent of the nurses had been disciplined for substance abuse and 40 percent for incompetence.

Nurses have also been disciplined or lost their licenses for failure to file tax returns and pay taxes, allowing the daughter of a nurse to pose as a nurse (Creighton, 1986a), and failing to comply with regulations for nurse midwives. Advanced nursing practice was the basis of a Missouri case on the role of nurse practitioners. An Idaho nurse named Jolene Tuma provided a client with information on alternative cancer therapies and retained her license after the Idaho board sought to remove it for unprofessional conduct. The Idaho court ruled that the nurse practice act was sufficiently vague on what constituted unprofessional conduct (Cushing, 1986).

You may be disciplined or have your licensed revoked for behavior that occurs within or even outside the scope of your employment. For example, a male nurse anesthetist lost his license after he was found guilty of photographing the male genitalia of three corpses. The court decided that his conduct was such that there was sufficient likelihood that he might invade the privacy and offend the dignity of patients entrusted to his care (Tammelleo, 1992a). Another male nurse lost his license after being convicted of sexual assault of 11- and 12-year-old girls.

As part of maintaining your clinical skills, you are expected to acquire and maintain current knowledge of nursing practice. This is accomplished by:

- attending educational programs presented by your employer or outside seminar companies.
- reading journals and books.
- listening to audiotapes.
- reading self-learning modules.
- watching videotapes.
- using a computer-assisted program.
- utilizing experts in clinical nursing.

• OBJECTIVE TEST

Part I. After reading this selection, fill in the blanks.

1. The ______________________ principle of law seeks to protect the rights of one party from infringement by the actions of another party.

2. The rights of individuals are protected by ______________________.

3. The state board of nursing is appointed by the ______________________.

4. A nursing license is issued by the ______________________.

5. The expectations of professional conduct are defined by the ______________ and other organizations.

Part II. Match the letters in column B with the numbers in column A.

A	B
1. Murphy and Connell study____	a. Reason for discipline
2. Nursing license ____	b. Responsibility of State Board of Nursing
3. Failure to pay taxes ____	c. Requirements to pay for license
4. Good health ____	d. Legal document
5. Approval of nursing school curriculum ____	e. 100 records of Arizona nurses

Part III. Answer the multiple-choice questions based on the passage you have read.

1. A nursing license is:
   a. unlawful
   b. required for practice
   c. automatically renewed
   d. issued upon request
2. A practicing nurse must:
   a. have her initial license
   b. apply for a new license each year
   c. reapply for nursing school each year
   d. have a current license
3. If a nurse has an impairment, disciplinary action is taken by:
   a. the national board.
   b. the physicians
   c. the state board
   d. the local board
4. Nursing boards have dealt with 70% of cases of:
   a. alcohol abuse
   b. legal substance abuse that impaired practice
   c. illegal substance abuse
   d. mental impairment
5. The percentage of cases of alcohol abuse dealt with by state boards was:
   a. 20%
   b. 99%
   c. 76%
   d. 70%
6. In Murphy and Connell's study the percent of Arizona nurses disciplined for incompetence was:
   a. 40%
   b. 60%
   c. 100%
   d. 76%
7. The basis of a Missouri case was:
   a. tax fraud
   b. substance abuse
   c. alternative cancer therapies
   d. advanced nursing practice
8. The nurse who provided her client with alternative cancer therapies was from:
   a. Arizona
   b. Idaho
   c. Colorado
   d. Missouri
9. The number of responsibilities listed for the state board is:
   a. five
   b. one
   c. two
   d. ten
10. Competency for nurses is determined by:
    a. the state board
    b. the hospital administration
    c. patients
    d. physicians

Part IV. Read the following statements. In the space provided write "T" if the statement is true or "F" if the statement is false.

1. State boards of nurses consist only of nurses. ___
2. Nurses are required to hold state licenses in order to practice. ___
3. The board of nurses takes disciplinary action when a nurse has a drug problem. ___
4. Eight-nine percent of the boards have dealt with illegal substance abuse. ___
5. Nurses can lose their licenses for not filing tax returns. ___

EXERCISE 15–6

Directions. Read the following excerpt from a nursing textbook (Iyer et al., 3rd ed., pp. 328–330). Create your own objective test based on the selection. Create five short answers, five matching, five true-false, and 10 multiple-choice questions.

A NURSE'S ACTIONS ARE JUDGED ON THE BASIS OF WHAT A SIMILARLY EDUCATED REASONABLE AND PRUDENT PERSON WOULD HAVE DONE IN A SIMILAR SITUATION

This fourth principle refers to the concepts that are applied in nursing malpractice cases. In a society that has increasingly turned to the courts for resolution of disputes, standards are needed to judge nursing performance.

Reasons for Lawsuits

The number of lawsuits being filed against nurses is increasing, although physicians are sued with greater frequency. According to the ANA, 6.2 nurses per 10,000 are sued each year. This is in contrast to 1,800 physicians per 10,000 (How likely is a lawsuit, 1990). Despite the relatively small number of nurses who are sued each year, nurses need to continue to be concerned with the legal aspects of nursing practice. Lawsuits against nurses are on the increase for a number of reasons:

1. The consumer has become better educated on what to expect from the health care system and nursing care.
2. Plaintiff attorneys (who represent the client) are becoming more able to identify the case that has merit.
3. Plaintiff attorneys are likely to name as many people as possible when filing a lawsuit. This allows them to potentially tap the pocket of the hospital's and the nurse's insurance companies, as well as the physician's insurance carrier.
4. Plaintiff lawyers are more aware that nurses are professionals and accountable for their own actions.
5. Many nurses are providing increasingly specialized and complex care that exposes the client and the nurse to greater risk (Godkin et al, 1987).

Definitions

The terms negligence and malpractice are often used to describe the *standard of care*. The standard of care is a concept that defines the expected and appropriate actions should occur. For example, if you take your car to the garage because the brakes are not working, the auto mechanic is expected to follow certain procedures to repair or replace the brakes. The mechanic who failed to properly fix the brakes would be considered negligent. *Negligence* is a general term referring to a deviation from the standard of care that a reasonably prudent person would follow in a particular set of circumstances. Any individual could be negligent in carrying out responsibilities. In the wintertime, if you do not clear the ice off your sidewalk and someone slips and breaks a hip, you could be judged to be negligent.

Malpractice is a specific type of negligence that occurs when a professional does not adhere to professional standards of care. If a doctor removes the wrong kidney or a nurse gives blood to the wrong client, they may be judged as having committed malpractice. Lawyers, doctors, dentists, and nurses are some of the professionals who are named in malpractice suits.

Outcomes of Lawsuits

Insurance studies show that of all medical malpractice cases filed, 50 percent are dropped, 40 percent are settled out of court, and 10 percent go to trial (Fig. 10–4). The 40 percent that settle out of court represent those cases that the team defending the nurse or physician believes would result in a verdict in favor of the plaintiff. The client who decides to file a malpractice suit is called the *plaintiff*. This person can be the client, a family member, or some other entity. The cases chosen for trial are either the ones that the defense believes it can win, or those that cannot be settled out of court because the plaintiff will not accept the dollar amount offered by the defense. The defense is successful in winning approximately 60 to 90 percent of the cases that get into court, although this varies from state to state. Daniels (1989) studied 1,886 malpractice cases in various geographical areas and found a 68 percent defense success rate.

A study by Taragin and others (1992) of 8000 cases involving New Jersey physicians found that physician care was considered defensible by the insurance company in 62 percent of the cases and indefensible in 25 percent. The remaining 13 percent of the cases were unclear as to the defensibility (Fig. 10–5). Payment to the plaintiff was made in 43 percent of all cases. Less than $50,000 was given to half of the plaintiffs. Only 15 percent received more than $200,000. It is difficult to find similar studies of nursing malpractice claims.

Student nurses are expected to provide nursing care as would a competent registered nurse. You are obligated to seek help when confronted with a new experience in which you are unclear how to proceed. While lawsuits against students are rare, the plaintiff could sue the student, instructor, facility, physician, and registered nurse staff.

Comprehending? Yes ____ No ____

• TAKING ESSAY TESTS

You can improve your grades on essay tests by learning the test-taking strategies for writing and revising essays. The first step in preparing for an essay test is to review your class notes and underlined material, outlines, and summaries of textbooks. Then you should organize all information into topics, main ideas, and major details. Organizing your information will help you to retain the material.

Writing strategies can help you to learn the information. These strategies, such as taking notes, composing questions, and writing summaries and outlines, will help you to prepare for your test.

Answering Essay Questions

BEFORE WRITING

Read the entire test, paying special attention to the directions.

- Find out how many questions you are required to answer.
- Notice the points given for each question. You will want to spend more time on a 30-point question than a 10-point question.

- Read the question carefully.
- Determine how you should organize your information. Is the question asking you to list, explain, compare, contrast, or sequence information?
- Think about approaches and construct an outline.

WHILE WRITING

- State main ideas in clear topic sentences.
- Support main ideas with relevant major details.
- Make sure you are answering the question that was asked.

AFTER WRITING

- Use an editing checklist to make necessary revisions in organization, word choice, and mechanics.
- Check to make sure that you have answered all the parts of each question.

EXAMPLE 15–5

Directions. Read the following example of an editing checklist. Apply this checklist when you write essay questions to improve your writing.

EDITING CHECKLIST	YES	NO
Content		
Is the main idea clearly expressed?	___	___
Do the details support the main idea?	___	___
Are the details organized according to your purpose?	___	___
Did you eliminate repetitive or unnecessary details?	___	___
Mechanics		
Did you check:		
• word choice?	___	___
• sentence structure?	___	___
• capitalization and punctuation?	___	___
• spelling?	___	___
Organization		
Is there a clear introduction, middle, and conclusion?	___	___
Did you write the ideas in the correct order?	___	___

EXAMPLE 15–6

Directions. Read the following excerpt from a nursing text (Bolander, 3rd ed., p. 91). Review the sample essay question and answer based on the selection.

EXAMPLES OF PRIMARY CARE AGENCIES

Ambulatory Care Centers

Ambulatory care centers provide a variety of services ranging from diagnostic to therapeutic; nurse practitioners and clinical nurse specialists may have pivotal roles in providing services in these centers.

Crisis Centers and Hotlines

Hospitals and communities typically offer services to assist citizens experiencing things like suicide, acquired immune deficiency syndrome, herpes, abuse, and psychiatric crisis. Hotlines generally provide information and support. Crisis centers may provide telephone hotlines, direct counseling, limited first aid, ongoing support, and guidance.

Day Care Centers

Formerly thought of for children only, day care centers now also serve the elderly and medically/emotionally impaired. Usually open during daytime hours, some may offer extended hours when there is a need. Respite care for families who need a break from caring for family members in the home or who need help while they work is also provided.

Employment Settings

As managers and employees recognize the benefits of healthy employees, nurses are much in demand to run employee health clinics at the worksite. Services may include histories/physicals, health teaching/promotion, health screens and occupational safety programs.

Home Health Care Agencies

Home health care agencies are a fast-growing service. Nurses and other health care team members (social workers, physical therapists, respiratory therapists, pharmacists, and others) render services traditionally provided in both the home and hospital; even acute care services (home ventilators, intravenous therapy, chemotherapy) are provided.

Managed Care Organizations

To hold down health care costs, many businesses use managed care organizations to provide health care to employees at a prearranged fee; examples of these are

HMOs: Health maintenance organizations are group health agencies providing basic and supplemental services to enrollees at a fixed rate; clients generally may not have much choice as to which physician will care for them; preventive care is stressed.

PPOs: Preferred provider organizations are groups of physicians/hospitals that provide services at a discounted rate; the client chooses which physician in the group they wish to see.

IPAs: Independent practice organizations are "middlemen" in the system; clients pay the IPA for services at a fixed rate, and the IPA pays the providers; profits are shared with the providers, and losses are absorbed by the IPA.

Neighborhood Health Centers

Neighborhood health centers are usually found in areas where citizens are underserved, financially stressed, and at risk; a variety of health care workers provide basic health care and social services support. A recent addition to this category is the health care center run primarily by volunteers to provide health services to the "working poor" (those who have jobs but cannot afford health care insurance).

Physicians' Offices

In general, people seek the services of the physician when they are ill; nurses working in these settings register clients, give medications, take vital signs, assist with examinations, and provide information and education.

Support Groups

Support groups assist individuals with ongoing coping and lifestyle changes. Reach for Recovery assists women who have had mastectomies, Alcoholics Anonymous helps alcoholics stop drinking through a 12-step program; the Dream Machine helps children who are terminally ill have one of their wishes come true; some of these are well funded by agencies, and others are purely voluntary.

Which of the health care services mentioned in the article do you think is most important? Why?

Sample Answer

NOTE: In the following paragraph the first sentence introduces the topic of the paragraph; the next three sentences provide the supporting details; and the final sentence supplies the conclusions.

An increase in home health care services is the most important trend in health care today. Many people cannot afford the staggering cost of hospitalization. Insurance companies and government funding for hospital care are being cut back. Some individuals respond better to home treatment because they are uncomfortable in the institutional setting of the hospital. If home care services were increased, health care costs would be reduced and patients would have the added comfort of their familiar home environment.

EXERCISE 15–7

Directions. Read the following excerpt from a nursing textbook (Iyer et al., 3rd ed., p. 323). Answer the following essay question based on the selection.

The estate of a New Jersey physician with AIDS won a six million dollar verdict against a hospital because the lab results of HIV positive were widely discussed within the hospital and community, resulting in the destruction of the physician's practice. The physician's family sued the hospital for breach of confidentiality. The verdict was upheld when the hospital appealed the case.

Question: Do you think the verdict should have been upheld? Why or why not?

EXERCISE 15–8

Directions. Read the following excerpt from a nursing text (Iyer et al., 3rd ed., p. 322). Create your own essay question based on the selection. Answer your question.

Right to Expect that All Communications and Records Pertaining to Care Will Be Kept Confidential. The ethical aspects of this issue will be discussed later in this chapter. Nurses are prohibited from sharing information about a client with anyone other than health care professionals directly responsible for the client's care. There are additional stringent rules that protect the privacy of clients who receive treatment for mental health disorders and drug and alcohol addictions. In these cases laws protect their confidentiality to prevent others from knowing that treatment is being received for these problems.

The principle of confidentiality applies to family members who are seeking detailed information. It is best to ask the client's permission before giving information to friends and family. Be sure to determine the procedure to follow if a family member wants to see the client's record. Most facilities require the client to give written permission and expect the nurse to notify the physician of the request.

Do not discuss the client's condition in public areas. The elevator is one such place in which a casual comment could be overheard by a family member or friend. You should be aware that certain information is so sensitive that it should not be discussed at all.

Comprehending? Yes ___ No ___

• MONITORING TIME

Students worry that they will not finish their exam, whether objective or essay, in the allotted time. For both objective and essay tests, the following strategies will help you to finish the test:

- Be aware of time. Do not spend too much time on any one question.
- Answer the questions you are sure of first. You can return to the more difficult questions.
- On essay tests, if you run out of time, construct an outline of the remaining main points and major details you would have included in your answer. You may then get partial credit.

• EVALUATING TEST RESULTS

Once your paper is returned, use your test results to evaluate what you have already learned in the subject and what you still need to study. Save all your test papers. Use your textbooks and notes to correct any errors. You can use all these corrected tests to review for your final exam. If you still need help in understanding the subject, schedule a conference with your instructor, your study partner, or your study group. Completed tests can be an effective study tool for future exams.

• VOCABULARY CHECK

Directions. Below are 10 words taken from the key words section of this chapter. Circle the letter of the best definition from the four choices.

1. Hallucinations
 a mind-reading or other extrasensory perception
 b psychosis, especially that which occurs after adolescence
 c accurate sensory impressions based on external stimuli
 d sensory impressions that have no basis in external stimuli

2. Construct
 a consider
 b confuse
 c destroy
 d compose

3. Scoliosis
 a lateral deviation of the spine
 b a normally straight spine
 c a ruptured disc
 d a fracture of the spine

4. Deficit
 a lacking interest
 b unplanned
 c leaning toward an idea
 d impairment in functional capacity

5. Resuscitate
 a to restore health
 b to rehabilitate
 c to restore to life
 d to regain strength

6. Revisions
 a choices
 b alterations
 c behaviors
 d alternatives

7. Sensory
 a pertaining to sight
 b pertaining to sensations
 c extremely sensitive
 d referring to clotting

8. Myths
 a mystery stories
 b false notions
 c nightmares
 d intentional lies

9. Malnutrition
   a loss in weight
   b poor nourishment
   c using food properly
   d diet control

10. Exotic
   a strikingly different
   b extremely beautiful
   c highly dangerous
   d very mysterious

• CRITICAL THINKING LOG

List the strategies you learned in this chapter.	Select the strategy that is most useful for your school success.	How can you apply this strategy to your nursing studies?

• SUMMARY

Test-taking strategies will help you improve your grades on both objective and essay tests in nursing school. Find out whether the test will be objective or essay. Take practice tests from end-of-chapter questions or create your own questions. Carefully read all directions on the exam before starting. Check over your paper to make necessary revisions. A positive attitude, careful preparation, and practice will ensure your success.

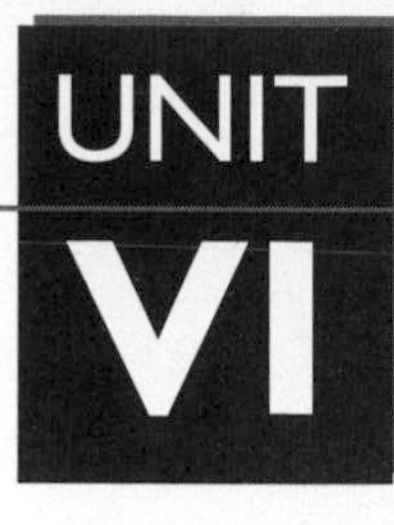

UNIT VI READING SELECTIONS

In Unit VI, "Reading Selections," you will have the opportunity to apply the strategies for reading nursing textbooks that you have learned in Units I through V.

Each of the 15 reading selections is an excerpt taken from an actual chapter in a nursing text. The reading selections are designed to give you practice in prereading strategies, improving your comprehension through active reading, and monitoring comprehension through summarizing and answering multiple-choice questions.

These reading selections can be used on a weekly basis or at the end of the semester as a culmination of your studies.

With the successful completion of Unit VI, "Reading Selections," you should be able to read your nursing textbook assignments confidently, with improved concentration, comprehension, and retention. Reading your nursing texts with competency will ensure your success in nursing school.

Reading Selection I

• PREVIEW QUESTION

Considering your own experiences, what do you know about people's reactions to their own dying?

• VOCABULARY

Underline any medical terminology or general vocabulary words you may need to learn in order to understand the ideas in the reading selection.

Theories of Loss, Dying, and Grieving

The theories that are used in discussing loss, dying, and grieving have been derived through research. These theories are not meant to be prescriptive; rather, they serve as general guides to alert the nurse to what may occur and, therefore, what to look for and how to proceed when a response is indicated. Using these findings to help guide client care is similar to using the systematic protocols of signs and symptoms of disease that help guide all nursing observations. For example, not all people with cholecystitis show all of its possible clinical manifestations, nor does the disease follow the same clinical course in all people. Knowing what can occur helps the nurse make observations and devise early interventions to prevent complications.

RESPONSES TO DYING

In 1969, Elisabeth Kübler-Ross, a psychiatrist, described a series of stages through which people may pass in response to their living through the dying process. She described the first stage as *shock and disbelief.* People could not believe that they were dying. The second stage was described as *denial.* People might say, "Yes, most people with this disease are dying, but not me!" The third stage was called *anger,* often characterized by the question "Why me?" or "What did I do to deserve this?" The fourth stage was termed *bargaining.* In this stage, characteristic responses were, "I'll do anything if . . ." or "Just let me live until my son gets married . . . or my daughter graduates." The next stage, when the person's deteriorating physical condition led to the realization that death was inevitable, was identified as *depression.* The final stage was termed *acceptance.* Acceptance, according to Kübler-Ross, was a stage of self-actualization, of feeling at peace with oneself and with one's imminent death.

From Ignatavicius, Workman, and Mishler, pp. 197–198.

PATTERNS OF LIVING-DYING

When death from a known fatal illness is preceded by several years of life, the use of the term "dying" from the time of diagnosis until the moment of death is paradoxical. These people frequently not only look healthy but also enjoy full activity for prolonged periods. They are living, yet dying, and in these cases, the living-dying period has the characteristics of a chronic illness.

Martocchio (1982), a nurse researcher, described four patterns of living-dying that are useful for understanding the uncertainties of living with life-threatening illness:

- **Peaks and valleys,** in which the person experiences hopeful highs and terrible lows
- **Descending plateaus,** in which the person experiences successive cycles of rehabilitation, loss, and rehabilitation
- **Downward slope,** in which there is a lack of time to prepare for death
- **Gradual slant,** in which the person is barely living and presents placement problems

These patterns, which all have a general downward course concluding in death, reflect the natural history of various diseases, such as some cancers and many cardiovascular, renal, and hepatic conditions. They also describe the effects of specific therapeutic regimens. The categories remain consistent regardless of the type of disease or treatment.

Peaks and Valleys. This pattern is characterized by a series of peaks and valleys, or remissions and exacerbations. The peaks represent periods of well-being, and the valleys represent times of loss of well-being. Clients describe "hopeful highs" and "terrible lows." They see previous highs as indicators of hope that they can rally one more time. They see the lows as threats to any expectation of recovery.

Descending Plateaus. The descending plateaus pattern is a series of steps. Each downward step represents a tangible reduction in functional ability, and each plateau represents a leveling-off or stable period. The plateaus and drop-offs can last for an indeterminate period and may occur any number of times. This pattern creates marked frustration as dying clients and their families try, again and again, to take part in rehabilitation programs to maintain a level of function in the client that is relentlessly but unpredictably declining.

Downward Slope. The third pattern of living-dying is the downward slope. This pattern, frequently observed in critical care units, is represented by a continuous and usually rapid downward course. In these cases, in which there are relatively short-term illnesses or unexpected deaths, clients and family members have little time to prepare for death.

Gradual Slant. The gradual slant pattern is characterized by a gradual decline over time. Toward the end, it is difficult to know whether the ill person is alive or dead. Difficulties regarding quality of life and definitions of death become issues of concern. Family members and caregivers begin to see the unresponsive client as a biologically living creature but also as a nonexistent person. As there is less meaningful interaction, the client is considered to be socially dead.

Regardless of the pattern, the direction is downward. As the dying person declines and draws nearer to death, all the people involved undergo losses. For each person, the loss is different: The mother loses her son; the wife, her husband; the children, their father; the business partner, his colleague. Each person manifests the loss both in a universally recognized pattern and in his or her unique way.

• SUMMARY

Directions. In the space provided, rewrite the above selection in your own words, focusing on the main idea and major details.

• COMPREHENSION QUESTIONS

Directions. Below are 10 multiple-choice questions. Circle the letter of the best answer from the four choices.

1 In 1969, Kübler-Ross described:

a what it is like to die

b nurse's responses to dying

c stages of the dying process

d ways to aid a dying patient

2 Stage one of Kübler-Ross' theory is characterized by:
- **a** disbelief
- **b** anger
- **c** withdrawal
- **d** defiance

3 According to Kübler-Ross, another response to dying is:
- **a** confrontation
- **b** excessive talking on the subject
- **c** seeking vengeance
- **d** denial

4 As the patient moves closer to death, Kübler-Ross says the patient asks:
- **a** Can you help me?
- **b** Why me?
- **c** Would you help me die quicker?
- **d** How can I stop dying?

5 The final stage of Kübler-Ross' theory is:
- **a** bargaining
- **b** concern for relatives
- **c** continuous denial
- **d** acceptance

6 Martocchio's patterns talk about:
- **a** the uncertainties of living with life-threatening illnesses
- **b** how nurses should treat dying patients
- **c** how patients have near-death experiences
- **d** the survivors' grieving patterns

7 Which is not a heading in this section?
- **a** peaks and valleys
- **b** gradual slant
- **c** ascending plateaus
- **d** downward slope

8 In Martocchio's research the peaks and valleys pattern is characterized by:
- **a** highs and lows
- **b** acceptance and denial
- **c** rehabilitation and deterioration
- **d** gains and losses

9 The four patterns of living-dying describe:
- **a** when death is preceded by many years of life
- **b** the ways of dying from a long illness
- **c** the uncertainties of living with a chronic illness
- **d** all of the above

10 The four patterns of living-dying:
- **a** sometimes lead to death
- **b** always lead to death
- **c** can be reversed
- **d** allow family members to have a lot of time to prepare for the death

Comprehending? Yes ___ No ___

• CRITICAL THINKING/EVALUATION

Were you successful in applying active reading strategies to this selection? Explain.

____

____

____

____

Reading Selection 2

• PREVIEW QUESTION

What questions can you create from the boldface headings?

• VOCABULARY

Underline any medical terminology or general vocabulary words you may need to learn in order to understand the ideas in the reading selection.

Impaired Skin Integrity and Impaired Tissue Integrity

Planning: Client Goals. The primary goal is that the client will experience minimal skin and tissue impairment and contamination as a result of surgery.

Interventions. Surgery is an invasive procedure that places the client at risk for complications related to:

- The surgical wound, such as incisional tears and lacerations
- Bacterial contamination
- Loss of body fluids from the wound during and after surgery

Sterile surgical technique and the use of protective drapes, skin closures, and dressings help to minimize complications and promote wound healing.

Plastic Adhesive Drapes. If a sterile plastic adhesive drape is used, the scrub nurse helps the surgical assistant apply the drape after the surgical site has been cleaned and dried. The plastic drape is applied directly to the client's skin to prevent shifting and exposure of skin edges. The surgeon makes the incision through the plastic drape. The cut edge remains adherent to the skin and keeps the surgical incision sealed from the migration of bacteria into the wound. The scrub nurse and surgical assistant *gently* remove the drape after closure of the surgical incision. The nurse pays special attention to the elderly and to clients with fragile skin to prevent skin tearing when the adhesive drape is removed.

Skin Closures. Skin and tissue closures, such as sutures and staples, are used for several reasons:

- To approximate wound edges until wound healing is complete
- To occlude the lumen of blood vessels, preventing hemorrhage and loss of body fluids
- To prevent wound contamination

The quality of the approximated tissue and the type of closure material are two factors that determine the strength and integrity of the closure. The wound is usually closed in layers to maintain tissue integrity and promote healing with minimal scarring. The surgeon selects the method and type of closures to be used on the basis of the surgical site, the tissue involved, the size and depth of the surgical wound, and the age and medical history of the client. A combination of sutures and clips is commonly used for closure of internal layers of the wound. Staples, stay and retention sutures, and skin closure tapes (Steri-Strips) are used for closure of superficial wounds of the epidermis. Figure 20–13 illustrates commonly used wound closures.

A suture consists of one or more strands of material and is designated by its size or gauge. The size designation sequence, from largest diameter to smallest is 5, 4, 3, 2, 1, 0, 2-0, 3-0, 4-0, and so forth, to 11-0. Size 5 may be used to close the deep layers of an abdominal wound; 11-0 is the smallest-diameter suture and is used in plastic surgery and ophthalmology. Other characteristics of the suture material, such as type (nylon, silk, Vicryl), color (e.g., green, blue, black, white, violet), and structure (twisted, braided) are often listed on the package (Fig. VI–1).

Suture material can be absorbable or nonabsorbable. *Absorbable* sutures are digested over time by body enzymes. These sutures first lose strength and then gradually disappear from the tissue. Catgut suture, such as "plain gut" and "chromic gut," was a common type of absorbable suture material that is still in use today, although not as frequently as it once was. Other absorbable sutures are made of synthetics and are labeled as such on the package. The client's physical status, the presence of inflammation, and the type of suture used all influence the rate of absorption, usually up to about 2 weeks.

Nonabsorbable sutures are not affected by body enzymes. Nonabsorbable sutures become encapsulated in the tissue

---

From Ignatavicius, Workman, and Mishler, pp. 402–404.

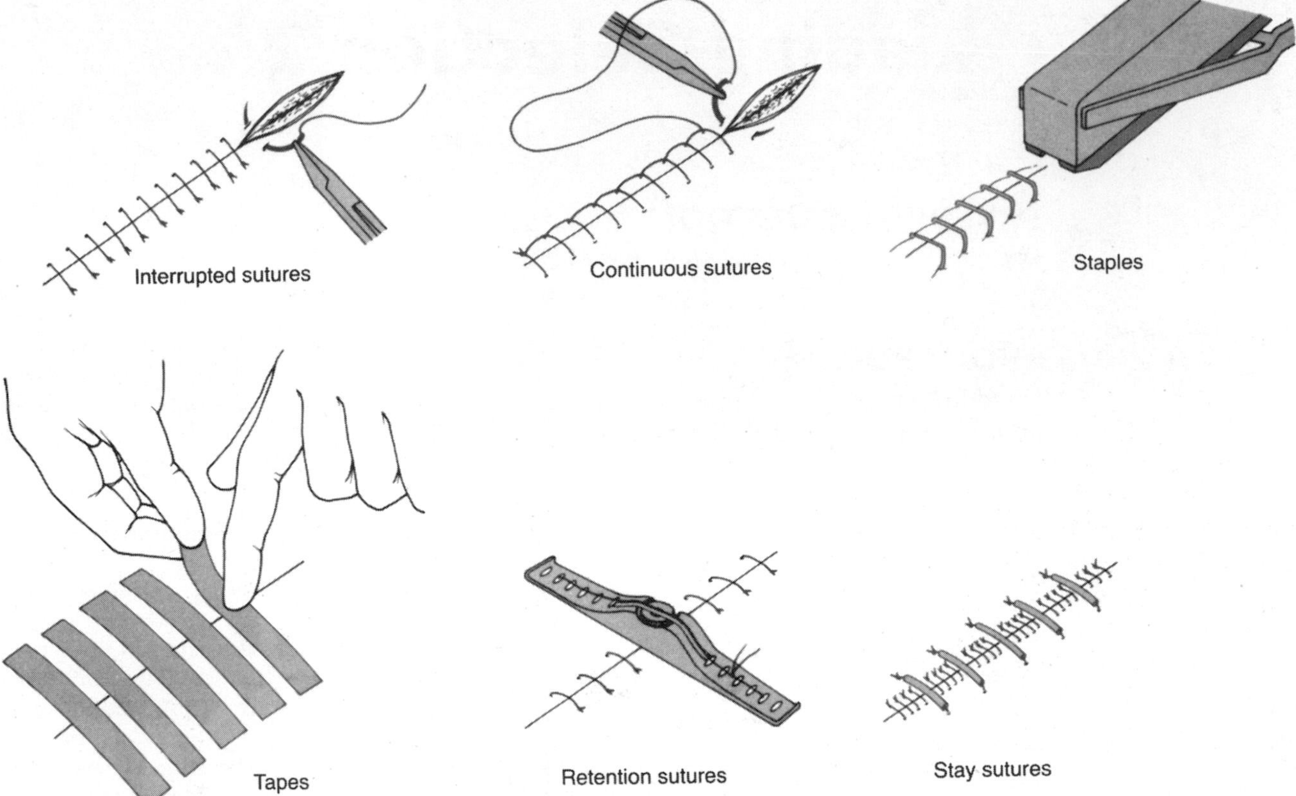

Figure VI–1 Common skin closures. (Reprinted with permission from Ignatavicius, D.D., Workman, L., and Mishler, M.A.: Medical-Surgical Nursing: A Nursing Process Approach, 2nd ed. Philadelphia, W.B. Saunders, 1995.)

during the healing process and remain embedded in the tissue unless they are removed. These sutures are made of silk, cotton, steel, nylon, polyester, or other synthetic material. Nonabsorbable sutures are used for vascular anastomosis, "wiring" the sternum together after open heart surgery, and closing external wounds. The surgeon may use a double or interlocking stitch to increase the integrity of the closure. Retention and stay sutures (see Fig. 20–13) may be used in addition to standard suture material for high-risk clients (those having major abdominal surgery, obese clients, diabetic clients, and clients taking steroids, which inhibit wound healing).

After the incision is closed, the physician may inject a local anesthetic or instill an antibiotic into the wound. A gauze or spray dressing may be applied to protect it from contamination. A variety of dressings may also be used to absorb drainage and provide support to the incision. A pressure dressing may be applied to prevent or stop a vascular area from bleeding postoperatively. One or more drains may be inserted to prevent the accumulation of secretions within tissues around the surgical area. These secretions, if not drained, impede healing and serve as a medium for bacterial growth, which could result in wound infection.

After the dressing is secure, the nurse coordinates the surgical team in repositioning and transferring the client as indicated. A roller board or a lift sheet is used to transfer the client safely from the operating bed to a stretcher or bed. The circulating nurse and anesthesiologist or CRNA accompany the client to the postanesthesia care unit (PACU) and give a report of the client's intraoperative experience to the PACU nurse. Important information to be relayed includes the following:

- The client's level of anxiety before anesthesia
- The type and length of the surgical procedure
- The location of incisions and drains
- Blood loss
- Intravenous fluids infused
- Medications given
- The client's previous reactions to anesthesia
- Respiratory dysfunctions
- Joint or limb immobility
- The client's primary language
- Any special requests the client may have verbalized

Evaluation

On the basis of identified nursing diagnoses, the nurse evaluates the care of the intraoperative client and ensures that the client:

- Is safely anesthetized without complications
- Does not experience any injury related to intraoperative positioning or equipment
- Is free of skin or tissue contamination during surgery
- Is free of skin tears, bruises, redness, abrasion, or maceration over pressure points and elsewhere

• SUMMARY

Directions. In the space provided, rewrite the above selection in your own words, focusing on the main idea and major details.

• COMPREHENSION QUESTIONS

Directions. Below are 10 multiple-choice questions. Circle the letter of the best answer from the four choices.

1 During surgery, which of the following helps minimize complications?
a plastic adhesive drapes
b skin closures
c sterile surgical techniques
d all of the above

2 The nurse helps to apply the adhesive drape:
a after surgical site has been cleaned and dried
b before the surgical site has a chance to dry
c immediately before cleaning surgical site
d none of the above

3 The purpose of skin closures is to:
a allow the surgeon to inspect the surgery site
b approximate wound edges until the wound is healed
c keep the surgery site flexible
d allow for gradual loss of body fluids

4 The strength of the closure is determined by:
a the size of the surgery site
b the age and skin condition of the patient
c the age and weight of the patient
d the quality of the approximated tissue

5 The two classifications of suture material are:
a reusable and nonreusable
b flexible and nonflexible
c absorbable and nonabsorbable
d strong and delicate

6 To promote proper healing, the wound is:
a inspected hourly
b usually closed in layers
c always closed with clamps
d never closed with clamps

7 Some types of sutures:
a are digested by body enzymes
b become encapsulated in the tissue
c a but not b
d both a and b

8 After the incision is closed the physician may:
a inject local anesthetic
b apply gauze
c use a drain
d all of the above

9 Right after the dressing is in place, the nurse's responsibility is to:
a coordinate the surgical team in repositioning and transferring the patient
b examine the surgical site frequently
c remain with the patient in the operating room before transfer
d reposition and transfer client himself or herself

10 The primary nursing ensures that the client is:
a not experiencing injury
b free of skin contamination
c neither a nor b
d both a and b

Comprehending? Yes ___ No ___

• CRITICAL THINKING/EVALUATION

Were you successful in applying active reading strategies to this selection? Explain.

____

____

____

____

Reading Selection 3

• PREVIEW QUESTION

Name the three stages of inflammatory responses.

• VOCABULARY

Underline any medical terminology or general vocabulary words you may need to learn in order to understand the ideas in this reading selection.

Sequence of Inflammatory Responses

Inflammatory responses for protecting the body against the effects of tissue injury or invasion by foreign proteins occur in a predictable sequence. The sequence is the same regardless of the initiating stimulus. Responses at the tissue level elicit the five cardinal physical manifestations of inflammation: warmth, redness, swelling, pain, and decreased function. Tissue and cellular events that cause these physical manifestations are described as part of the different stages of inflammation (Table VI–1). The inflammatory response can occur in three distinct functional stages, although the timing of the stages may overlap.

STAGE I (VASCULAR)

In stage I of the inflammatory response, most of the early effects involve changes at the blood vessel level. When inflammation is an effect of tissue injury, this stage has two phases.

Phase I

The first phase is an immediate but short-term vasoconstriction of arterioles and venules as a direct result of physical trauma to vascular smooth muscle. This phase lasts only seconds to minutes and may be so short that the person undergoing the response is unaware of the vasoconstriction.

Phase II

The second phase is characterized by increased blood flow to the area (hyperemia) and swelling (edema formation) at the site of injury or invasion. Injured tissues and the leukocytes in this area secrete vasoactive amines (histamine, serotonin, and kinins) that cause constriction of the small veins and dilation of the arterioles in the immediate area. The effects of these changes in blood vessel dilation cause the symptoms of redness and increased warmth of the tissues. This response increases the supply of nutrients at the tissue level by increasing the blood flow.

Some of these vasoactive amines increase capillary permeability, allowing blood plasma to leak into the interstitial space. This response causes the symptoms of swelling and pain. Pain, although an uncomfortable sensation, is somewhat beneficial to the person experiencing inflammation. Pain increases the person's awareness that a problem exists and encourages action to avoid further injury or inflammation. Edema formation at the site of injury or invasion is an overall helpful event. This swelling protects the area from further injury by creating a cushion of fluid. The extra fluid can also dilute the concentration of any toxins or microorganisms that entered the area. The duration of these responses depends on the severity of the initiating event.

The major leukocyte involved in stage I of inflammation is the tissue macrophage. The response of tissue macrophages is immediate because they are already in place at the site of injury or invasion. However, this response is limited because the number of such macrophages is so small. In addition to functioning in phagocytosis, the tissue macrophages secrete several cytokines to enhance the inflammatory response. One cytokine is colony-stimulating factor, which stimulates the bone marrow to reduce the time of leukocyte production from 14 days to a matter of hours. In addition, tissue macrophages secrete substances that increase the release of neutrophils from the bone marrow and attract them to the site of injury or invasion, which leads to the next stage of inflammation.

STAGE II (CELLULAR EXUDATE)

Stage II of inflammation is characterized by neutrophilia (an increase in the percentage and number of circulating neutrophils), secretion of many factors into the interstitial fluid, and formation of exudate.

The most active leukocyte in this stage is the neutrophil. Under the influence of chemotactic agents and substances

From Ignatavicius, Workman, and Mishler, pp. 442–444.

TABLE VI–1 Stages of Inflammation*

Stage	Onset	Cells Involved	Actions
Stage I: Vascular stage	• Minutes after injury or invasion	• Tissue macrophages	• Limited phagocytosis of invading micro-organisms or cell debris from injured tissues • Secretion of vasoactive amines (histamine, bradykinin, serotonin) to dilate blood vessels and increase capillary leak; this action results in redness, warmth, swelling, and pain at the site but also increases blood flow to the area; more nutrients are available to the tissues; plasma proteins moved into the tissues clot and "wall off" micro-organisms, limiting their spread • Secretion of chemotaxins to draw more leukocytes into the area to sustain the inflammatory response • Secretion of cytokines to increase bone marrow production of granulocytes
Stage II: Cellular exudate stage	• Hours after injury or invasion	• Granular myeloid cells • Neutrophils • Basophils • Eosinophils	• Increased phagocytosis • Secretion of slow-acting vasoactive amines to ensure a sustained inflammatory response • Secretion of substances to increase the rate of neutrophil maturation and macrophage maturation
Stage III: Tissue repair and replacement stage	• Begins at initial injury and continues until new tissues are formed and mature or are functional	• Neutrophils • Macrophages	• Stimulation of mitotically active cells to divide; stimulation of fibroblasts in blood vessels to grow and release collagen to form scaffold on which to build scar tissue

*Reprinted with permission from Ignatavicius, D.D., Workman, L., and Mishler, M.A.: Medical-Surgical Nursing: A Nursing Process Approach, 2nd ed. Philadelphia, WB Saunders, 1995.

that increase the number and rate of maturation of neutrophils, the neutrophil count can increase up to five times within 12 hours after the onset of inflammation. At the site of inflammation, the neutrophils attack and destroy foreign materials and remove dead tissue. Both of these functions are accomplished through phagocytosis.

During acute inflammatory responses, the healthy person can synthesize enough mature neutrophils to keep pace with the effects of injury and invasion and to eventually overcome the ability of invaders to multiply. At the same time, the leukocytes secrete *cytokines,* which increase reproduction of tissue macrophages and bone marrow production of monocytes. Although this reaction is slower to start, its effects are long lasting.

When infectious processes stimulating inflammation are longer or chronic, the bone marrow cannot synthesize and release enough mature neutrophils into the blood to keep pace with the ability of micro-organisms to multiply. In this situation, the bone marrow begins to release immature neutrophils, many of which cannot complete maturation and phagocytose. Such a reduction in the number of functional phagocytic neutrophils limits the effectiveness of the inflammatory response and increases the susceptibility of the person to microbial infections.

STAGE III (TISSUE REPAIR AND REPLACEMENT)

Although stage III is completed last, it begins at the time of injury and is critical to the ultimate function of the inflamed area.

Some of the leukocytes involved in inflammation are capable of stimulating replacement and repair of lost or damaged tissues by inducing the remaining healthy tissue to divide. In tissues that are not mitotically active (nondividing tissues), leukocytes stimulate revascularization and the laying down of different types of collagen to form scar tissue. Because scar tissue does not behave like normal differentiated tissue, functional loss occurs where damaged tissues are replaced with scar tissue. The extent of the functional loss is determined by the percentage of tissue that is replaced by scar tissue.

Inflammation alone cannot confer immunity; however, the interaction of specific components of inflammation with other leukocytes and tissues assists in providing long-lasting immunity against re-exposure to the same micro-organisms. Long-lasting immune actions are those generated by antibody-mediated immunity and cell-mediated immunity.

• SUMMARY

Directions. In the space provided, rewrite the preceding selection in your own words, focusing on the main ideas and major details.

• COMPREHENSION QUESTIONS

Directions. Below are 10 multiple-choice questions. Circle the letter of the best answer from the four choices.

1 In the inflammatory response:
- **a** the sequence is the same regardless of the initiating stimulus
- **b** the sequence is determined by the initiating stimulus
- **c** there is no set sequence
- **d** there is sometimes a set sequence and sometimes not

2 The vascular stage is characterized by:
- **a** one phase
- **b** two phases
- **c** three phases
- **d** four phases

3 The purpose of changes in blood vessel dilation in phase II is to:
- **a** stop bleeding
- **b** fight invading foreign protein
- **c** make the individual aware of injury
- **d** increase the supply of nutrients

4 Edema in Phase II is helpful because:
- **a** it prevents further injury
- **b** it dilutes concentration of toxins
- **c** neither a nor b
- **d** both a and b

5 Pain, as part of the inflammatory response:
- **a** increases the individual's awareness of injury
- **b** exacerbates the healing process
- **c** is not yet understood
- **d** none of the above

6 The function of neutrophils is to:
- **a** evoke the pain response
- **b** cause the dilation of the vascular system
- **c** promote formation of scar tissue
- **d** none of the above

7 One problem with chronic infections is that:
- **a** tissue microphages are produced
- **b** too many neutrophils are released
- **c** the bone marrow releases immature neutrophils
- **d** the bone marrow production of monocytes is increased

8 Stage III:
- **a** begins at the time of injury
- **b** begins after stage I
- **c** begins after stage II
- **d** is not always a part of the inflammatory response

9 Scar tissue is formed:
- **a** in mitotically active tissue
- **b** in nondividing tissue
- **c** only in dividing tissues
- **d** before the inflammatory response

10 The table accompanying this selection describes
- **a** the stages of inflammation
- **b** the structure of the immune system
- **c** methods of tissue destruction
- **d** the function of lymphocytes

• CRITICAL THINKING/EVALUATION

Were you successful in applying active reading strategies to this selection? Explain.

___

___

___

___

Reading Selection 4

• PREVIEW QUESTION

An assessment of the skeletal system consists of assessing which parts of the body?

• VOCABULARY

Underline any medical terminology or general vocabulary words you may need to learn in order to understand the ideas in this reading selection.

Physical Assessment

Although bones, joints, and muscles are usually assessed simultaneously in a head-to-toe approach, each subsystem is described separately for emphasis and understanding. For physical assessment of the musculoskeletal system, the nurse incorporates inspection, palpation, active range of motion, and special techniques for specific problems. A general assessment is described in this chapter. More specific assessment techniques are discussed in the interventions chapters that follow for each musculoskeletal problem.

GENERAL INSPECTION

The nurse observes the client's posture, gait, and mobility for gross deformities and impairment.

Posture

Posture includes the person's body build and alignment when standing and walking. The nurse observes the curvature of the spine and the length, shape, and symmetry of extremities. Figure VI–2 illustrates some common musculoskeletal deformities. Muscle mass is also inspected for size and symmetry.

Gait

Most clients with musculoskeletal problems eventually have a problem with gait. The two phases of normal, automatic gait (Fig. VI–3) are:

- The stance phase
- The swing phase

The nurse evaluates the client's balance, steadiness, and ease and length of stride; a limp or other asymmetric leg movement or deformity is noted. An abnormality in the stance phase of gait is called an antalgic gait. When part of one leg is painful, the person shortens the stance phase on the affected side. An abnormality in the swing phase is called a lurch. This abnormal gait occurs when the muscles in the buttocks and/or leg are too weak to allow the person to change weight from one foot to another. In this case, the shoulders are moved either side-to-side or front-to-back for help in shifting the weight from one leg to another. Some clients, such as those with chronic hip pain and muscle atrophy from degenerative joint disease, have a combination of the antalgic gait and lurch.

Mobility

The nurse observes the client's need for or use of ambulatory devices, such as canes and walkers, during transfer from bed to chair and while walking and climbing stairs. The nurse also assesses mobility by asking the client to perform simple activities of daily living (ADL), such as putting on shoes. Pain and deformity may limit physical mobility and function.

After performing a functional assessment, the nurse assesses major bones, joints, and muscles by inspection, palpation, and determination of range of motion (ROM). A goniometer (used by physical therapists and clinical specialists) provides an exact measurement of ROM, but the nurse can estimate the degree of joint mobility by having the client put each joint through its ROM. As long as the client can function to meet personal needs, a limitation in ROM may not be significant. For each anatomic location, the nurse observes the skin for color, elasticity, and lesions that may relate to musculoskeletal dysfunction.

ASSESSMENT OF THE HEAD AND NECK

The nurse inspects and palpates the skull for shape, symmetry, tenderness, and masses. The temporomandibular joints (TMJs) are best evaluated by palpation. The client is asked to open his or her mouth while the nurse palpates the TMJs. Common abnormal findings are:

- Tenderness or pain
- Crepitus (a grating sound)

From Ignatavicius, Workman, and Mishler, pp. 1399–1401.

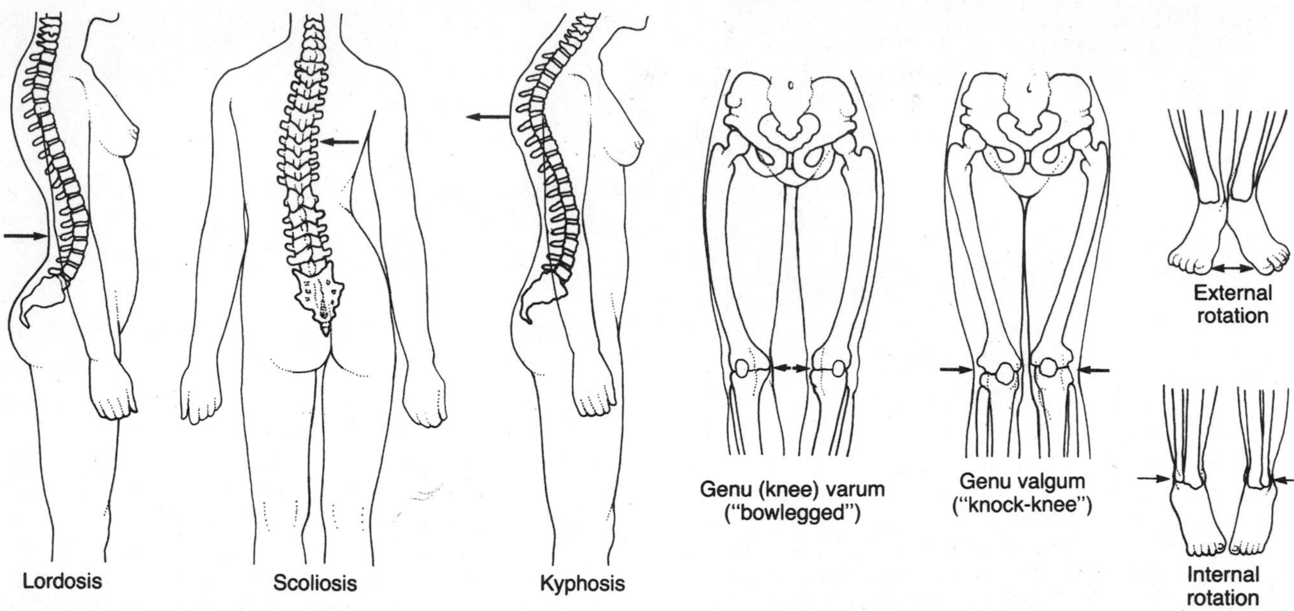

Figure VI–2 Common musculoskeletal deformities. (Reprinted with permission from Ignatavicius, D.D., Workman, L., and Mishler, M.A.: Medical-Surgical Nursing: A Nursing Process Approach, 2nd ed. Philadelphia, W.B. Saunders, 1995.)

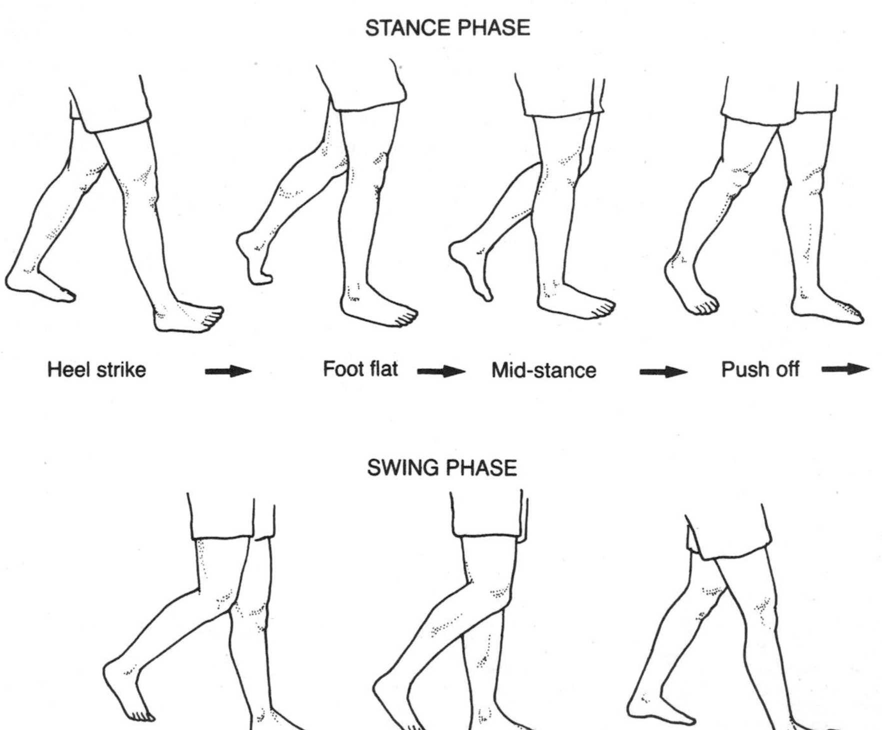

Figure VI–3 The phases of gait. (Reprinted with permission from Ignatavicius, D.D., Workman, L., and Mishler, M.A.: Medical-Surgical Nursing: A Nursing Process Approach, 2nd ed. Philadelphia, W.B. Saunders, 1995.)

- A spongy swelling caused by excess synovium and fluid, which can be palpated

The nurse then inspects and palpates each vertebra of the spine in the neck. Clinical findings may include:

- Malalignment
- Tenderness
- Inability to flex, extend, and rotate the neck as expected

ASSESSMENT OF THE VERTEBRAL SPINE

The thoracic spine, lumbar spine, and sacral spine are evaluated in the same manner as the neck. Spinal alignment problems are common (see Fig. VI–2). In addition, the nurse places both hands over the lumbosacral area and applies pressure with the thumbs to elicit tenderness. Many clients do not complain of discomfort until the area is palpated.

ASSESSMENT OF THE UPPER EXTREMITIES

The nurse assesses both extremities concurrently. For example, both shoulders are inspected and palpated for size, swelling, deformity, malalignment, tenderness or pain, and mobility. A shoulder injury may prevent the client from combing his or her hair with the affected arm, but severe arthritis may inhibit movement in both arms. The elbows and wrists are assessed in a similar way.

Because the hand has multiple joints in a single digit, assessment of hand function is perhaps the most critical part of the examination. The nurse inspects and palpates the metacarpophalangeal (MCP), proximal interphalangeal (PIP), and distal interphalangeal (DIP) joints. The same digits are compared on the right and left hands. The nurse also determines ROM for each joint by observing active movement, if it is possible. For a quick and easy assessment of ROM, the nurse asks the client to make a fist and then oppose each finger to the thumb. If the client can perform these maneuvers, ROM of the hand is not seriously restricted.

ASSESSMENT OF THE LOWER EXTREMITIES

Evaluation of the hip joint relies primarily on determination of its degree of mobility because the joint is deep and difficult to inspect or palpate. The client with hip pain experiences pain in the *groin* area. The pain may radiate to the knee. The knee is readily accessible for nursing assessment, particularly when the client is sitting and the knee is flexed. Fluid accumulation, or effusion, is easily detected in the knee joint; limitations in movement with accompanying pain are common findings. The ankles and feet are often neglected in the physical examination, yet they contain multiple bones and joints that can be affected by disease and injury. The nurse observes and palpates each joint and tests for range of motion.

• SUMMARY

Directions. In the space provided, rewrite the preceding selection in your own words, focusing on the main ideas and major details.

• COMPREHENSION QUESTIONS

Directions. Below are 10 multiple-choice questions. Circle the letter of the best answer from the four choices.

1 Figure VI–2 shows:
- **a** common difficulties of the vertebral spine
- **b** common musculoskeletal deformities
- **c** lower and upper extremities deformations
- **d** assessment of the head and neck

2 Figure VI–3 shows:
- **a** directions for assessing mobility
- **b** directions for assessing upper extremities
- **c** the vertical spine
- **d** the two phases of gait

3 Posture refers to:
- **a** curvature of the spine
- **b** an individual's body build and alignment
- **c** only how you stand
- **d** only how you walk

4 Muscle mass is inspected for:
- **a** strength and size
- **b** size and symmetry
- **c** strength and symmetry
- **d** strength and flexibility

5 Gait is evaluated for all but:
- **a** endurance
- **b** balance
- **c** ease and length of stride
- **d** steadiness

6 The function of the goniometer is to provide measurement of:
- **a** bone strength
- **b** bone length
- **c** joint range of motion
- **d** spinal alignment

7 The nurse inspects the skull for:
- **a** smoothness, rotation, and misalignment
- **b** deformity, swelling, size, mobility
- **c** rotation, shape, mass, mobility
- **d** shape, symmetry, tenderness, masses

8 The nurse needs to apply pressure to the lumbosacral area because:
- **a** the nurse needs to assess for swelling
- **b** the patient does not complain of discomfort until pressure is applied
- **c** the nurse needs to assess for flexibility
- **d** the patient has complained of tenderness

9 In an assessment of the upper extremities, the most critical part is the assessment of:
- **a** hand function
- **b** shoulder flexibility
- **c** elbow function
- **d** wrist function

10 Evaluation of the hip joint relies on determining hip:
- **a** strength
- **b** density
- **c** injury
- **d** mobility

Comprehending? Yes ___ No ___

• CRITICAL THINKING/EVALUATION

Were you successful in applying active reading strategies to this selection? Explain.

____

____

____

____

Reading Selection 5

• PREVIEW QUESTION

Review the headings and subheadings, then answer the following question. The cranial nerves are located in what part of the body?

• VOCABULARY

Underline any medical terminology or general vocabulary words that you may need to learn in order to understand the ideas in this reading selection.

Assessment of Cranial Nerves

CRANIAL NERVE I: OLFACTORY

With the client's eyes closed, the nurse tests one of the client's nostrils at a time; the client occludes the other with a finger. The nurse asks the client to identify familiar odors, such as coffee, tobacco, mint, or soap. Alcohol sponges and ammonia are not used because they stimulate the trigeminal nerve rather than the olfactory nerve. Lack of or decreased smell sensation may not be significant. Loss or decrease occurs with age, smoking, colds, and allergies. It is more significant if the client reports that smell was suddenly lost without a predisposing factor or that odors are distorted.

CRANIAL NERVE II: OPTIC

Each eye is tested alone with the other eye covered but open. The nurse tests *central vision,* or visual acuity, using the Snellen chart. The client reads out loud from a pocket reader card, a magazine, or a newspaper. Clients should wear their glasses if glasses are used for far or near vision.

The nurse can assess the client's visual fields or peripheral vision by asking the client to focus his or her eye on the examiner's nose. The nurse wiggles one finger of each hand in the superior visual field, asking the client to indicate where the movement is. The client should see movement on both sides. The nurse then repeats the test in the inferior visual field. For testing the second eye, the nurse wiggles the finger of only one hand to prevent the client from repeating the previous answers. The nurse then tests the superior and inferior fields using a finger of each hand. If the client cannot see the fingers in one or more of the fields, further testing is required. The fundus, or optic disk, is inspected with the ophthalmoscope to check for vascular problems, retinal disease, papilledema, or optic atrophy. Nurses require special training to use the ophthalmoscope.

From Ignatavicius, Workman, and Mishler, pp. 1102–1105.

CRANIAL NERVE III: OCULOMOTOR

Pupil constriction is tested with the room darkened, if possible. The nurse brings the penlight in from the side or from above or below and shines the light in the client's eye. The pupil should constrict, and it should stay constricted (*direct* response). The nurse also watches for *consensual* response in the eye not being tested (consensual response is less than direct response). *P*upils should be *e*qual in size, *r*ound, *r*egular, and react to *l*ight and *a*ccommodation (PERRLA). Using a millimeter ruler or other measuring device, the nurse estimates the size of both pupils.

As a person ages, the pupils become less regular and round. The pupils should react to light with the same rate of speed and to the same degree. Glaucoma, cataract surgery, and iridectomy may influence the shape and size of the pupil as well as its reaction to light. With the light stimulus still present, a pupil may dilate slightly after constricting (hippus); this reaction may be normal. In a few people, one pupil may be larger than the other (anisocoria); this may also be normal if there are no other eye symptoms. The client is usually aware of the size difference. The client with Adie's pupil has one pupil that is larger than the other; in addition to the size difference, the pupil is slow to react to light.

The nurse assesses accommodation by bringing an object from far to near the client's eyes. The pupils should constrict and the eyes converge (turn in to focus on the object). Accommodation need not be tested if constriction to light is normal. Some medications may affect constriction and dilation.

The nurse assesses lid elevation. The upper eyelid should rest approximately at the top or slightly below the top of the pupil. The strength and closure of the lid are a function of cranial nerve VII (see later) but can be tested with the eye examination.

The nurse evaluates eye movement (upward, downward, and medial) by assessing cranial nerve VI.

CRANIAL NERVE IV: TROCHLEAR

Eye movement (inferior and medial) is tested with assessment of cranial nerve VI.

CRANIAL NERVE V: TRIGEMINAL

The client's eyes are closed for the sensory portion of trigeminal nerve testing. The nurse asks the client to indicate when touch is felt by saying "now." By stroking a piece of cotton over the client's face (light touch), the nurse tests all three branches of the trigeminal nerve (ophthalmic branch—forehead; maxillary branch—cheek; mandibular branch—jaw). The nurse alternates sides for comparison. Next, by use of an object that has sharp and dull components, such as a safety pin, the nurse asks the client to indicate whether the sensation is sharp or dull and then repeats the process. The motor aspect can be tested with the client's eyes open. The nurse palpates the temporal and masseter (jaw) muscles (with one hand on each side) for strength and equality.

The corneal reflex has traditionally been tested by using a wisp of cotton and touching the edge of the cornea, which normally causes blinking. However, this procedure can cause abrasion to the cornea. In a routine examination, the examiner will see blinking and need not test the corneal reflex. If there is concern that the corneal reflex is absent, there are two safer tests. One is to bring a hand quickly toward the client's face in a threatening motion. If the client has vision, this will cause blinking. Alternatively, the nurse can use a syringe full of air and, while holding it 4 to 6 inches away from the client's eyes, expel it gently toward the eyes. The client will blink if the reflex is intact.

CRANIAL NERVE VI: ABDUCENS

Cranial nerve VI controls lateral eye movement. Together with cranial nerves III and IV, cranial nerve VI is tested by checking the six cardinal positions of gaze. The nurse asks the client to follow the examiner's finger or a held object while keeping his or her head still. The nurse starts at the 1 o'clock position and moves clockwise through the six positions shown in Figure VI–4. The nurse pauses in the horizontal and vertical positions to check for nystagmus (involuntary oscillation of the eyes) or deviation. Some nystagmus in the extreme lateral position is normal. Severe lateral nystagmus or nystagmus in any other position is abnormal. If there is weakness or paralysis of a particular muscle, the eye will not turn in that direction.

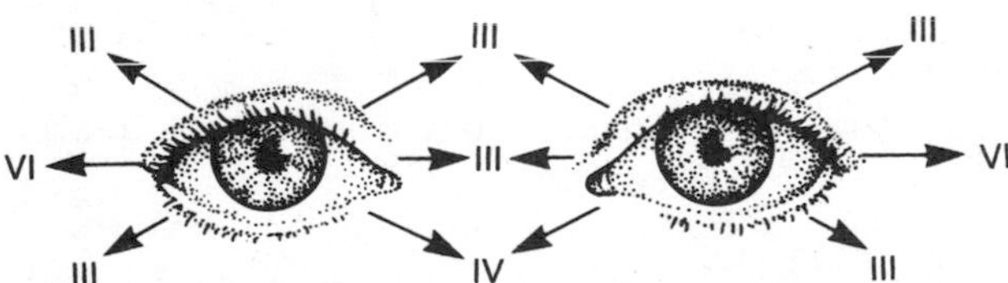

Figure VI–4 Checking extraocular movements in the six cardinal positions indicates the functioning of cranial nerves III, IV, and VI. (Reprinted with permission from Ignatavicius, D.D., Workman, L., and Mishler, M.A.: Medical-Surgical Nursing: A Nursing Process Approach, 2nd ed. Philadelphia, W. B. Saunders, 1995.)

CRANIAL NERVE VII: FACIAL

Only the motor portion of the facial nerve is tested. Taste on the anterior portion of the tongue is tested with cranial nerve IX. The nurse asks the client to frown, smile, wrinkle the forehead, and puff out the cheeks while looking for symmetry of both sides. The nurse tests eyelid closure and strength by asking the client to close the eyes tightly and keep them closed while the nurse tries to pry them open.

CRANIAL NERVE VIII: VESTIBULOCOCHLEAR (ACOUSTIC)

Hearing is tested initially with the client's eyes closed. The nurse rubs a thumb and finger together next to the client's ear and asks where sound is heard. The nurse then repeats this maneuver for the other ear. A watch can also be used, or the nurse can whisper close to each ear. (Quartz and electronic watches do not tick.)

The nurse may use the Weber and Rinne tests (with the client's eyes open) to check for conductive or sensorineural hearing loss.

- Conductive hearing loss is caused by external-ear and middle-ear problems, such as excessive cerumen, the presence of pus, ossicle fusion, or a damaged eardrum.
- Sensorineural hearing loss is due to cochlear or nerve damage.

In the *Weber* test, a vibrating tuning fork is placed on top of the client's head or forehead. The client should hear sound equally in both ears. (Touching the fork tines will stop the vibration; therefore, the fork must be held by the handle only.) With conductive loss, the sound is heard louder in the ear with the deficit because the sound bypasses the obstruction. With sensorineural loss, the sound is louder in the better ear. The *Rinne* test measures the difference between bone and air conduction. A vibrating tuning fork is placed on the mastoid bone until sound is no longer heard and then moved near the external ear canal. With a normal or *positive* test result, the client hears the sound about twice as long by air conduction as by bone. In conductive hearing loss, the client hears the sound longer through bone (*negative* Rinne test result). The sound is heard longer by air than by bone (positive test result) in sensorineural loss.

Equilibrium, although regulated by cranial nerve VIII, is generally tested with the cerebellum at the end of the examination to avoid having the client stand and sit excessively.

CRANIAL NERVE IX: GLOSSOPHARYNGEAL

The motor portion is tested with cranial nerve X assessment. Taste (the posterior third of the tongue) is often not tested unless the client reports loss of taste. When testing taste, remember that the tongue must be rinsed in between the sweet, sour, bitter, and salty samples. Taste occurs only when the substance is in solution, so the tongue must be moist for a true test result.

CRANIAL NERVE X: VAGUS

To test the motor portion, the nurse asks the client to say "Ah" when the examiner looks into the throat. The uvula and palate should rise bilaterally and equally. Stimulating the gag reflex with a tongue blade reflects sensitivity to a stimulus. The ability to swallow and normal phonation and articulation also imply intact nerves IX and X.

CRANIAL NERVE XI: SPINAL ACCESSORY

The nurse assesses the strength of the client's sternocleidomastoid and trapezius muscles by having the client turn his or her head against resistance (provided by the nurse's hand on the side of the face toward the turn). The test is then repeated in the other direction. In the second test, the client shrugs his or her shoulders upward against the resistance of the nurse's hands placed on the client's shoulders (Fig. 40–13).

CRANIAL NERVE XII: HYPOGLOSSAL

The nurse tests motor innervation to the tongue by asking the client to stick out his or her tongue. The nurse checks for deviation to one side or the other. The tongue deviates toward the same side where the lesion has occurred in the brain. The nurse can test the strength of the tongue by asking the client to push against a tongue blade held at one side of the tongue. The test is then repeated on the other side.

• SUMMARY

Directions. In the space provided, rewrite the above selection in your own words, focusing on the main ideas and major details.

• COMPREHENSION QUESTIONS

Directions. Below are 10 multiple-choice questions. Circle the letter of the best answer from the four choices.

1 When assessing for smell, it is permissible to use all of the following familiar odors except:

a mint

b ammonia

c soap

d coffee

2 When assessing the optic nerve, the nurse checks:
  a central vision only
  b peripheral vision only
  c both central and peripheral vision
  d neither central nor peripheral vision

3 Light touch perception is the function of the:
  a trochlear nerve
  b oculomotor nerve
  c abducens nerve
  d trigeminal nerve

4 When the facial nerve is assessed, the portion tested is:
  a motor
  b sensory
  c parasympathetic motor
  d none of the above

5 Hearing is the property of the:
  a facial nerve
  b vagus nerve
  c abducens nerve
  d vestibulocochlear nerve

6 The Weber test uses a:
  a syringe full of air
  b piece of cotton
  c tuning fork
  d tongue blade

7 The nerve assessed for taste is the:
  a glossopharyngeal
  b facial
  c hypoglossal
  d vagus

8 The nerve responsible for the gag reflex is the:
  a glossopharyngeal
  b facial
  c hypoglossal
  d vagus

9 When assessing the hypoglossal, the nurse is checking for:
  a ability to swallow
  b motor innervation to the tongue
  c strength of the sternocleidomastoid
  d normal phonation

10 The purpose of the nurse assessing the 12 cranial nerves is to:
- **a** judge reflex activity
- **b** judge cerebellar function
- **c** judge motor and sensory functioning
- **d** none of the above

Comprehending? Yes ___ No ___

• CRITICAL THINKING/EVALUATION

Were you successful in applying active reading strategies to this selection? Explain.

____

____

____

____

Reading Selection 6

• PREVIEW QUESTION

This selection is about uveitis, an eye disease. What, as a nursing student, do you think you need to know about uveitis?

• VOCABULARY

Underline any medical terminology or general vocabulary words you may need to learn in order to understand the ideas in this reading selection.

Uveal Tract Disorders: Uveitis

OVERVIEW

The uveal tract is composed of three separate but interrelated parts:

- The iris
- The ciliary body
- The choroid

The most common problem associated with these structures is inflammation, or uveitis.

Anterior Uveitis

Anterior uveitis can include inflammation of the iris, inflammation of the ciliary body, or both. The etiology of anterior uveitis is unknown but may be related to:

- Exposure to allergens (fungi, bacteria, viruses, chemicals)
- Surgical or accidental trauma
- Systemic diseases (rheumatoid arthritis, ankylosing spondylitis, herpes simplex, herpes zoster)

Symptoms include:

- Moderate periorbital aching
- Tearing
- Blurred vision
- Photophobia, caused by the pain that accompanies contraction of the inflamed iris in bright lights

A small, irregular, nonreactive pupil is caused by the adhesions that form between the iris and the lens during inflammation. Engorgement of the scleral vessels creates a purplish discoloration called *ciliary flush* (Boyd-Monk & Steinmetz, 1987). Fibrinous material or accumulation of purulent matter in the anterior chamber may be noted in severe cases.

Posterior Uveitis

Posterior uveitis is the common term for *retinitis,* inflammation of the retina, and *chorioretinitis,* inflammation of both the choroid and the retina. Posterior uveitis is usually associated with infectious processes, such as tuberculosis, syphilis, and toxoplasmosis.

The onset of symptoms is slow and insidious. Visual impairment in the affected eye is the primary symptom. It results from the exudation of protein-rich fluid, fibrin, and cells into the vitreous cavity. The location and extent of visual impairment depend on the size and site of inflammation. The vision loss appears to be more severe than the amount of choroid or retina involved.

On examination, the pupil is observed to be small, nonreactive, and irregularly shaped because of the adhesions that bind the iris to the lens. Black dots are visible against the red background of the fundus. Chorioretinal lesions appear as grayish-yellow, defined patches on the retinal surface.

COLLABORATIVE MANAGEMENT

Treatment of the client with anterior and posterior uveitis is symptomatic. The treatment plan includes putting the ciliary body to rest with a cycloplegic agent. The pupil is dilated to prevent adhesions between the iris and the lens. Steroid drops (e.g., prednisolone acetate [Ocu-Pred, Ophtho-Tate]) are administered every hour to decrease the inflammatory response of the eye and to prevent adhesions of the iris to the cornea and lens. Ointments such as dexamethasone phosphate (Maxidex) are also used. Subconjunctival injections of steroids may be used in posterior uveitis or when topical steroids have been ineffec-

From Ignatavicius, Workman, and Mishler, pp. 1336–1337.

tive. Analgesics such as acetaminophen (Abenol, Tylenol) or acetaminophen with oxycodone (Endocet, Percocet, Tylox) are ordered for pain. Antibiotics may be initiated for the client with posterior uveitis (Boyd-Monk & Steinmetz, 1987).

The nurse applies cool or warm compresses for ocular pain. Darkening the room and encouraging the client to wear sunglasses reduce the discomfort of photophobia. Because the client's vision is blurred from the use of cycloplegic drops, the nurse instructs the client not to drive or operate machinery. The nurse reviews the signs and symptoms of bacterial and fungal ulcers as well as indications of increased intraocular pressure.

• SUMMARY

Directions. In the space provided, rewrite the above selection in your own words, focusing on the main ideas and major details.

• COMPREHENSION QUESTIONS

Directions. Below are 10 multiple-choice questions. Circle the letter of the best answer from the four choices.

1 The uveal tract consists of:
- **a** iris, ciliary body, and choroid
- **b** the vitreous, iris, and ciliary bodies
- **c** optic nerve, iris, and vitreous
- **d** lens, iris, and choroid

2 Uveitis is a type of:
- **a** blindness
- **b** inflammation
- **c** hemorrhage
- **d** injury

3 Retinitis is:
- **a** hemorrhaging of the retina
- **b** injury to the retina
- **c** removal of the retina
- **d** inflammation of the retina

4 The two types of uveitis are:
a right eye and left eye
b interior and exterior
c anterior and posterior
d dorsal and ventral

5 One possible cause of uveitis is:
a aging
b bacteria
c poor nutrition
d heredity

6 One symptom of uveitis is:
a hemorrhaging
b photophobia
c headaches
d bleeding

7 Treatment of uveitis includes:
a putting the ciliary body to rest
b dilating the pupil
c using ointment
d all of the above

8 A common treatment of uveitis is:
a laser therapy
b surgery
c steroids
d agents that enhance pupillary constriction

9 When an individual complains of ocular pain relating to uveitis, the nurse should:
a darken the patient's room
b validate the patient's concerns
c advise the patient to avoid driving
d use warm compresses

10 Because the client's vision is blurred the nurse should:
a tell the client not to drive or operate heavy machinery
b identify for the patient those activities that cause uveitis
c remind the patient not to wash her/his face
d encourage the patient to change eyeglass prescriptions

Comprehending? Yes ____ No ____

• CRITICAL THINKING/EVALUATION

Were you successful in applying active reading strategies to this selection? Explain.

____

____

____

____

Reading Selection 7

• PREVIEW QUESTIONS

What features of the ear does this selection discuss? What do you already know about these features?

• VOCABULARY

Underline any medical terminology or general vocabulary words you may need to learn in order to understand the ideas in this reading selection.

The ear is the sensory organ of hearing and balance. Hearing impairment is common, and onset may be insidious. Many clients who seek health care for another problem may not even be aware of an existing hearing problem. In addition, many medications affect hearing. Therefore, to conduct an adequate health assessment, nurses need to understand the structure of the ear and the nature of hearing.

Anatomy and Physiology Review

STRUCTURE

The ear consists of three structural parts: external, middle, and inner. Each of these structures and their functions are integral to the hearing process.

External Ear

The external ear develops in embryonic life at the same time as the kidneys and urinary tract. Therefore, any person with a defect of the external ear must be examined for possible malformations of the renal and urinary systems (Moore, 1991).

The external ear is embedded in the temporal bone bilaterally at the level of the eyes. It is attached to the head by skin and cartilage at approximately a 10-degree angle. The external ear extends from the pinna through the external canal to the tympanic membrane, or eardrum (Fig. VI–5). The external ear canal is slightly S-shaped and lined with *cerumen* (wax)-producing glands, sebaceous glands, and hair follicles. The hair follicles and cerumen protect the tympanic membrane and the middle ear. In the adult, the distance from the opening of the external canal to the tympanic membrane is approximately 2.5 to 3.75 cm (1 to 1 1/2 inches). The external ear includes the *mastoid process,* the bony ridge located over the temporal bone behind the pinna.

From Ignatavicius, Workman, and Mishler, pp. 1351–1353.

Middle Ear

The middle ear begins at the medial side of the tympanic membrane. It consists of the *epitympanum,* a compartment containing the three bony *ossicles* (Fig. VI–6):

- Malleus
- Incus
- Stapes

In addition, the proximal end of the eustachian tube opens in the middle ear. The *tympanic membrane* is a thick, transparent sheet of tissue providing a barrier between the external and middle ear. The landmarks on the tympanic membrane include (Fig. VI–7) the:

- Annulus
- Pars flaccida
- Pars tensa

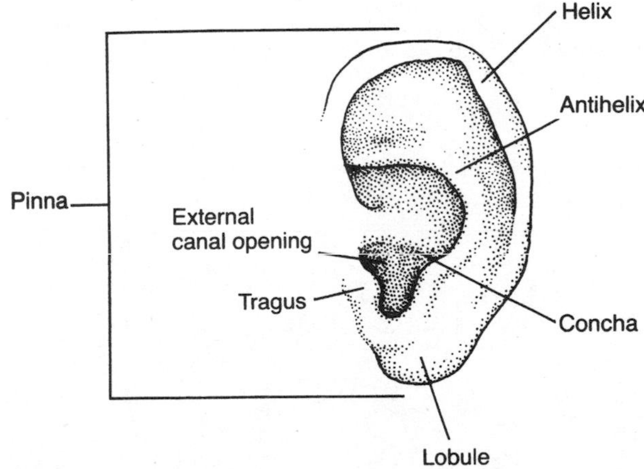

Figure VI–5 Anatomic features of the external ear. (Reprinted with permission from Ignatavicius, D.D., Workman, L., and Mishler, M.A.: Medical-Surgical Nursing: A Nursing Process Approach, 2nd ed. Philadelphia, W. B. Saunders, 1995.)

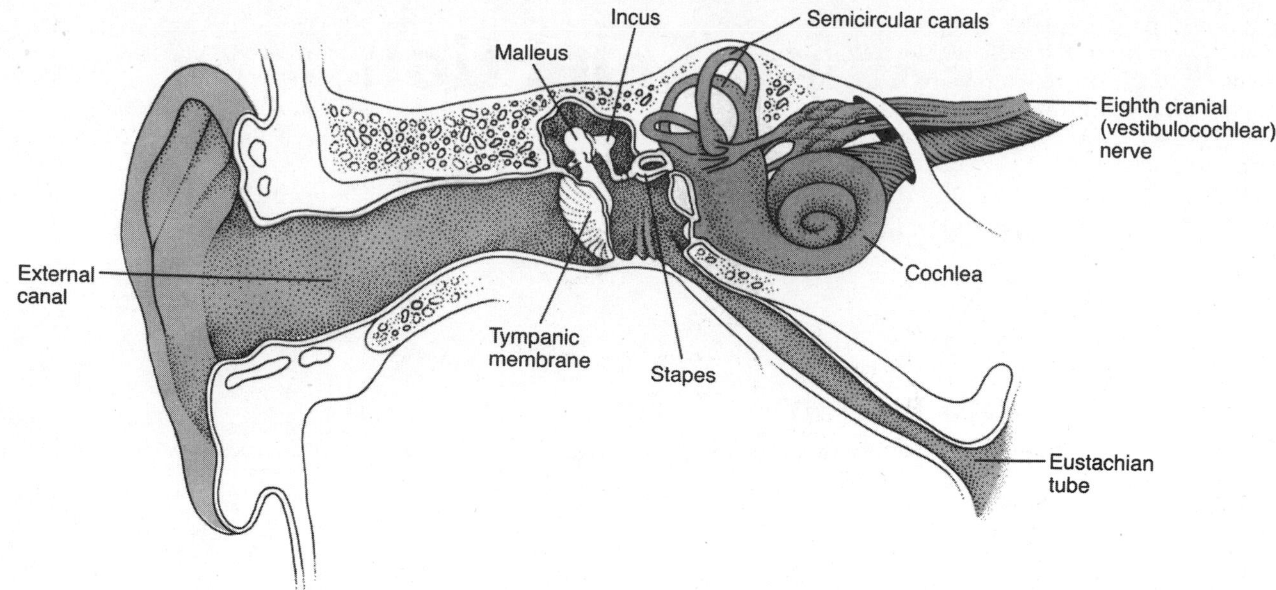

Figure VI–6 Anatomic features of the internal ear. (Reprinted with permission from Ignatavicius, D.D., Workman, L., and Mishler, M.A.: Medical-Surgical Nursing: A Nursing Process Approach, 2nd ed. Philadelphia, W. B. Saunders, 1995.)

The tympanic membrane is attached to the first bony ossicle, the *malleus,* at the *umbo* (see Fig. VI–7). The bony ossicles behind the tympanic membrane are joined, although not rigidly, which allows vibratory movement.

The pars flaccida and pars tensa are parts of the tympanic membrane. The *pars flaccida* is that portion of the tympanic membrane above the short process of the malleus. The *pars tensa* is that portion of the tympanic membrane surrounding the long process of the malleus. It is usually described as transparent, opaque, or pearly gray and is mobile when air is injected into the external canal. The umbo is seen through the tympanic membrane as a

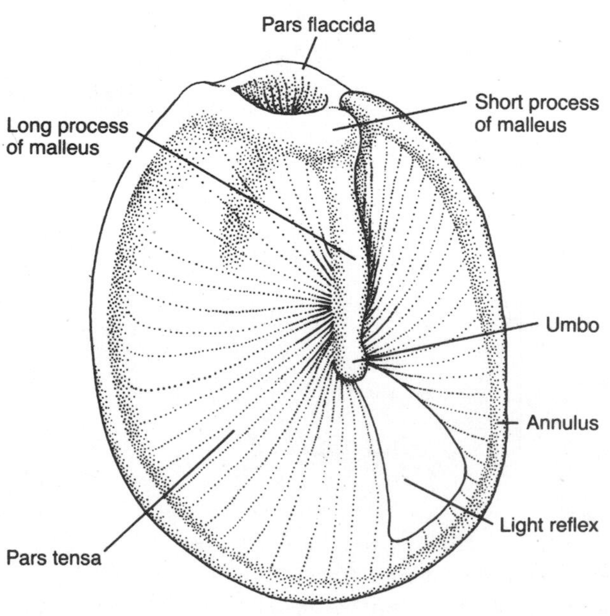

Figure VI–7 Landmarks of the tympanic membrane. (Reprinted with permission from Ignatavicius, D.D., Workman, L., and Mishler, M.A.: Medical-Surgical Nursing: A Nursing Process Approach, 2nd ed. Philadelphia, W. B. Saunders, 1995.)

white dot at the end of the long process of the malleus. The short process of the malleus, the long process of the malleus, and the umbo are structures seen *through* the transparent tympanic membrane.

The middle ear is separated from the inner ear by the round and the oval windows. The eustachian tube originates from the floor of the middle ear at the proximal end and opens at the distal end in the nasopharynx. The distal opening in the nasopharynx is surrounded by adenoid lymphatic tissue (Fig. VI–8). The eustachian tube allows equalization of pressure on both sides of the tympanic membrane. Secretions from the middle ear drain through it.

Inner Ear

The inner ear, lying on the other side of the oval window, contains (see Fig. VI–6):

- The semicircular canals
- The cochlea
- The distal end of the eighth cranial nerve

The *semicircular canals* contain fluid and hair cells connected to the sensory nerve fibers of the vestibular portion of the eighth cranial nerve. They help to maintain a person's sense of balance.

The *cochlea* is the spiral organ of hearing. It is divided into two parts, the scala tympani and the scala vestibuli. Reissner's membrane stretches across the scala vestibuli and forms the duct of the cochlea, or the scala media. The scala media is filled with *endolymph,* a fluid that is similar to intracellular fluid. The scala tympani and scala vestibuli are filled with *perilymph.* Endolymph and perilymph protect the cochlea and the semicircular canals. These structures literally float in the fluids, which cushion against abrupt movements of the head.

The *organ of Corti* is the receptor end-organ of hearing located on the basilar membrane of the cochlea. The cochlea contains hair cells that detect vibration from sound and stimulate the eighth cranial nerve.

FUNCTION

The main function of the ear is hearing. Hearing is accomplished when sound is delivered through the air to the external ear canal and the temporal bone covering the mastoid air cells. The sound waves strike the mastoid and the movable tympanic membrane, which is connected to the first bony ossicle, the malleus. The sound wave vibrations are transferred from the tympanic membrane to the malleus, the incus, and the stapes. From the stapes, the vibrations are transmitted to the cochlea. Receptors there transduce (change) the vibrations into action potentials, which are conducted to the brain as neural impulses by the cochlear portion of the eighth cranial nerve. Thus, sound is processed and interpreted by the brain.

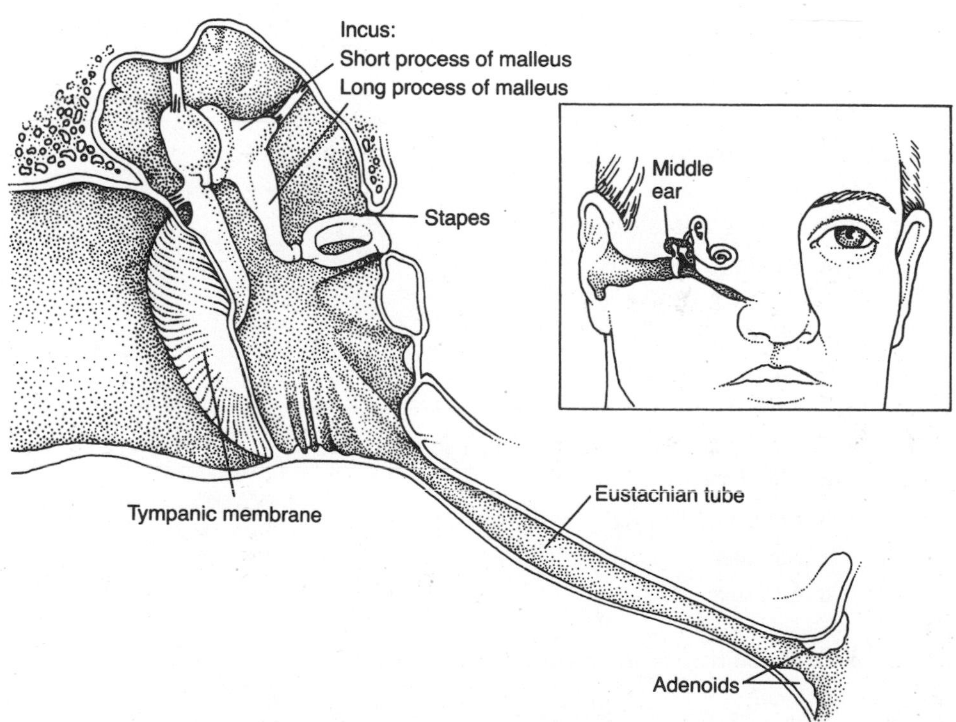

Figure VI–8 Anatomic features and attached structures of the middle ear. (Reprinted with permission from Ignatavicius, D.D., Workman, L., and Mishler, M.A.: Medical-Surgical Nursing: A Nursing Process Approach, 2nd ed. Philadelphia, W. B. Saunders, 1995.)

• SUMMARY

Directions. In the space provided, rewrite the above selection in your own words, focusing on the main ideas and major details.

• COMPREHENSION QUESTIONS

Directions. Below are 10 multiple-choice questions. Circle the letter of the best answer from the four choices.

1 The external ear is located:
a bilaterally at the level of the eyes
b at a 25-degree angle with the head
c bilaterally at the level of the nose
d at a 20-degree angle with the head

2 The shape of the external canal is:
a slightly V shaped
b slightly L shaped
c slightly T shaped
d slightly S shaped

3 The common name for the tympanic membrane is:
a hair follicle
b ear drum
c ear lobe
d ear canal

4 The tube that opens in the middle ear is the:
a incus
b malleus
c eustachian
d stapes

5 The function of the tympanic membrane is to:
- **a** provide a barrier between the external and the middle ear
- **b** cover the mastoid air cells
- **c** produce cerumen
- **d** equalize pressure

6 Three major features of the middle ear are:
- **a** tragus, concha, helix
- **b** stapes, incus, helix
- **c** concha, malleus, incus
- **d** malleus, incus, stapes

7 The pars flaccida is a feature of the:
- **a** external ear
- **b** tympanic membrane
- **c** inner ear
- **d** middle ear

8 The eustachian tube:
- **a** maintains balance
- **b** allows vibratory movement
- **c** equalizes pressure on both sides of the tympanic membrane
- **d** is connected to sensory nerve fibers

9 The semicircular canals help people maintain:
- **a** a sense of balance
- **b** a sense of high tones
- **c** a sense of low tones
- **d** a sense of both soft and low tones

10 The inner ear contains:
- **a** semicircular canals
- **b** cochlea
- **c** part of the eighth cranial nerve
- **d** all of the above

Comprehending? Yes ___ No ___

• CRITICAL THINKING/EVALUATION

Were you successful in applying active reading strategies to this selection? Explain.

____

____

____

____

Reading Selection 8

• PREVIEW QUESTION

What is Figure VI–9 illustrating?

• VOCABULARY

Underline any medical terminology or general vocabulary words you may need to learn in order to understand the ideas in this reading selection.

• SUMMARY

In the space provided, rewrite the main features of Figure VI–9 in your own words.

• COMPREHENSION QUESTIONS

Directions. Below are 10 multiple-choice questions. Circle the letter of the best answer from the four choices.

1 In the diagram unoxygenated blood is represented by a:
  - **a** black dotted line
  - **b** white dotted line
  - **c** red (or dark) arrow
  - **d** white arrow

From Ignatavicius, Workman, and Mishler, p. 777.

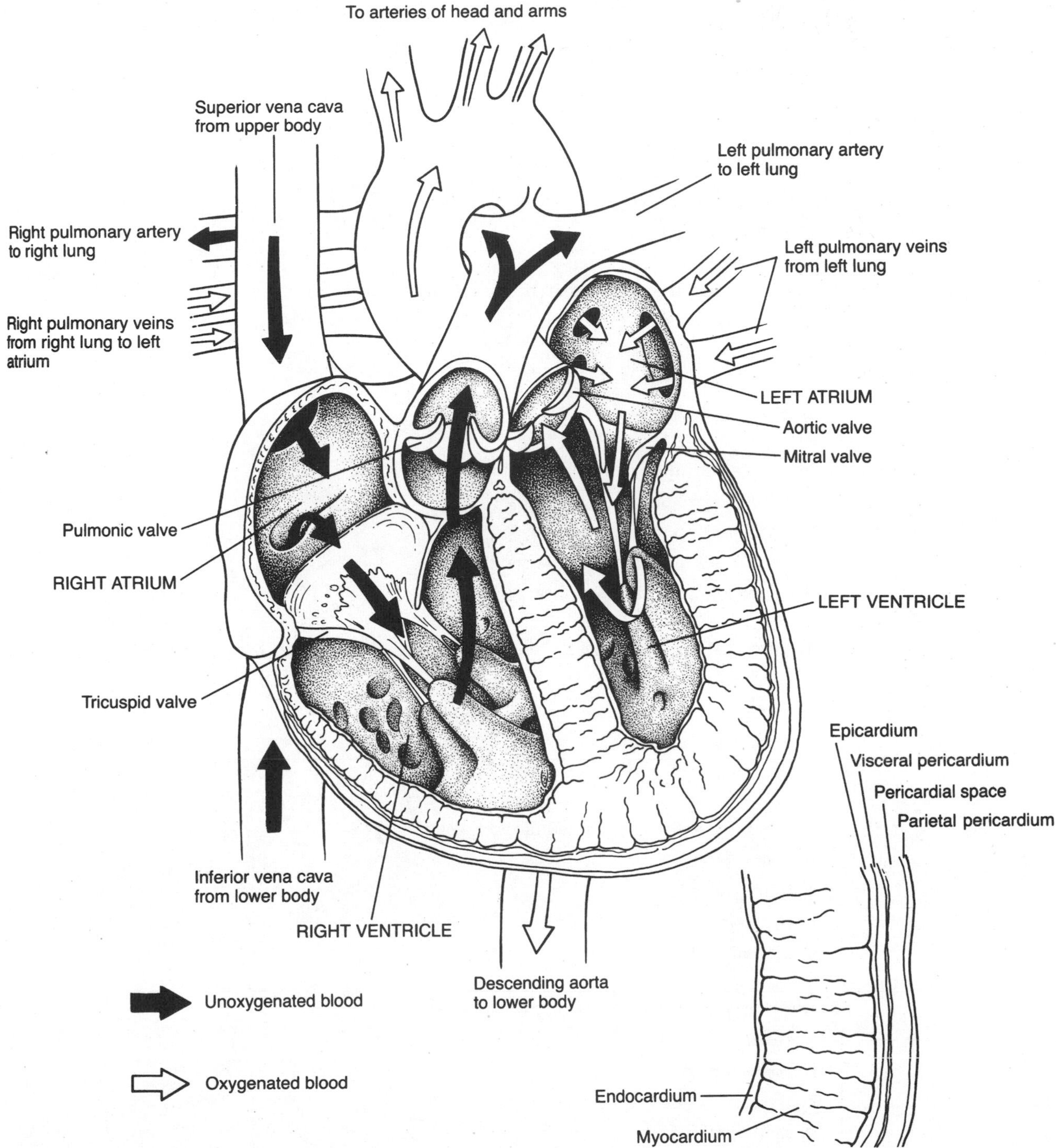

Figure VI–9 Blood flow through the heart. (Reprinted with permission from Ignatavicius, D.D., Workman, L., and Mishler, M.A.: Medical-Surgical Nursing: A Nursing Process Approach, 2nd ed. Philadelphia, W. B. Saunders, 1995.)

2 In this diagram oxygenated blood is represented by a:
a black dotted line
b white dotted line
c black arrow
d white arrow

3 Blood from the upper body enters the heart via the:
a superior vena cava
b inferior vena cava
c left pulmonary artery
d right pulmonary artery

4 The first valve the unoxygenated blood flows through is the:
a aortic valve
b tricuspid valve
c mitral valve
d bicuspid valve

5 In the diagram the left ventricle is located in the:
a bottom right portion of the heart
b upper right portion of the heart
c bottom left portion of the heart
d upper left portion of the heart

6 The first part of the heart the newly oxygenated blood flows through is the:
a right ventricle
b aorta
c pulmonary artery
d pulmonary veins

7 The first valve the oxygenated blood flows through is the:
a aortic valve
b mitral valve
c tricuspid valve
d bicuspid valve

8 After leaving the left ventricle, the blood flows into the:
a aorta
b aortic valve
c arteries to head and arms
d right ventricle

9 Blood in the aorta flows into arteries in the:
a upper and lower body
b left pulmonary artery
c right pulmonary artery
d lungs

10 The blood enters the lungs through the right and left:

a atria
b ventricles
c pulmonary arteries
d pulmonary veins

Comprehending? Yes ___ No ___

• CRITICAL THINKING/EVALUATION

Were you successful in applying active reading strategies to this selection? Explain.

____

____

____

____

Reading Selection 9

• PREVIEW QUESTION

Primary head injuries include injuries to which three areas?

• VOCABULARY

Underline any medical terminology or general vocabulary words you may need to learn in order to understand the ideas in this reading selection.

• HEAD TRAUMA

Injuries to the Scalp, Skull, or Brain

RISK FACTORS

The major factor contributing to the occurrence of head injury is alcohol consumption. Alcohol slows reflexes and alters cognitive processes and perception. These physiologic changes increase the chances of being involved in an accident or altercation.

Primary prevention centers on the education of clients of all ages. Children should be taught the importance of safety restraints in cars and of bicycle helmets. The use of motorcycle helmets and the dangers of driving after drug or alcohol ingestion are necessary information for older children and adults. Secondary prevention is not an issue in head trauma because other health conditions do not increase the incidence of head trauma. Pre-existing conditions may have an impact on recovery from head injury.

Tertiary prevention focuses on preventing or minimizing the complications of head trauma. At-the-scene care by trained professionals, stabilization, and transportation to tertiary care centers improve outcomes. At the time of an accident, many clients suffer primary, irreversible brain injury, which ultimately causes death. The most common causes of such deaths are brain stem hemorrhage and diffuse axonal injury throughout the brain due to the impact.

PATHOPHYSIOLOGY

Primary head injuries include injuries to the scalp, skull, or brain or all of these. The injuries result from the original impact.

Scalp Injuries

Scalp injuries can cause lacerations, hematomas, and contusions or abrasions to the skin. These injuries may be unsightly and bleed profusely. Clients with minor scalp injuries not accompanied by damage to other areas do not require hospitalization.

Skull Injuries

Skull fractures are often caused by a force sufficient to cause both fracture and brain injury. The fractures in themselves do not mean brain injury is also present. However, skull fractures often cause serious brain damage. Depressed skull fractures injure the brain by bruising it (abrasion) or by driving bone fragments into it (lacerations). The site of a fracture and the extent of brain injury may not correlate.

There are three types of skull fracture.

Linear Skull Fractures. Linear skull fractures appear as thin lines radiographically and do not require treatment. They are important only if there is significant underlying brain damage.

Depressed Skull Fractures. Depressed skull fractures may be palpated and are seen radiographically. Surgery may be required within the first 24 hours after injury if the depression is as deep as the skull thickness. Depressed fractures may be associated with bone fragments penetrating into brain tissue. When this occurs, the area is usually surgically explored and debrided.

Basilar Skull Fractures. Basilar skull fractures occur in bones over the base of the frontal and temporal lobes. They are rarely seen radiographically.

Basilar skull fractures, depressed fractures, and other open (compound) fractures all allow communication between the exterior environment and the brain. Infection is therefore a possible complication. (See later discussion of brain abscess and meningitis.)

Brain Injuries

There is a wide variety of brain injuries (see Mechanisms of Injury). A single classification of brain injuries does not exist. However, the terms open, closed, contusion, and concussion are often applied to brain injuries. Open head injuries are those that penetrate the skull. Closed injuries are from blunt trauma.

From Black and Matassarin-Jacobs, pp. 743–745.

Concussions. A concussion is head trauma that may result in loss of consciousness for 5 minutes or less and retrograde amnesia. There is no break in the skull or dura, and no visible damage on the CT or MRI is seen. The client usually presents with headache and dizziness and may complain of nausea and vomiting. The duration of amnesia may directly correlate with severity of the concussion.

Contusions. Contusions cause more extensive damage than do concussions. Contusions damage the brain substance itself, causing multiple areas of petechial and punctate hemorrhage and bruised areas. Diffuse axonal injury resulting in anatomic disruption of the white matter may result from serious contusions. Microscopic nerve fiber lesions also occur. Abnormalities may be mainly in one area of the brain, but other areas may also be injured. This is particularly true of brain stem contusions, which are a very serious type of lesion.

Nuchal rigidity (involuntary stiffness of neck muscles) may indicate cervical spine (C-spine) injuries, meningeal irritation, or subarachnoid bleeding after head injury.

CLINICAL MANIFESTATIONS

Skull Fractures

Other than a history of head injury, clients with skull fractures may not have clear symptoms of their injury. They may develop other clinical signs including (1) CSF or other drainage from the ear or nose, (2) various cranial nerve injuries, (3) blood behind the eardrum, (4) periorbital ecchymosis (bruise around the eyes), and (5) later, a bruise over the mastoid (Battle's sign).

Indications of cranial nerve damage may occur at the time of the initial injury or may develop later. They include

- vision loss (e.g., blindness, blurred vision) from optic nerve damage
- hearing loss with postural vertigo and nystagmus from auditory nerve damage
- loss of the sense of smell (bilaterally or unilaterally) from olfactory nerve damage
- squint or fixed dilated pupil and loss of some of the eye movements from oculomotor nerve damage
- facial paresis/paralysis (unilateral) from facial nerve damage.

Contusions

There are various clinical manifestations in clients with contusions. This is partly because of the numerous areas of damage. Contusions are often associated with other serious injuries, including cervical fractures. Secondary effects (e.g., brain swelling and edema) accompany serious contusions. Increased ICP and herniation syndromes may result.

Contusions may be divided into cerebral contusions and brain stem contusions.

Cerebral Contusions. These contusions can be diagnosed only if the client is alert, although they may be present in comatose patients. Assessment findings vary, depending on which areas of the cerebral hemispheres are damaged. An agitated, confused head-injured client who remains alert may have a temporal lobe contusion. Hemiparesis in an alert head-injured client may indicate a frontal contusion. An aphasic head-injured client may have a frontal-temporal contusion. Other findings indicate contusions in other areas. Remember that although these findings correlate with cerebral contusion, they do not rule out other abnormalities such as a developing mass or lesion. Adverse changes in the client's condition require immediate medical attention. They may indicate treatable complications.

Brain Stem Contusions. Brain stem contusions render a client immediately unresponsive or partially comatose because of significant brain stem disruption. Typically, an altered LOC continues for at least several hours and usually days or weeks. The client may regain partial consciousness within hours or remain in a coma.

Damage to the reticular activating system may render the client permanently comatose. Other neurologic abnormalities are present and are usually symmetric (i.e., on both sides of the body). Some may be lateralized (asymmetric, on one side of the body only), indicating development of a secondary event such as a hematoma.

In addition to the altered LOC that is always present with brain stem contusion, respiratory, pupillary, eye movement, and motor abnormalities may occur.

- Respirations may be normal, ataxic, periodic, or very rapid.
- Pupils are usually small, equal, and reactive. Damage to the upper brain stem (third cranial nerve) may cause pupillary abnormalities.
- Loss of normal eye movements may occur because pathways controlling eye movements traverse the midbrain and pons.
- The client may respond to light or noxious stimuli by purposeful movements, pushing the stimulus away. Or the client may have no response to stimuli, that is, may be flaccid. In the presence of profound LOC alterations, flexion and extension posturing may be elicited with or without noxious stimuli.

Brain stem contusions do not usually injure the brain stem alone. Swelling or direct injury to the hypothalamus may produce autonomic nervous system effects. The client has a high temperature, has rapid pulse and respiration, and perspires profusely. These effects may wax and wane but, if sustained, can lead to serious complications.

These clinical manifestations often vary from one observation to another (whereas findings indicating a developing hematoma are more consistent). Careful documentation of assessment findings is important to identify patterns or trends in the client's condition.

Diagnostic Assessment

There is a high association of cervical fracture with head injury; therefore, lateral cervical spine radiographs are obtained before the client's head is moved. CT scans and radiographs are also obtained to assess for fractures and areas of bleeding or brain shift. Lumbar puncture can also be used to assess for bleeding within the subarachnoid space.

MEDICAL MANAGEMENT

A complete history is taken of the mechanism of injury. These data allow the physician to determine the probable extent of injury. Diagnostic findings are reviewed.

Open head wounds should be covered and pressure applied to control bleeding unless there appears to be underlying depressed or compound skull fracture. Do not attempt to remove foreign objects or any penetrating objects from the wound. Uncomplicated scalp wounds (that do not lie over depressed or compound skull fractures) are anesthetized locally, cleansed, and sutured.

Simple skull depressions are electively treated by surgically elevating the depressed bone fragment and repairing the dura if it is lacerated. All bone fragments are removed. Compound depressed skull fractures are immediately treated surgically. The scalp, skull, and devitalized brain are débrided, and the wound is cleansed thoroughly. Unless all foreign material is removed, a brain abscess develops. Débridement of a penetrating wound or depressed skull fracture frequently leaves a cranial defect that is cosmetically unsightly. The defect is surgically corrected by cranioplasty.

Severe Head Injury

Major goals in the care of severely head-injured clients are (1) the prompt recognition and treatment of hypoxia and acid-base disturbances that can contribute to cerebral edema increasing ICP resulting from factors such as cerebral edema or expanding hematoma and (2) stabilization of other conditions.

Few clients die instantly from head injury. However, many head-injured clients die within the first few minutes after injury from shock or impaired respiration. Early death may also result from brain stem damage. Rigorous intervention is started immediately because severe brain trauma is associated with high morbidity and mortality rates.

Some clients survive initial head trauma only to develop intracranial mass lesions such as expanding hematomas (e.g., epidural and subdural hemorrhages), which may be fatal unless promptly diagnosed and treated. Severe cerebral swelling often follows brain injury. It is probably the most common cause of death in clients who survive the initial injury and who do not develop intracranial mass lesions.

Clients with traumatic head injuries often have other major injuries. These include facial fractures, lung and heart injuries, cervical fractures, abdominal injuries, and musculoskeletal injuries. Facial fractures and lung injuries may contribute to respiratory insufficiency. Airway obstruction and decreased ability to breathe (e.g., from pulmonary contusion, flail chest, pneumothorax) contribute to respiratory insufficiency and poor oxygenation of the brain and other tissues. Brain death may result.

Hemorrhagic shock in clients with multiple trauma is rarely caused by head injury alone. Frequently it relates to (1) ruptured abdominal organs or (2) musculoskeletal injuries (e.g., fractured femur and pelvis). Circulation may be further compromised by cardiac contusion and associated arrhythmias. Head injuries can also cause arrhythmias and further complicate the client's recovery.

The medical management of severely head-injured clients focuses on supporting all organ systems while recovery from the injuries takes place. This involves ventilatory support, management of nutrition and gastrointestinal function, and management of fluid balance and elimination. Head trauma has impact on all systems of the body, and managing these effects requires a holistic perspective. Clinical manifestations must be evaluated as stemming from the head injury or arising from a complicating process.

Fluids are usually managed carefully for avoidance of either over- or underadministration. Parameters such as central venous pressure and urinary output are used to guide fluid intake. Because severely head-injured clients are given nothing by mouth, potassium is commonly given through the intravenous line.

• SUMMARY

Directions. In the space provided, rewrite the above selection in your own words, focusing on the main ideas and major details.

• COMPREHENSIVE QUESTIONS

Directions. Below are 10 multiple-choice questions. Circle the letter of the best answer from the four choices.

1 A skull fracture:
- **a** always is an indication of brain injury
- **b** is often accompanied with brain injury
- **c** does not cause brain injury
- **d** is caused by an insufficient force

2 Blindness may occur from damage to the:
- **a** frontal lobe
- **b** scalp
- **c** optic nerve
- **d** auditory nerve

3 Nuchal rigidity is:
- **a** hearing loss
- **b** loss of sense of smell
- **c** involuntary stiff neck
- **d** vision loss

4 Simple skull depressions are treated by:
- **a** mandatory surgery
- **b** observation
- **c** medicine
- **d** elective surgery

5 Contusions cause:
a more extensive damage than concussions
b less extensive damage than concussions
c no damage
d the same damage as concussions

6 Amnesia means:
a loss of consciousness
b confusion
c brain damage
d memory loss

7 A fracture that does not require treatment is a:
a depressed skull fracture
b linear skull fracture
c cranial nerve damage
d contusion

8 A bruise is:
a an abrasion
b a laceration
c a hematoma
d a contusion

9 Primary head injury sites include the:
a skull and scalp
b scalp and brain
c skull and brain
d arteries and tissues

10 A person has to be alert to diagnose a:
a concussion
b vision loss
c linear skull fracture
d cerebral contusion

Comprehending? Yes ___ No ___

• CRITICAL THINKING/EVALUATION

Were you successful in applying active reading strategies to this selection? Explain.

____

____

____

____

Reading Selection 10

• PREVIEW QUESTIONS

Is Alzheimer's disease part of the normal aging process? Why or why not?

• VOCABULARY

Underline any medical terminology or general vocabulary words you may need to learn in order to understand the ideas in this reading selection.

Alzheimer's Disease

DEFINITION

Alzheimer's disease is a form of dementia. Dementia involves progressive decline in two or more areas of cognition, usually memory and one or more of the following: language, calculation, visual-spatial perception, constructional praxis, judgement, abstraction, and personality change. Dementia of the Alzheimer's type (DAT) comprises at least half of all dementias (see Chap. 29 for a general discussion of dementia).

PREVALENCE

Recent studies have shown that the prevalence of DAT is higher than previously expected.[6, 23] DAT occurs in 10 to 15 percent of people over age 65, 19 percent of people over age 75, and 47 percent of people over age 85. The incidence of DAT increases greatly with increasing age.

ETIOLOGY/RISK FACTORS

The cause of DAT has not been found, although several risk factors have been identified. As can be seen by the statistics listed earlier, increasing age is a risk factor. DAT can be a genetic disorder. A defect associated with chromosome 21 has been found in some families with early-onset DAT, and a defect associated with chromosome 19 has been found in some families with late-onset DAT. However, the lack of 100 percent concordance in studies of identical twins implies that environmental, metabolic, and other factors also may play a role. Head trauma, lack of education, and myocardial infarction have been shown to be risk factors,[14] although the reasons for their being risk factors are not fully understood. Some have postulated that aluminum intoxication, disordered immune function, and viral infection are causes of DAT; however these factors have not yet been proved.[3]

From Black and Matassarin-Jacobs, pp. 773–778.

PATHOPHYSIOLOGY

Alios Alzheimer first described presenile dementia in 1907. He used a new staining technique of human brain tissue to demonstrate the pathology. The changes he noted are now termed *neurofibrillary tangles* and *neuritic plaques* (Figure 31–1). These are abnormal proteins that accumulate in the brain. The neuritic plaque is a cluster of degenerating nerve terminals, both dendritic and axonal, that contains amyloid protein. The precursor of this protein, amyloid precursor protein, is coded by a gene on chromosome 21 and an adjacent "housekeeping" gene that regulates the daily functioning of cells. A hypothesis, based on studies of clients with Down syndrome (who develop the characteristic pathologic features of DAT), proposes that accumulation of amyloid protein leads to DAT.[14] Neurofibrillary tangles are abnormal neurons in which the cytoplasm is filled with bundles of abnormal protein called *paired helical filaments.* Neuritic plaques and neurofibrillary tangles are located in areas of cell loss in the brain of the person with DAT. These areas are the association areas of the neocortex and the hippocampus, which account for the cognitive decline. The term "association" is used to describe all the intellectual activities of the cerebral cortex. These functions include learning and reasoning, memory storage and recall, language abilities, and even consciousness.

In addition to structural changes, there are neurotransmitter changes in the brains of clients with DAT. A decline in cholinergic neurons in the basal nucleus leads to loss of choline acetyltransferase in the neocortex and hippocampus. Also affected are neuronal systems that project to the neocortex: the noradrenergic locus ceruleus and the serotonergic dorsal raphe nucleus in the brain stem. These two areas also contain neurofibrillary tangles. Involved neurons in the neocortex include those using corticotropin-releasing factor, somatostatin, and glutamate.[14]

CLINICAL MANIFESTATIONS

Clinically, Alzheimer's disease is characterized by a relentless impairment of decision making that generally begins insidiously and can progress for a decade or so. The onset of DAT typically occurs in late middle age (age 65 and older), although some familial cases occur in the fifth and sixth decades. The clinical progression of symptoms is usually divided into three stages. The sequence of loss of higher cognitive functions is a helpful clue for establishing the clinical diagnosis. Memory disturbance is usually the first feature of the disease. Family members or co-workers often notice the memory loss before the individual does. The individual may demonstrate poor judgement and problem-solving skills and become careless in work habits and household chores. He or she may do well in familiar surroundings and be able to follow well-established routines but lack the ability to adapt to new challenges. The person may become irritable, suspicious, or indifferent.

In the second stage of illness, the client may demonstrate language disturbance, characterized by impaired word finding and circumlocution (talking around a subject rather than directly about it). Later, spontaneous speech becomes increasingly empty and paraphasias (words used in the wrong context) are used. The person may repeat words and phrases used by him- or herself (palilalia) or others (echolalia). Motor disturbance (apraxia) is characterized by difficulty in using everyday objects like a toothbrush, comb, razor, and utensils. Apraxia combined with forgetfulness can create serious safety problems. The individual may leave a burner on in the kitchen or forget to extinguish a cigarette. Indifference worsens and restlessness with frequent pacing appears. Hyperorality (the desire to take everything into the mouth to suck, chew, or taste) may develop. Swallowing may become difficult. Depression and irritability may worsen, and delusions and psychosis may appear. The person fears personal harm, theft of property, or infidelity of the spouse. He or she may see bugs crawling in the bed or throughout the house. Wandering at night is common. Occasional incontinence may occur.

In the final stage, virtually all mental abilities are lost, including speech. Voluntary movement is minimal, and the limbs become rigid with flexor posturing. Urinary and fecal incontinence is frequent. The person has lost all ability for self-care.

Diagnostic Assessment

Because there is no definitive test for DAT, the diagnosis is made by exclusion of known causes of dementia (e.g., toxic/metabolic alterations, drug side effects, cerebrovascular disease, neoplasm, and infection). Diagnosis of DAT requires the presence of dementia involving two or more areas of cognition, insidious onset, steady progression, and normal alertness.[17] When these criteria are applied, 9 of 10 individuals given this diagnosis have DAT confirmed at autopsy. Postmortem examination of the brain is the only way DAT can be definitively diagnosed. The brain is viewed under the microscope for the presence of neuritic plaques and neurofibrillary tangles.

Diagnostic assessments such as the electroencephalogram (EEG), computerized tomography (CT), and magnetic resonance imaging (MRI) are sometimes used in the diagnosis of DAT. In general, these studies rule out other causes of dementia, such as seizures and cerebral bleeding, but do not diagnose DAT. Changes on EEG, CT, and MRI do not appear until the later stages of DAT. Finally, laboratory studies are currently being performed to assist in the diagnosis of DAT looking at beta-amyloid protein.

MEDICAL MANAGEMENT

There is no cure for DAT. Results of studies in which acetylcholine precursors (choline, lecithin, and deanol) and anticholinesterase agents (physostigmine and tetrahydroaminoacridine) are used to enhance memory and cognitive function have been disappointing. Pharmacologic therapy is primarily aimed at treating behavior problems, although behavioral and environmental manipulations are often more effective (see later). Low-dose antipsychotic agents, like haloperidol, can be effective for agitation and confusion. The lowest effective dose should be used and should be given just before bedtime. Sometimes, twice-a-day dosing is required. Adverse side effects such as akathisia (motor restlessness), parkinsonian symptoms, tardive dyskinesias, orthostatic hypotension, anticholinergic symptoms (urinary retention and confusion), and sedation should be monitored. Antidepressants (e.g., nortriptyline and desipramine) that have few anticholinergic side effects, fluoxetine, and trazadone are helpful for depression.[14]

NURSING MANAGEMENT

Assessment

When DAT is suspected, a complete history should be taken to assess for other causes of dementia. Data should be obtained from the client, family, and co-workers (if possible). Secondary sources are used because the client is often unaware of a problem with thought processing and minimizes it. The nurse should ask specific questions about difficulties with activities of daily living, increasing forgetfulness, and changes in personality. Past medical history should be assessed for previous head injury or surgery, recent falls, headache, and family history of DAT. A mini-mental state examination may provide objective data for ongoing evaluation of the client.

DAT has a profound impact on psychosocial behaviors. The nurse should ask about the client's reactions to changes in routine or in the environment. It is not uncommon for a client with DAT to become very agitated over small changes. Likewise, apathy, social isolation, and irritability may be noted. As the brain continues to atrophy and the limbic system becomes dysfunctional, the client displays paranoia, uses abusive language, and becomes suspicious of others.

DAT also has a profound impact on the family. The nurse needs to assess the family for strengths and weaknesses, the ability to provide care for the client, and financial concerns. In large centers, the assessment of the client and family is performed through a team approach.

Nursing Intervention

Nursing Diagnosis. Communication, Impaired Verbal R/T neuronal degeneration.

Planning: Expected Outcomes. The client's needs will be communicated effectively, as evidenced by making his or her needs known and interacting meaningfully with others.

Implementation. In the initial stage of DAT, the client's receptive and expressive language skills are relatively intact. The nurse must be prepared to adapt to the communication level of the client. If the client speaks only single words or short phrases, the nurse should do likewise. It is best to speak slowly and simply, with firm volume and low pitch. The tone of voice should always be calm and reassuring and project control of the situation. However, when language becomes impaired in the second stage of the illness, the nurse must be prepared to apply new techniques for communicating with the client.

Bartol[2] wrote in 1979 a very useful guide for nurses that is still appropriate today. Nonverbal behavior can provide the nurse with clues. Clients with DAT often avert their eyes, look down, back away, and increase hand gesturing when they do not understand. If they are frustrated, angry, or hostile, they may increase motor activity by pacing, rattling door knobs, waving their arms or shaking their fists, frowning, raising their voice volume and pitch, or tightening their face muscles. These behaviors should signal staff to increase their alertness, search for the cause of the distress, and prepare to intervene. Interventions can include (1) decreasing environmental stimuli, (2) approaching the client calmly and with assurance, (3) taking care not to place any more demands on the client, (4) distracting the client, (5) making sure that all verbal and nonverbal communication cues are concordant, and (6) using multiple sensory modalities (visual, auditory, and tactile) to send the message. The client's memory loss can be an advantage in distracting him or her from the stressful situation. If removed from the situation and provided a calm, nonthreatening environment, the client may forget why he was upset. Bartol suggested that nurses can elicit listening behavior from DAT clients by reaching out and touching, holding a hand, putting an arm around the waist, or in some way maintaining physical contact with the client. Dementia sufferers can perceive nonverbal behavior from others and can become agitated or upset if they sense negative nonverbal behavior from others.

The identification of pain or discomfort in clients with advanced DAT is also difficult. Hurley[12] has developed a tool to facilitate assessment. Behavioral indicators of discomfort include noisy breathing, negative vocalization (constant muttering, making noise with a negative quality), sad or frightened facial expression, frown, tense body language, and fidgeting.

Nursing Diagnosis. Thought Processes, Altered R/T neuronal degeneration.

Planning: Expected Outcomes. The client will have improved thought processing, as evidenced by exhibiting retention of information to maximal capacity, maintaining orientation to maximal capacity, and sharing meaningful life experiences.

Implementation. Because memory deficit occurs in all stages of DAT, the nurse must continually apply interventions to enhance memory. The nurse should reorient the client as necessary by placing a calendar and clock in obvious places. Because DAT clients' long-term memory is retained longer than their short-term memory, the nurse should allow clients to reminisce. The nurse should be aware of a client's past so experiences can be shared meaningfully. Repetition is useful for ensuring maximal retention of information by the client.

Nursing Diagnosis. Injury, High Risk for R/T impaired judgement and forgetfulness.

Planning: Expected Outcomes. The client's physical and environmental safety will be maintained, as evidenced by the absence of physical injury and the existence of a safe living environment.

Implementation. Impaired judgement, forgetfulness, and motor impairment can make any environment unsafe for the client with DAT. In the home, electrical devices, toxic substances, loose rugs, hot tap water, inadequate lighting, and unlocked doors can be sources of injury. Family members should be educated on how to eliminate these safety hazards. In the inpatient setting, nurses should ensure that clients cannot leave the premises without being noticed, that they wear an identification badge in case they become lost, and that doors and windows be secured. Dangerous objects should be kept out of reach, and potentially dangerous activities, like cooking, should be supervised.

Nursing Diagnosis. Self-Care Deficit R/T loss of memory and motor praxis.

Expected Outcomes. The client will have activities of daily living (ADLs) completed, as evidenced by completing the tasks he or she is capable of performing and receiving assistance with ADLs he or she is incapable of performing.

Implementation. The client with DAT should be encouraged to do as much as possible, as long as it is safe and appropriate. The nurse must carefully balance helping the client with maintaining his or her autonomy. This will boost the client's confidence and self-respect, which can be very fragile during the early and middle stages of the disease. The client should be given plenty of time to complete a task. Constant encouragement, urging, and reminding the client in a step-by-step approach is necessary.

Nursing Diagnosis. Incontinence, Urge R/T neuronal degeneration and forgetfulness.

Planning: Expected Outcomes. The client will have optimal continence of bladder and bowel, as evidenced by having clean, dry clothing and bedding as much as possible; having intact skin; and voiding appropriately in the bathroom.

Implementation. DAT clients develop urge incontinence as cortical neurons degenerate and no longer provide inhibition of the micturition and defecation responses. Anticipation of elimination needs and scheduled voiding and defecation times can help in the initial stages. The client may show nonverbal signs of needing to void or defecate, like restlessness, grasping the genital area, or picking at clothing. Sometimes, the client may forget where the bathroom is located. Having clear, bright signs indicating where the bathroom is and frequently taking the client there may help control incontinence. Fluid intake after the dinner meal can be restricted to help maintain continence during the night. A bowel program can be arranged to coincide with the client's usual pattern. In the later stages of DAT, clients may need to wear incontinence pads during the day and external urinary drainage devices at night. Indwelling catheters should be avoided because of the risk of infection and injury.

Nursing Diagnosis. Care Giver Role Strain R/T grieving the loss of a family member to DAT, change in social role, and intense demands for time commitment and provision of care.

Planning: Expected Outcomes. The family will demonstrate decreased role strain, as evidenced by voicing their emotional concerns, seeking appropriate assistance, and providing adequate care for the client.

Implementation. Family members and especially care givers (usually a spouse or adult child) of clients with DAT face a great deal of emotional and physical burden. Family members grieve the loss of the person they used to know. Each decline in cognitive function becomes another source of grief. Jones and Martinson[13] describe two stages of grief in the family. The process of grief begins during the care giving stage and continues after the client's death. Normal family routines are lost, and the relationship between the family member and the dementia sufferer changes. Morris et al.[19] summarized studies of the factors that affect the emotional well being of care givers of dementia sufferers. The behavior problems most likely to be reported by care givers are incontinence, overdemanding behavior, and the need for constant supervision. Wives tend to experience a higher degree of emotional burden as care givers than do husbands. Paradoxically, the closer the emotional bond between care giver and dementia sufferer, the less the strain for the care giver. Conversely, a low past level of intimacy is associated with an increased level of both perceived strain and depression in the spouse care giver. Care givers are most likely to be depressed if they feel a loss of control over their spouse's behavior, if they feel unable to cope with the impact of care giving, and if they perceive the situation to be stable and to affect everything. Studies have not determined that formal support of the care giver (home visits by special practitioners, chore workers, and day care) relieves the care giver's burden more than informal support (family member visits and support groups). The Alzheimer's Disease and Related Disorders Association has local chapters that offer support groups in many major cities in the United States. The toll free number is 1-800-272-3900 for information on nearby local chapters.

A variety of options are available to care givers. Chore service workers can help with household chores and relieve the care giver of these duties. Other paid help can provide in-home respite care by observing the dementia sufferer while the care giver tends to business outside the home, seeks social interaction, or meets recreational needs. Adult day care provides time away from home for the dementia sufferer. Day care usually offers a lunchtime meal as well as several hours of scheduled activities that are tailored to the client's abilities. These activities may include games, crafts, music, and exercise. Respite care involves admission to an extended care facility for a few days to a few weeks to allow the care giver time to recover from the demands of providing 24-hour care. Nursing home care is usually the final, and most difficult and trying, option for a care giver. This decision creates guilt, self-doubt, and anxiety. However, it is often the only option when the care giver suffers burnout and becomes unable to provide adequate care.

When the person with DAT reaches the terminal stage of illness, questions about end-of-life treatments arise. Should a feeding tube be used to provide nourishment? Should antibiotics be used to treat pneumonias or other infections? Should cardiopulmonary resuscitation be used? Ideally, decisions about these questions are raised and discussed with the client, before he or she loses decisional capacity, and with family members. Two forms of advance directives (means of expressing one's wishes about life-sustaining treatment after losing mental capacity to make informed decisions) are available. One is the living will, a written document, signed by the individual (while he or she is still mentally capable of making informed decisions) in the presence of a witness, that lists conditions under which the person wishes life-sustaining treatments to be withheld or withdrawn. The other is a durable power of attorney for health care. This is a legal document in which the individual (while still mentally capable) assigns a person to act on his or her behalf in matters of health care decisions if the individual loses decisional capacity (e.g., becomes demented).

Evaluation

The nurse continually evaluates the degree of expected outcome attainment. In the case of the client with DAT, this includes evaluation of outcomes focused on improving verbal communication; facilitating memory; preventing injury; enhancing self-care; maintaining continence; and, perhaps most important, bolstering care giver and family coping strategies. Most of the nursing care of persons with DAT is provided in an outpatient setting or in a nursing home.

POST-HOSPITAL CARE

Discharge Teaching

Family members should be interviewed to determine their understanding of the diagnosis and prognosis of DAT and to allow them to discuss their concerns about caring for the client. Do they know about community resources? Do they have someone to call when they can no longer cope with care giving? The home environment should be evaluated before the client is sent home from the hospital to ascertain safety issues (see Bridge to Home Health Care). Is the home on a busy street? Can doors be secured so that the client cannot get out without supervision? Are potentially dangerous appliances out of reach?

• SUMMARY

Directions. In the space provided, rewrite the above selection in your own words, focusing on the main ideas and major details.

• COMPREHENSION QUESTIONS

Directions. Below are 10 multiple-choice questions. Circle the letter of the best answer from the four choices.

1 The primary feature of Alzheimer's disease is:

a appetite loss
b memory loss
c weight loss
d aging

2 Alzheimer's disease is:

a reversible
b irreversible
c cured by environmental factors
d the leading cause of death in the United States

3 Dementia is:

a a deterioration in intellectual functioning
b an increase in intellectual functioning
c unrelated to intellect
d always caused by infection

4 Dementia of the Alzheimer's type are:
a 15% of the population
b 75% of the people older than 65 years of age
c 50% of all dementias
d 47% of people older than 75 years of age

5 Indications of Alzheimer's disease often appear during:
a young adult years
b old age
c middle age
d late middle age

6 The cause of Alzheimer's disease is:
a unknown
b environmental hazards
c dehydration
d depression

7 Alzheimer's disease is:
a a sudden decline
b a progressive disorder
c stable
d not life threatening

8 The patient can usually function independently:
a during the first stage of Alzheimer's disease
b during the second stage of Alzheimer's disease
c during the third stage of Alzheimer's disease
d after recovering from Alzheimer's disease

9 The final option for the care of patients with Alzheimer's disease is usually:
a physicians
b family members
c nursing homes
d hospital administrators

10 Pharmacologic therapy for the patient with Alzheimer's disease is aimed primarily at:
a curing the patient
b treating behavior problems
c eliminating behavior problems
d eliminating depression

• CRITICAL THINKING/EVALUATION

Were you successful in applying active reading strategies to this selection? Explain.

____

____

____

____

Reading Selection II

• PREVIEW QUESTION

What is an advantage of open heart surgery?

• VOCABULARY

Underline any medical terminology or general vocabulary words you may need to learn in order to understand the ideas in this reading selection.

Cardiac Surgery

Cardiac surgery is performed when the probability of survival with a useful life is greater with surgical treatment than with nonsurgical treatment. The first heart surgery was performed in 1923 by Cutler and Levine.[27] That procedure was repair of a stenosed mitral valve. Since that time, heart surgery has been revolutionized by the development of open-heart techniques that allow surgeons to visualize the heart directly while they explore, incise, repair, and suture. These improved operating conditions have enabled today's surgeons to replace diseased valves with prosthetic valves, repair severe congenital lesions, and perform heart transplants. Today, under ideal conditions, cardiac surgery should have a hospital mortality approaching zero. However, a description of the results of cardiac surgery by hospital mortality alone is not sufficient. The preoperative condition of the client's heart and other body systems greatly influences the results of cardiac surgery. The identification of incremental risk factors will continue to improve results.

TYPES OF HEART SURGERY

There are three types of cardiac surgery: (1) reparative, (2) reconstructive, and (3) substitutional. Reparative surgeries are likely to produce cure or excellent and prolonged improvement. These operations include closure of patent ductus arteriosus, atrial septal defect, and ventricular septal defect; repair of mitral stenosis; and simple repair of tetralogy of Fallot. Reconstructive procedures are more complex. They are not always curative procedures, and reoperation may be needed. Reconstructive procedures include coronary artery by-pass grafting and reconstruction of an incompetent mitral, tricuspid, or aortic valve. Substitutional surgeries are not usually curative because of the preoperative condition of the client. Examples of substitutional surgeries include valve replacement, cardiac replacement by transplantation, ventricular replacement or assistance, and cardiac replacement by mechanical devices.

VALVULAR SURGERY

The repair or replacement of cardiac valves with acquired stenosis or incompetence is not considered curative, but generally good and long-lasting palliation results. Cure is usually unable to be obtained because of the preoperative condition of the heart or other body systems. Indications for surgery include

- progressive impairment of cardiac function due to scarring and thickening of the valve with either (1) impaired narrowing of the valvular opening (stenosis) or (2) incomplete closure (insufficiency, regurgitation)
- gradual enlargement of the heart with symptoms of decreased activity, shortness of breath, and congestive heart failure.

Surgical therapy for mitral valve stenosis can include valve commissurotomy or valve replacement. Commissurotomy or valve reconstruction can be accomplished if the preoperative assessment indicates that the valve is quite pliable. If the valve is nonpliable, valve replacement is necessary. In clients with mitral regurgitation, valve reconstruction or annuloplasty may be done. This may include the use of a flexible ring that is sewn into the valve for stabilization. Clients experiencing aortic stenosis may be surgically treated with valve replacement or balloon aortic valvuloplasty. The valvuloplasty procedure uses a catheter with a balloon to dilate the valve orifice.[4] Surgical treatment for the client with aortic regurgitation is not always the treatment of choice but may be considered.

Artificial cardiac valves are continuing to show improvements in design, safety, function, and durability. Mechanical and tissue prosthetic valves are currently available. The type of valve prosthesis used is based on a number of considerations. The surgeon primarily considers the client's tolerance of anticoagulation and the dura-

---

From Black and Matassarin-Jacobs, pp. 1238–1242.

bility of the valve. Clients with mechanical valves require continuous anticoagulation therapy for the remainder of their lives. Therefore, if the client has a preoperative history of bleeding or noncompliance with pharmacologic regimens, the surgeon may decide to use a tissue valve. The overall advantages and disadvantages of tissue and mechanical valves are almost equal. The mechanical valves are very durable but require anticoagulant therapy; the tissue valves may not require anticoagulation therapy but are less durable. Some physicians generally recommend mechanical valves in clients under 65 or 70 years of age and tissue valves in clients 70 years or older.[7]

Potential complications of heart valves include a risk of thrombus formation, especially in mechanical valves. Newer types of heart valves have reduced rates of thrombus. Most clients require long-term anticoagulation. The major risk with tissue valves is durability. The leaflets of these valves may degenerate, calcify, or develop structural abnormalities. Mitral valves tend to fail most often because of the higher stress on the valve. The rate of tissue valve failure is 2 to 5 per cent for the first 6 years, and then the rate accelerates. Almost every client with a tissue valve will require replacement eventually.[51]

Management of the client after heart surgery is discussed later in this section.

HEART TRANSPLANTATION

Cardiac transplantation is now a standard and effective treatment for clients with end-stage cardiac disease. The clinical use of transplantation is now in its third decade. The first successful human heart transplant was performed in 1967 in South Africa by Dr. Christiaan Barnard. Much publicity and discussion throughout the world has surrounded heart transplantation since that time. Between 1967 and 1970, about 150 heart transplantations were performed with a dismal 85 per cent mortality rate.[73] Almost all institutions stopped performing the operation for several years while advances in the laboratory continued.

In the 1980s, heart transplants were being performed on a routine basis (see Ethical Issues in Nursing). The survival rate has improved dramatically as a result of advances in technique and better control of the rejection process. At Stanford University, the mean life expectancy for clients awaiting transplantation (surgery not performed) is about 3 months. More than 80 per cent of clients who receive transplanted hearts survive for at least 1 year. Approximately 60 per cent of these clients are alive at 5 years. Another important statistic is that 85 per cent of those 1-year survivors have been rehabilitated and have returned to work or school.

Technique. The current orthotopic technique for heart transplant retains a large portion of the right and left atrium in the recipient and implants the donor heart to the atria. Cardiopulmonary bypass is used during the operation. Temporary pacemaker wires and chest drainage catheters are inserted.

Another type of heart transplant is the heterotopic transplant. In this form the donor heart is placed parallel to the recipient's heart. The right side of the client's heart can continue to function while the dysfunctional left side of the heart is bypassed.

THE ARTIFICIAL HEART

The artificial heart is a commercially made device implanted in place of the failing heart. These hearts are made of rubber, silicone, and Teflon and are air-powered through a life-support console. The artificial heart is attached surgically in an operation similar to that described in the heart transplant procedure. Major complications (hemorrhage, infection, acute tubular necrosis, and neurologic disturbances) have been frequently encountered, and the permanent use of the artificial heart is currently not recommended. There is some use of the artificial heart as a bridge to transplantation, helping patients survive until a donor heart can be transplanted.

The greatest single problem in performing heart transplants is not the surgical procedure itself but the rejection process by which the client's body rejects the donor heart. Allograft rejection, discussed in Chapter 24, remains poorly understood. The recipient forms antibodies against the foreign heart tissue, which leads to an antigen-antibody reaction. As a result, the heart's lining hemorrhages, walls thicken, and myocardium assumes a mottled appearance. Because of rejection, the new heart fails to function altogether, and circulatory collapse ensues.

MEDICAL MANAGEMENT

Clients may enter the health care facility a few days before surgery for a thorough medical evaluation. Preoperative laboratory tests include urine tests and blood electrolytes, enzymes, and coagulation studies. Important diagnostic studies that give valuable information about cardiac status include the ECG, phonocardiogram, echocardiogram, vectorcardiogram, chest x-ray films, and cardiac catheterization.

Any physiologic imbalance or problem in cardiac or respiratory status is corrected when possible by means of rest, diet, medication, or other appropriate therapy. Physiologic baselines should be established for postoperative comparison of vital signs, weight, and laboratory values.

• SUMMARY

Directions. In the space provided, rewrite the above selection in your own words, focusing on the main ideas and major details.

• COMPREHENSIVE QUESTIONS

Directions. Below are 10 multiple-choice questions. Circle the letter of the best answer from the four choices.

1 Open heart surgery allows the surgeon to:
  a always cure the patient's heart problems
  b prevent any recurrence of heart disease
  c prevent the spread of disease
  d directly visualize the heart during the operation

2 The first heart surgery was performed in:
  a 1967
  b 1923
  c 1970
  d 1980

3 The first successful human heart transplant was performed by:
  a Dr. Cutter
  b Dr. Levine
  c Dr. Barnard
  d doctors at Stanford University

4 ECG is:
  a open heart surgery
  b a treatment for reversing heart disease
  c a diagnostic study about cardiac status
  d an anesthetic used only during heart surgery

5 The number of types of heart surgery is:
a 3
b 2
c 4
d 1

6 The type of surgeries that are likely to produce a cure or excellent improvement are:
a substitutional
b transplantation
c reconstructive
d reparative

7 An example of reconstructive surgery is:
a repair of mistral stenosis
b coronary artery bypass grafting
c valve replacement
d cardiac replacement by mechanical devices

8 The percentage of clients who survive for at least 1 year after a heart transplant is:
a 80
b 60
c 85
d 50

9 The greatest problem in performing heart transplant is:
a the surgical procedure
b the patient's age
c surgical error
d the rejection process

10 A complication that results from the artificial heart is:
a hemorrhage
b donors
c mechanical failure
d age of patient

• CRITICAL THINKING/EVALUATION

Were you successful in applying active reading strategies to this selection? Explain.

____

____

____

____

Reading Selection 12

• PREVIEW QUESTION

Who would be especially prone to hip fractures?

• VOCABULARY

Underline any medical terminology or general vocabulary words you may need to learn in order to understand the ideas in this reading selection.

Management of Specific Fractures

HIP FRACTURES

Definition

Hip fractures are generally divided into three types: (1) femoral neck, (2) intertrochanteric, and (3) subtrochanteric (Fig. VI–10). Fractures of the femoral neck and intertrochanteric regions constitute 97 per cent of hip fractures.[14]

Incidence

Hip fractures are the leading traumatic injury in the elderly, and with degenerative arthritis increasing in frequency with age, hip surgery is a very common orthopedic procedure. In 1980, 267,000 hip fractures were reported in the United States; 90 per cent of these fractures occurred in clients over 65 years of age. This figure is expected to rise to 500,000 per year by the early 1990's.[14]

Etiology

Hip fractures result from two major changes seen with aging. The most significant loss in the aged is the loss of postural stability, leading to an increased incidence of falls. The amount of bone mass has been shown to be equal in clients who fall and age-matched controls. This leads to the conclusion that falling is the more significant etiology.

Decreased bone mass does contribute to hip fractures, however. Bone mass decreases linearly with age. The combination of decreased bone mass and tendency toward falls explains why the incidence of hip fracture doubles every 5 years after the age of 50.

From Black and Matassarin-Jacobs, pp. 1923–1927.

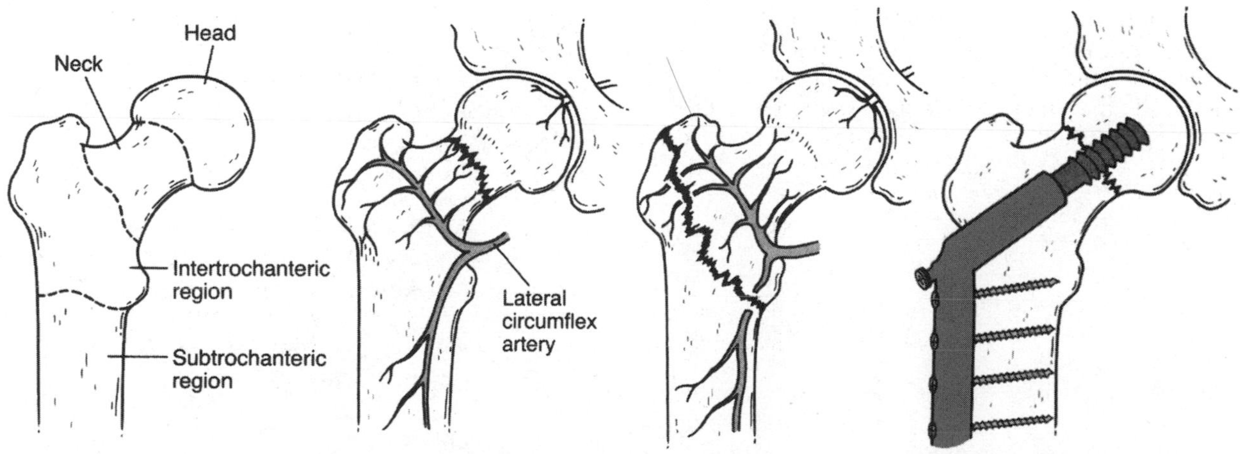

Figure VI–10 *A*, Normal proximal end of the femur. *B*, Intracapsular fracture of the proximal end of the femur. Note the blood supply. *C*, Extracapsular intertrochanteric fracture. Note the effect of the fracture on the blood supply. *D*, Femoral neck fracture with a compression screw inserted for reduction. (Reprinted with permission from Black, J.M. and Matassarin-Jacobs, E.: Luckmann and Sorensen's Medical-Surgical Nursing: A Psychophysiologic Approach, 4th ed. Philadelphia, W.B. Saunders, 1993.)

Pathophysiology

The pathophysiology of fracture injury was discussed earlier in this chapter.

Femoral neck fractures are often called the unsolved fracture because there is a significant failure rate after primary fixation.[14] For the most part, complications are due to the anatomic features of the proximal femur. The femoral neck and head lie entirely within the joint capsule and, therefore, have no periosteum. Secondly, the arterial supply to the femoral head is usually disrupted by fracture fragments. These facts often lead to nonunion and avascular necrosis (tissue death due to a lack of blood supply) of the femoral head.

Intertrochanteric fractures are usually comminuted and more osteoporotic, leading to difficulty with good anatomic reduction of the fragments and fixation. Because this section of bone has a periosteum and the vascular supply is not affected, avascular necrosis and nonunion are uncommon complications.

Clinical Manifestations

The client or family reports a history of a fall. Even accidents that seem relatively minor, such as slipping out of a chair onto the floor, can produce hip fracture in the aged. Objective findings include a shortened, externally rotated hip and sometimes deformity along the lateral side of the hip. There may also be ecchymosis and tissue trauma from the fall. Other sites of tissue trauma may also be present, such as forehead or hand lacerations.

Diagnostic Assessment

Hip fracture is confirmed by x-ray study. Other diagnostic tests may be used to assess the client's readiness for surgery and anesthesia. A complete blood count, electrolyte levels, urinalysis, chest x-ray study, and electrocardiogram are the most common tests.

Medical Management

Treatment plans vary depending on the type of fracture, other injuries sustained during the fall, and concurrent medical conditions. While the client is being stabilized for surgery, perhaps with blood transfusions or correction of underlying disorders such as heart failure, skin traction is commonly applied to the leg. Traction assists to realign the fractures and reduce muscle spasms in the extremity. In general, the client is taken for surgical repair quickly, because placing an elderly person at bed rest increases the risks of immobility.

The number of disorders the client has (concomitant illnesses) increases the risk of morbidity and mortality with hip fracture. Nursing home residents with hip fractures are at increased risk of perioperative complications. These clients often have preoperative limitations in mobility and can seldom return to any form of ambulation. Because of the limited progress clients can make and their surgical risk, sometimes hip fractures in these clients are not surgically repaired.

Surgical Management

The primary goal of surgery is to provide a solid union of fracture sites to allow for early weight bearing and functional recovery.

Femoral Neck Fractures. Four surgical procedures are common to repair femoral neck fractures: (1) a Knowles pin; (2) a Jewett nail; (3) a sliding nail or compression screw; and (4) hemiarthroplasty or total hip arthroplasty. Following fixation with a Knowles pin, full weight bearing is not allowed because the pin does not pull the fracture fragments together (a process called compression). The Jewett nail also does not provide compression of the fragments, but it is a stronger device and the client can usually bear weight after surgery. The compression screw is the most commonly used device and has an advantage of drawing the fracture fragments together. The alignment of the fractures increases healing and allows for weight bearing. A hemiarthroplasty, with replacement of the femoral component of the hip with a noncemented metallic prosthesis, can be performed. This procedure allows the client to have full weight bearing. But when the hip prosthesis is used, there is a risk of postoperative dislocation. Because of the problems with nonunion after hip fracture, a complete hip replacement can also be performed.

Intertrochanteric Fractures. The most widely used device for repair of intertrochanteric fractures is the sliding nail or compression screw. Following surgery, clients cannot bear weight. These clients also have a poorer functional outcome and higher mortality than clients with fractures of the femoral neck.

Postoperative Complications. There are several complications that can result from both the surgery and the postoperative immobility; three will be discussed here. They include deep vein thrombosis, pressure ulcers, and delirium.

DEEP VEIN THROMBOSIS

The incidence of deep vein thrombosis in clients not receiving prophylaxis is reported to be 40 to 60 per cent following hip surgery. Because approximately 20 per cent of clients with deep vein thrombosis develop pulmonary embolus, the prevention of thrombosis is essential. Measures to decrease the risk of deep vein thrombosis include the use of aspirin, heparin, warfarin, low molecular weight dextran, and external pneumatic compression devices. Antiembolism stockings are also commonly used.

PRESSURE ULCERS

Pressure ulcers occur in 20 to 70 per cent of clients following hip fracture. It should be recognized that significant pressure has often been applied to the skin before the client is admitted to the nursing unit, from lying on a hard floor or hard surfaces in ambulances and emergency departments and x-ray departments. Prevention of ongoing ischemia is critical and can be accomplished by decreasing the risk of pressure through the use of eggcrate mattresses, excellent skin care, early ambulation, and elevation of the heels from the bed with rolled towels. Identification of high-risk clients can be made through the use of assessment tools such as the Braden tool, presented in Chapter 18.

DELIRIUM

Postoperative confusion usually occurs in response to systemic stressors rather than the result of central nervous system disorders. Medications, infection, impaction, and hypoxemia are common causes of delirium.

REHABILITATION

Physical therapists teach the client how to ambulate, and most clients are moved to a chair the day after surgery. Eventual recovery of clients after the repair of hip fractures is influenced by premorbid dementia, preoperative immobility, presence of intertrochanteric fracture, and advanced age.[1] Several large series report that of clients surviving 1 year after a fracture, only 50 per cent achieve prefracture functional status.[14]

Nursing Management

Assessment

On admission, the client is usually weighed before being placed in bed. A complete assessment is performed, including the assessment of abrasions or other injuries from the fall.

Nursing Diagnosis. Physical Mobility, Impaired R/T prescribed limitations in movement and pain.

PLANNING: EXPECTED OUTCOMES

The client will maintain adequate strength to regain physical mobility once able to ambulate, as evidenced by performing exercises while bedridden, transferring to the chair with decreasing need for assistance once ambulatory, and walking with a walker safely.

IMPLEMENTATION

The client is encouraged to perform various exercises for the upper and lower extremities. A trapeze is placed above the bed to facilitate upper arm and shoulder strength. Exercises such as quadriceps setting, gluteal setting, and leg movements up and down in bed maintain some muscle strength. Passive and active range-of-motion exercises should also be implemented.

When the client is allowed to be in the chair, the nurse assists the client to the edge of the bed while keeping the legs abducted. The client is assisted by at least two nurses to stand and then balance with the walker. The degree of weight bearing that the client can safely use must be reinforced as the client stands. If the client is unable to stand, a complete lift is usually performed to assist the client to the chair.

Collaborative Problem. High risk for dislocation of the hip R/T inappropriate stress on the joint and surrounding tissues.

PLANNING: EXPECTED OUTCOMES

The nurse will monitor the client for clinical manifestations of hip dislocation and position the client to decrease the risk of dislocation.

IMPLEMENTATION

Handle the operated leg gently following hip surgery. Before moving the client, explain what is going to happen and how the client can help. An overbed trapeze helps with moving. Teach the client how to use the trapeze. Avoid extremes of position following hip surgery. Keep the leg abducted, i.e., out to the side, at all times. Never adduct the leg past the body's midline (e.g., over the other leg), or the head of the femur (or prosthesis) may dislocate out of the acetabulum. Place a pillow or A-frame between the client's legs to help maintain abduction and to remind the client not to cross the legs.

Avoid acute flexion of the operated hip. This can be caused by excessive elevation of the head of the bed. Check the physician's instructions about how high the head of the bed can be safely elevated. Some can have the head of the bed raised 35 to 40 degrees. If the head of the bed can be somewhat elevated, instruct the client not to lean farther forward, because this practice further flexes the hip and may cause dislocation.

Prevent external rotation of the leg on the operated side by placing a trochanter roll beside the external aspect of the thigh. Without this intervention, the operated leg may tend to lie slightly externally rotated when the person is supine.

Turn the client only with the physician's order following hip surgery. Commonly after hip surgery the client can be turned to the unoperated side. Following hip pinning, some people are permitted to turn to either side. However, after other types of hip surgery, such as total hip replacement, turning is not permitted for several days. When helping a client to turn following internal fixation, (1) avoid adduction of the operated leg and excessive movement, (2) prevent strain on the hip, and (3) keep the leg and hip in proper alignment. If the client is permitted to turn onto the operated side, roll the client gently toward you after placing pillows between the legs. The bed acts as a splint for the injured leg. If it is not permitted to turn to either side, the client may be able to lift straight up off the bed by using a trapeze for back care and linen changes.

Commonly following an anterior surgical approach, the operated limb is positioned so it is internally rotated and in a neutral or an abducted position. The individual may be permitted to sit up unless the capsule has been removed. With a posterior approach the operated leg is positioned in slight abduction and external rotation (a change from "typical" positioning) and the client lies fairly flat.

Do not position the bed too low when a client is getting up after hip surgery. Less hip strain and bending occur if the bed is somewhat elevated. Be sure the bed is locked so it will not move while the client is getting up. For the same reasons, elevated toilet seats are needed following hip surgery once the client can go to the bathroom.

Usually when a client first gets up in a chair following hip surgery, the operated leg is kept extended, well supported, and elevated. Once the operated leg may be lowered, the client should sit with hips even with knees. Tell the client not to cross the legs but to keep both feet on the floor. Crossing the legs adducts the operated leg and can dislocate the hip. The first few times the leg is lowered, assess for swelling and discoloration.

Collaborative Problem. High risk for compartment syndrome R/T leg edema and bleeding.

PLANNING: EXPECTED OUTCOMES

The nurse will monitor the client for clinical manifestations of compartment syndrome.

IMPLEMENTATION

The nurse monitors the color, capillary refill, warmth, movement, sensation, pedal pulses, and ability to dorsiplantar flex the operative leg using the nonoperative leg as a control. Clinical manifestations of compartment syndrome include pallor, pulselessness, paresthesias, pain, and paralysis of the leg. These findings must be reported to the physician immediately. Compartment syndrome was discussed earlier.

Nursing Diagnoses. Pain R/T trauma and surgical repair of a fractured hip.

PLANNING: EXPECTED OUTCOMES

The client will experience improved comfort, as evidenced by less facial grimacing and guarding with movement, ability to transfer to the chair or ambulate without reports of pain, and using a decreasing amount of narcotics for pain relief.

IMPLEMENTATION

Most surgical and traumatic pain is managed with narcotic analgesics until the pain subsides somewhat. Usually within 3 to 4 days, less potent narcotics and non-narcotic analgesics are used for pain relief.

The treatment of clients with discomfort from lying in one position (supine) can be decreased by placing a small folded bath towel beneath the lumbar spine and by moving the legs slightly in bed.

EPIDURAL ANALGESIA

Some clients are being pain managed with epidural narcotics. Epidural narcotics relieve most or all of the pain but carry some significant side effects. If the client is receiving epidural narcotics, the nurse must closely monitor the client for respiratory depression, hypotension, loss of motion and sensation in the legs, and infection at the catheter site. Before ambulating a client with an epidural infusion, the nurse closely assesses for sensation by asking about numbness and by touching the client's legs with an alcohol wipe. The ability to lift the legs from the bed is also assessed. Once the client is moved to the chair, the blood pressure measurement should be reassessed to detect orthostatic hypotension. Clients with epidural anesthetics have decreased venous return due to the lack of muscle activity in the legs. They can very quickly develop orthostasis and faint.

Nursing Diagnosis. Constipation, High Risk for R/T side effects of narcotics and immobility.

PLANNING: EXPECTED OUTCOMES

The client will decrease risk of constipation by consuming high-fiber and bulk foods, adequate fluids, and having a bowel movement every 2 to 3 days.

IMPLEMENTATION

The nurse determines the client's usual defecation pattern and monitors for the return of bowel sounds after surgery. Once the client is eating, foods with fiber such as bran and prunes should be encouraged. Some clients find that hot fluids such as coffee stimulate the bowels. Bowel programs should be instituted in the morning after breakfast because the gastrocolic reflex is strongest at that time. Docusate sodium (Colace) and other stool softeners are commonly prescribed. In addition, the client may require suppositories or enemas to maintain a normal bowel movement schedule. When possible, the client should be placed on a bedside commode to facilitate moving the bowels.

Evaluation

The degree of expected outcome attainment is assessed frequently, usually daily. Some of the expected outcomes for mobility may require extended periods of time to accomplish, depending on the status of the client before surgery.

Post-Hospital Care

Discharge Teaching

Since many of the clients with fractured hips are covered by Medicare, their hospital stay is very short and only a portion of rehabilitation can be accomplished. Finding a location for ongoing rehabilitation is a collaborative effort among all members of the health care team, the client, and family.

Many clients benefit from transfer to an extended care facility, where they can complete their rehabilitation. Ochs[14] questions whether the clients see as much benefit when transferred to a community nursing home where little rehabilitation is offered. Many clients remain as nursing home residents after a year because rehabilitation was incomplete and the client cannot maintain self-care.

Follow-Up Care

At the time of dismissal, most clients cannot walk more than a few feet and transfer from bed to chair or wheelchair. In addition to ongoing rehabilitation, these clients need complete care to provide food, hygiene, and other needs for daily living. If the client is sent home, the nurse and social worker ascertain that the client's family can safely move the client and that other activities of daily living are provided for the client.

• SUMMARY

Directions. In the space provided, rewrite the above section in your own words, focusing on the main ideas and major details.

• COMPREHENSION QUESTIONS

Directions. Below are 10 multiple-choice questions. Circle the letter of the best answer from the four choices.

1 97% of hip fractures are:
- **a** femoral neck
- **b** femoral neck and intertrochanteric
- **c** intertrochanteric regions
- **d** subtrochanteric

2 Even minor accidents can cause a fractured hip in:
- **a** babies
- **b** teenagers
- **c** elderly people
- **d** women of all ages

3 Letter D in Figure VI–10 depicts:
- **a** anatomic regions
- **b** osteoporosis
- **c** complications of surgery
- **d** compression screen

4 The goal of surgery is:
- **a** 100% recovery
- **b** functional recovery
- **c** delayed healing
- **d** delayed weight bearing

5 Clients with deep vein thrombosis may develop:
- **a** urinary tract infection
- **b** sharp hip pain
- **c** pulmonary embolus
- **d** dislocation

6 After a hip fracture the percent of clients who achieve prefracture function status is:
- **a** 30%
- **b** 50%
- **c** 70%
- **d** 85%

7 Following hip surgery a patient should be turned:
- **a** routinely
- **b** every few days
- **c** only at the patient's request
- **d** only at the doctor's request

8 A common procedure to repair femoral neck fractures is with a:
- **a** Jewett nail
- **b** plate
- **c** graft
- **d** hip prosthesis

9 The patient may become discouraged after hip surgery because of:
- **a** swelling of the lower leg
- **b** difficult exercises
- **c** slow healing
- **d** foot pain

10 After surgery the hip may become dislocated by:
- **a** staying in bed
- **b** acute hip flexion
- **c** placing a pillow between the patient's legs
- **d** using an overbed trapeze

• CRITICAL THINKING/EVALUATION

Were you successful in applying active reading strategies to this selection? Explain.

Reading Selection 13

• PREVIEW QUESTION

What are possible side effects of strong analgesics?

• VOCABULARY

Underline any medical terminology or general vocabulary words you may need to learn in order to understand the ideas in this reading selection.

Strong Opiate (Narcotic) Analgesics. Opiates are generally used when other methods of pain relief are not feasible, have failed, or the pain is moderate to severe. Although physical dependence and tolerance can occur when potent analgesics are given, this does not mean that these medications should be withheld. Tolerance and physical dependence are very unlikely to occur in short-term pain therapy.

Examples of opiate analgesics are morphine and various morphine-like agents, such as opiate agonists. Agonists are opiates that stimulate the activities of selected pain receptor sites. Antagonists are drugs that counteract both the CNS and analgesic effects of opiates. Some drugs are combinations of agonists and antagonists, such as butorphanol (Stadol) and pentazocine (Talwin). The morphine-like drugs differ from morphine only in individual characteristics such as rate of onset, duration of action, route of administration, adverse side effects, and chemical configuration.

NARCOTIC AGENTS

The pharmacologic action of all opiate agonists is similar to those of their parent compound, morphine. They all share certain desirable and undesirable characteristics.

NARCOTIC ANTAGONISTS

A pure antagonist, naloxone, reverses the effects of narcotics, both side effects and analgesia. It has no agonist effects, that is, it produces no analgesia or CNS depression. This drug would be used only to counteract against an overdose of a narcotic.

NARCOTIC AGONIST-ANTAGONISTS

The combined agonist-antagonist drugs act in two ways. When they are given following long-term use of narcotics, they will reverse the narcotic and can precipitate acute withdrawal. When the combination agents are given alone, they produce analgesia and the positive effects of opioids without as many side effects. They are less likely to produce respiratory depression, although many of them are more likely to produce psychomimetic effects.

METHADONE

Methadone is a potent, long-acting narcotic analgesic that gained popularity in the management of cancer pain before the development of the newer long-acting forms of morphine. Unlike most morphine preparations, methadone has a long plasma half-life. This long plasma half-life, when repeated doses are given, may account for methadone's longer duration of analgesic action. The long plasma half-life of methadone also poses certain problems. Elderly clients and individuals with compromised hepatic and renal function should be monitored closely for signs of overdosage. The long plasma half-life also necessitates close monitoring of any client receiving repeated doses of this medication because cumulative effects develop. If the client becomes oversedated, the dosage should be reduced or the intervals between administration lengthened.

Complications of Opiate Analgesics. Respiratory depression, one complication of narcotic analgesic therapy, is caused by diminished sensitivity of the respiratory center to carbon dioxide. All narcotics can potentially produce respiratory depression, but this does not have to be a life-threatening problem, because this effect can be rapidly reversed with a narcotic antagonist. This potential problem should not interfere in any way with the proper use of narcotics to relieve pain in clients of all ages. The development of respiratory depression is not necessarily dose related because even lesser amounts of a narcotic may produce respiratory depression. The problem is related more to individual differences and the type of pain being experienced rather than the medication used. Narcotic agonist-antagonists cause respiratory depression to a lesser degree than do narcotics. Narcotic antagonists, such

From Black and Matassarin-Jacobs, pp. 341–342.

as butorphanol and nalbuphine, also cause respiratory depression, although the extent of respiratory depression is limited. Rather than limit the use of narcotic analgesics, the nurse must carefully assess each client after giving the pain medication for the occurrence of any side effects.

Deaths that occur secondary to narcotic poisoning are usually due to respiratory depression. With morphine, maximal respiratory depression usually occurs within 7 minutes of intravenous administration, within 30 minutes of intramuscular administration, and within 90 minutes of subcutaneous administration.[95] It is very important to remember these time ranges when assessing the client's respiratory status following administration of narcotics. For poisoning to occur, however, doses well above the therapeutic level would have to be given.

Treatments for respiratory depression include arousing the client, establishing a patent airway, administering an opiate antagonist such as naloxone, and providing artificial ventilation as necessary.

Circulatory depression is a second complication of opiate analgesics. In a supine client, therapeutic dosages of morphine or synthetic opioids have very little effect on blood pressure and cardiac rate or rhythm. However, some clients experience orthostatic hypotension when moving from a supine position to a head-up or standing position. This hypotension is secondary to a direct dilating action on the peripheral blood vessels caused by the opiates, which reduces the capacity of the cardiovascular system to respond to gravitational shifts. Avoid abrupt body position changes in clients who have received opiates. For this reason, opiates are used very cautiously in clients with decreased blood volume.

Opiates may precipitate *nausea and vomiting* owing to their action on the brain stem centers. Morphine-like drugs also affect the vestibular system, which also can produce these symptoms. Changing the type of opiate used may stop the side effect, or the addition of an antiemetic agent may help.

Constipation, another complication of morphine and other opiates, results from increased smooth muscle tone and decreased motility of the gastrointestinal tract. Opiates diminish the propulsive peristaltic contractions in the small and large intestine and delay the passage of gastric contents through the duodenum. Tolerance does not develop to constipation as it does to the other side effects of opiates. Clients taking opiate analgesics need to follow some type of bowel regimen to prevent constipation. A diet high in roughage with plenty of fluids and stool-softening medications (such as Colace or Pericolace) is common prophylactic treatment. It is better to prevent constipation than to begin treatment after it develops.

Paresthesias may complicate the use of intramuscular opiate analgesics. The intramuscular injection of analgesic agents is generally not irritating to the local tissues. However, two exceptions are meperidine and methadone. Subcutaneous methadone may cause local tissue irritation. Both subcutaneous and intramuscular meperidine cause local tissue irritation and induration, and frequent administration can lead to severe fibrosis of muscle tissue.

If any analgesic is deposited in the region of a nerve when it is injected intramuscularly, paresthesia and paresis may result along the course of the nerve. Proper injection techniques prevent nerve injury.

Physical dependence, another complication of opiate analgesics, is defined as the altered physiologic state produced by repeated administration of a drug. When the drug is stopped abruptly, physiologic symptoms of withdrawal occur. Continued administration of the drug is necessary to prevent withdrawal syndrome. Physical dependence on opioids can develop as well as dependence on other substances such as alcohol, barbiturates, and nicotine.

Physical dependence is not an addiction, but it is an involuntary physiologic response that is an expected effect of the drug when it is taken for a time and then stopped. The nurse must observe the client for these physiologic symptoms. Gradual withdrawal of the medication can usually prevent this response.

Clients who receive a therapeutic dose of morphine several times a day develop some physical dependency in approximately 2 weeks. This means that if morphine were suddenly discontinued, a withdrawal syndrome would occur. Assessment findings that indicate a withdrawal syndrome include diarrhea, lacrimation, sweating, dilated pupils, restlessness, tremor, and anorexia. Most symptoms, if untreated, subside in 5 to 10 days. Withdrawal symptoms can be avoided by gradually (over 1 to 2 weeks) reducing and, finally, by discontinuing a client's opiate intake as the pain decreases.

Tolerance to opioid analgesics, another of their complications, is characterized by a shortened duration of pain relief, a decrease in peak analgesic effect, and an increase in the amount of opiate needed to relieve pain. An example of tolerance is when pain has been adequately controlled by a particular dosage of opiate, but it begins to be less effective for the same length of time. A higher dose is needed to obtain the desired effects. The usual treatment for tolerance when pain relief is necessary is to increase the analgesic dose or decrease the interval between doses.

Addiction, another complication of opioid analgesics, is a behavioral pattern of drug use characterized by (1) overwhelming involvement with the use of a drug (compulsive use) and securing a supply of it, and (2) a high tendency to relapse after withdrawal from the drug, that is, to begin taking it again. The vast majority of clients who take opiate analgesic medication for pain do not become addicted.

• SUMMARY

Directions. In the space provided, rewrite the above selection in your own words, focusing on the main ideas and major details.

• COMPREHENSION QUESTIONS

Directions. Below are 10 multiple-choice questions. Circle the letter of the best answer from the four choices.

1 Respiratory depression is caused by:
- **a** increased sensitivity of the respiratory center to carbon dioxide
- **b** decreased sensitivity of the respiratory center to carbon dioxide
- **c** diminished insensitivity of the respiratory center to carbon dioxide
- **d** rejection by the respiratory system of carbon dioxide

2 Another term for narcotic overdose is:
- **a** narcotic poisoning
- **b** respiratory depression
- **c** narcotic intervention
- **d** artificial ventilation

3 A supine position is:
- **a** standing up
- **b** sitting
- **c** lying down
- **d** a change in position

4 Morphine:
- **a** increases smooth muscle tone
- **b** increases motility
- **c** decreases smooth muscle tone
- **d** decreases motility

5 If a patient receives a therapeutic dose of morphine several times a day, a physical dependence will develop in about:
- **a** 2 hours
- **b** 2 days
- **c** 2 weeks
- **d** 2 months

6 Nerve injury is prevented by:
- **a** all injection techniques
- **b** proper injection techniques
- **c** intramuscular injection
- **d** paresis

7 The usual treatment for tolerance when pain relief is necessary is to:
- **a** increase the analgesic dose
- **b** decrease the analgesic dose
- **c** increase the time between doses
- **d** eliminate the interval between doses

8 If withdrawal symptoms are untreated, they:
- **a** continue at least 10 days
- **b** disappear in 1 week
- **c** last over 2 weeks
- **d** subside in 5 to 10 days

9 Physical dependence is implied by:
- **a** a withdrawal syndrome
- **b** addiction
- **c** tolerance
- **d** overdose

10 Addiction is characterized by:
- **a** taking narcotics
- **b** requiring analgesic medicine for pain
- **c** compulsive drug use
- **d** opioid tolerance

Comprehending? Yes ___ No ___

• CRITICAL THINKING/EVALUATION

Were you successful in applying active reading strategies to this selection? Explain.

___

___

___

___

Reading Selection 14

• PREVIEW QUESTION

What does the gate-control model of pain explain?

• VOCABULARY

Underline any medical terminology or general vocabulary words you may need to learn in order to understand the ideas in this reading selection.

Theories of Pain

SPECIFICITY THEORY

The specificity theory was described by Descartes in the 17th century. This theory is based on a belief that specialized pathways for pain transmission exist. It was thought that free nerve endings existed in the periphery that acted as pain receptors. These nerves were believed to be capable of receiving painful stimuli and transmitting the impulses on highly specific nerve fibers. The sensation would then be transmitted through the dorsal horns and SG to the thalamus and finally to the higher cortical areas. Pain would be interpreted in these higher areas, and a response would occur.

This theory did not address the multidimensional characteristics of pain, viewing it simply as a sense like all the other senses. It is mainly a biologic explanation of a highly complex process.

GATE-CONTROL THEORY

The physiology of pain transmission and perception is less well understood than the underlying physical structure (anatomy). There are various theoretical models that attempt to explain how neural units interact during the experience of pain. One such model is the gate-control theory, described more than 25 years ago and revised periodically. It explains many aspects of pain and how pain may be controlled by thoughts, emotions, and action.

In 1965, Melzack and Wall[75] presented the first version of the gate-control theory. They suggested the existence of a gate that could either facilitate or inhibit the transmission of pain signals. The gate is controlled by the dynamic function of certain cells in the spinal cord's dorsal horn. The fibers bringing information about pain from tissue synapse for the first time in laminae of the dorsal horns. Laminae II is known as the SG. The SG is visually distinct from other laminae when the spinal cord is inspected in cross section. Melzack and Wall proposed that the SG is the anatomic location of the gate. Both A-delta, small-diameter fibers that carry information about pain, and C fibers, large-diameter fibers that carry information such as touch, converge in the SG. Also, fibers sending their pain-inhibitory information down from the brain act here. They come from areas such as the PAG, hypothalamus, NMR, and locus ceruleus.

Melzack and Wall[75] proposed that a spinal cord transmission cell (T cell) exists in the SG. Depending on its input from other cells, the T cell either facilitates pain transmission (opens the gate) or inhibits pain transmission (closes the gate). The gate can be influenced (opened or closed) by information from various sources. Activity from large-diameter fibers (carrying information, such as touch) can inhibit pain transmission (close the gate); for example, one rubs one's elbow after banging it to ease the pain, thereby closing the gate.

Whether the gate is open or closed, it can be influenced by fibers carrying information from many different brain centers down to the T cells. According to this theory, information from non-pain fibers or information from the brain can reduce or totally block pain information before it is experienced. When the gate is open, pain information influences multiple centers in the brain. When working together, these centers produce the complex but integrated responses that occur in a client experiencing pain. The model suggests, however, that the brain also can influence whether or not the gate is open. Thus, factors such as attention, memory, thinking, and emotion may either inhibit or enhance the transmission of pain signals.

A recent version of the gate-control theory (called Mark II by Melzack and Wall[76]) is presented in Figure VI–11. The newer model emphasizes the probability that there is an inhibitory system within the brain stem that also acts as a gate inhibiting pain transmission. This brain stem inhibitory circuit has been described in detail by Basbaum and Fields[9] who believe that the system involves structures in the midbrain, medulla, and the spinal cord. Activation of cells in the mid-brain's PAG (by electric stimulation, opiate analgesic drugs, or possible psychological factors), in turn, stimulates structures in the medulla.

From Black and Matassarin-Jacobs, pp. 317–318.

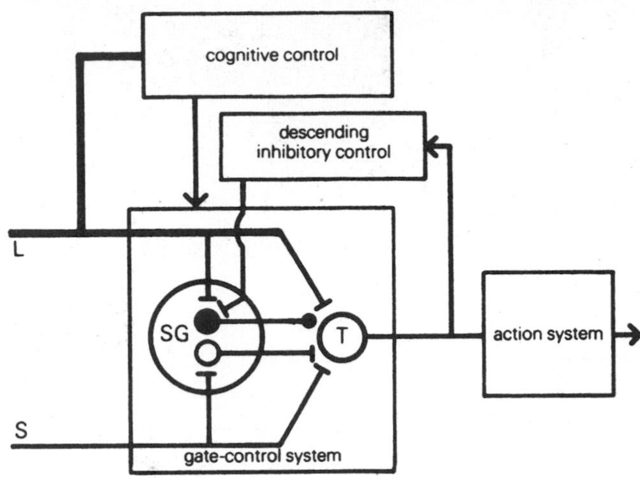

Figure VI–11 The gate-control theory: Mark II. The new model includes excitatory *(white circle)* and inhibitory *(black circle)* links from the substantia gelatinosa (SG) to the transmission (T) cells as well as descending inhibitory control from brain stem systems. The round knob at the end of the inhibitory link implies that its action may be presynaptic, postsynaptic, or both. All connections are excitatory, except the inhibitory link from SG to T cell. (From *The Challenge of Pain* by Ronald Melzack and Patrick D. Wall. Copyright © 1973 by Ronald Melzack. Copyright © 1982 by Ronald Melzack and Patrick D. Wall. Reprinted by permission of Basic Books, Inc., Publishers, New York.)

These medullary structures then project to and inhibit spinal pain transmission fibers. Pain itself might activate this system. Under some circumstances, it acts as a natural control mechanism that limits the severity of the pain experience, such as in the soldier severely injured in battle who is unaware of pain.

• SUMMARY

Directions. In the space provided, rewrite the above selection in your own words, focusing on the main ideas and major details.

• COMPREHENSION QUESTIONS

Directions. Below are 10 multiple-choice questions. Circle the letter of the best answer from the four choices.

1 The gate-control theory is a model of:
- **a** how thoughts affect the experience of pain
- **b** how emotions affect the experience of pain
- **c** how to eliminate pain
- **d** how neural units interact during the experience of pain

2 The gate-control theory was first presented in:
- **a** 1965
- **b** 1695
- **c** 1956
- **d** 1984

3 Laminae II is known as the
- **a** NMR
- **b** SG
- **c** PAG
- **d** T cell

4 Another name for the spinal cord transmission cell is the:
- **a** SG
- **b** DFL
- **c** T cell
- **d** PAG cell

5 The newer model of the gate-control theory is called:
- **a** Mark II
- **b** Marc 2
- **c** Basbaum and Fields
- **d** Pain inhibition

6 The newer model of the gate-control theory emphasizes the probability that:
- **a** a system exists within the brain stem
- **b** a system within the brain stem inhibits pain transmission
- **c** a system within the brain stem prevents pain
- **d** there is a gate that prevents all pain within the brain

7 The severity of pain is limited by a:
- **a** control of the midbrain structure
- **b** circuit in the medulla
- **c** transfer of pain from the spinal cord
- **d** natural control mechanism

8 Figure VI–11 indicates that the inhibitory link from SG to T cell is:
- **a** causing excitatory connections
- **b** causing pain to increase
- **c** excitatory
- **d** not excitatory

9 In Figure VI–11 the white circle is:
- **a** inhibitory
- **b** excitatory
- **c** the new model
- **d** a descending control of pain

10 Figure VI–11 presents:
- **a** Basbaum and Fields
- **b** Melzack and Wall
- **c** Mark II
- **d** the first gate-control theory

Comprehending? Yes ___ No ___

• CRITICAL READING/EVALUATION

Were you successful in applying active reading strategies to this selection? Explain.

____

____

____

____

Reading Selection 15

• PREVIEW QUESTION

What are the methods of ICP monitoring?

• VOCABULARY

Underline any medical terminology or general vocabulary words you may need to learn in order to understand the ideas in this reading selection.

Medical Management

INTRACRANIAL PRESSURE MONITORING

Continuous intracranial pressure (ICP) monitoring is used for clients experiencing conditions associated with potentially elevated ICP (e.g., head trauma, pre- and postoperative aneurysms, tumors, posterior fossa lesions). However, ICP monitoring supplements rather than replaces serial clinical observations of the client's condition.

There are several methods of ICP monitoring. The most common types measure CSF pressure in the ventricles or subarachnoid space. Each type works differently and has advantages and disadvantages. Most health care facilities have a standard procedure for setting up and maintaining the monitors.

Advantages of ICP monitoring are the following.

- Pressure increase may be recognized and treated before the onset of signs and symptoms.
- Some systems allow ventricular fluid drainage above a set pressure. The system becomes part of treatment as well as assessment.
- Delays in bringing the client to definitive treatment (e.g., surgery) can sometimes be avoided.
- The effectiveness of other types of treatment can be monitored.
- Sustained pressure waves (plateau waves) can be detected.
- Intracranial compliance can be measured.
- Level of ICP elevation can provide prognostic information.
- Cerebral perfusion can be calculated.
- ICP monitoring is of particular value for clients who require paralyzing drugs (e.g., curare for mechanical ventilation) or are being treated with barbiturate-induced coma or induced hypothermia, because key changes in the "neuro signs" of these clients are not easily assessed.
- The effect of nursing intervention on ICP can be monitored. The timing of procedures known to raise ICP (e.g., suctioning) can be altered to coincide with periods of "lower" pressure.

From Black and Matassarin-Jacobs, pp. 69–71.

Guidelines for Management of ICP

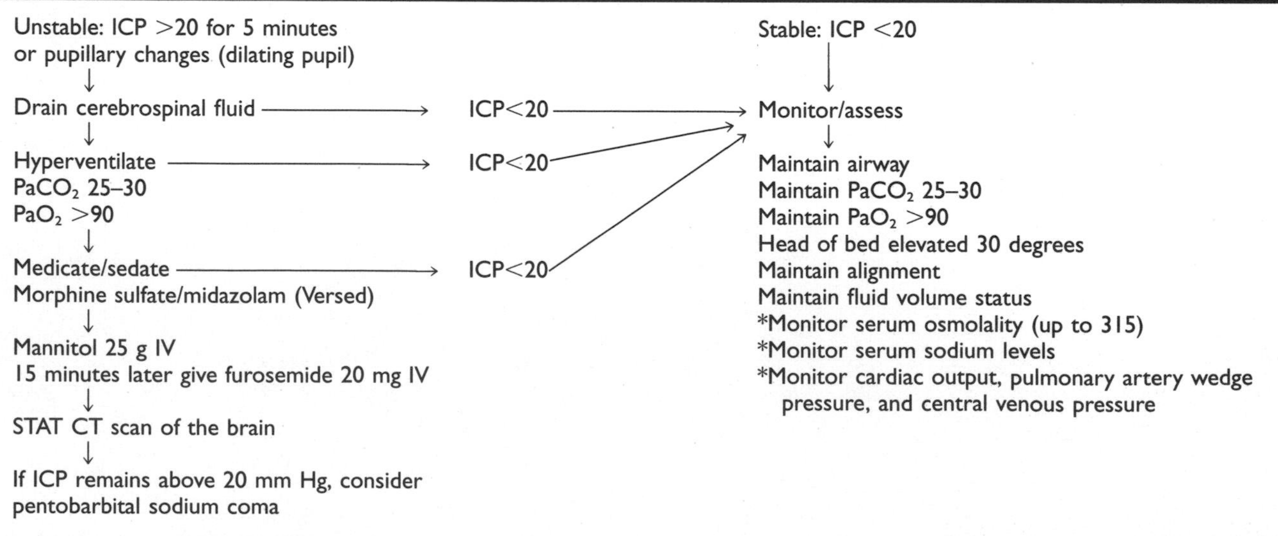
Unstable: ICP >20 for 5 minutes
or pupillary changes (dilating pupil)
Drain cerebrospinal fluid
ICP<20
Hyperventilate
PaCO2 25–30
PaO2 >90
ICP<20
Medicate/sedate
Morphine sulfate/midazolam (Versed)
ICP<20
Mannitol 25 g IV
15 minutes later give furosemide 20 mg IV
STAT CT scan of the brain
If ICP remains above 20 mm Hg, consider
pentobarbital sodium coma
Stable: ICP <20
Monitor/assess
Maintain airway
Maintain PaCO2 25–30
Maintain PaO2 >90
Head of bed elevated 30 degrees
Maintain alignment
Maintain fluid volume status
*Monitor serum osmolality (up to 315)
*Monitor serum sodium levels
*Monitor cardiac output, pulmonary artery wedge
pressure, and central venous pressure

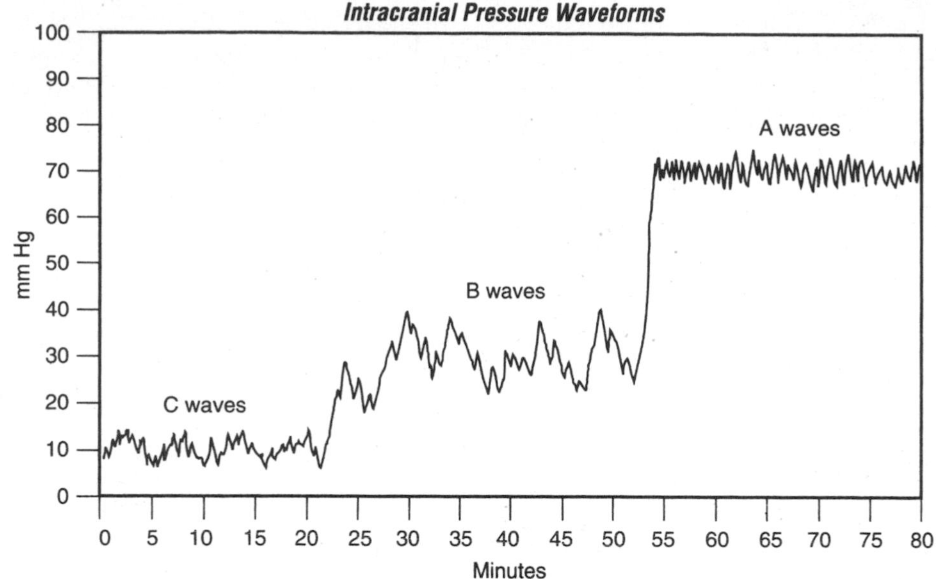

Measuring Compliance and Cerebral Perfusion. Monitoring ICP also allows another method of determining intracranial compliance. Compliance is a measure of how much "slack" is present, that is, how much intracranial contents can expand within the nondistensible skull before the fit becomes "tight" and intracranial contents are compromised. A very compliant system is one in which "slack" exists. A noncompliant system is tight or has little "slack." Measuring compliance identifies low compliance, that is, when a small increase in volume would produce a large increase in ICP.

Compliance is tested by introducing a known volume of fluid into the ventricle and measuring its effect on ICP. Detecting a change in the critical relationship between volume and pressure allows early treatment before the onset of signs and symptoms or sustained elevated ICP.

Measurements of cerebral perfusion pressure (CPP) can be made with ICP monitors. CPP is the amount of blood flow from the systemic circulation required to provide adequate oxygen and glucose for brain metabolism. A normal brain can survive with a CPP of 30 mm Hg, but an injured brain requires a CPP of 50 mm Hg. Because ICP is normally 0 to 15 mm Hg, the mean arterial pressure (MAP) needs to be at least 60 mm Hg to produce an adequate CPP. In cases of profound increased ICP, the MAP and ICP become the same, and brain perfusion ceases.

$$CPP = MAP - ICP$$

Nursing Responsibilities. An ICP monitor requires continuous observation. Nursing responsibilities include (1) observing for increased ICP, (2) intervening when this occurs, and (3) preventing infection. The client should be monitored continuously for ICP, MAP, and CPP. ICP should be less than 15 mm Hg, MAP above 70 mm Hg, and CPP above 50 mm Hg.

Increased ICP may be recognized by observing the number on the monitor or by noting elevated (plateau) waves continuing for 5 to 20 minutes. These periods of sustained pressure elevation may be followed or accompanied by signs and symptoms such as extension posturing or disorientation.

Plan nursing intervention so that activities known to increase ICP are not performed when elevations are present (e.g., suctioning, excessive hip flexion, turning the client). Administration of endotracheal lidocaine has been helpful in limiting the effect of suctioning on ICP. Space out interventions so that a stair-step rise in ICP does not occur. Other problems that may contribute to increased ICP are (1) excess water in the respirator tubing, (2) excess secretion production causing a rise in PCO_2, (3) an endotracheal tube taped tightly over the jugular veins, retarding venous circulation from the head, and (4) discussing the client's condition at the bedside (see Nursing Research).

Avoid ICP catheter infections by (1) keeping the area around the catheter site clean and dry, (2) documenting and reporting leakage from the catheter, and (3) maintaining a closed system from the catheter to the monitor. If CSF drainage is required, most systems have a stopcock where the tubing and a drainage bag are attached. To drain fluid from the ventricles, the stopcock is turned to the drainage tubing. The system is therefore opened only to change the drainage bag.

PHARMACOLOGIC MANAGEMENT

Osmotic Diuretics. The most commonly used diuretic is mannitol, which removes fluid from the normal brain tissue and not from edematous tissue. Side effects of large doses of mannitol include (1) production of hyperosmolar states, (2) decreased effectiveness with repeated use, and (3) aggravation of edema in some clients.

Loop Diuretics. Treatment with a nonosmotic diuretic like furosemide (Lasix) inhibits reabsorption of sodium and chloride at the proximal portion of the ascending loop of Henle. This drug is often given in varying doses ranging from 10 to 40 mg, alone or in combination with hyperosmolar agents to control cerebral edema. For older clients at risk for congestive heart failure, furosemide may improve the cardiovascular status. Watch for electrolyte disturbances, ototoxic effects, nausea, and vomiting. Monitor vital signs carefully.

Steroids. Steroids, such as dexamethasone (Decadron), may be used. The exact mechanism by which steroids work is unknown, but some physicians believe they are useful in controlling edema, especially brain tumor edema. Their use is controversial. Antacids or H_2-blockers may also be prescribed to control gastrointestinal irritation and hemorrhage.

Antihypertensives. Sustained arterial hypertension over 160 mm Hg is treated. Caution is used to avoid agents that cause peripheral vasodilation along with cerebral vasodilation. Beta blockers have been used in conjunction with other antihypertensives to block effects on cerebral vessels.

Anticonvulsants. Treatment of seizures after head injury requires anticonvulsants. Seizures increase metabolic requirements, cerebral blood flow, cerebral blood volume, and ICP even in paralyzed patients. Phenytoin (Dilantin) and phenobarbital are the usual agents. Seizures are discussed in Chapter 30.

Barbiturate Therapy for Uncontrolled ICP. Some clients require large doses of barbiturates for treatment of uncontrolled ICP. The use of this treatment requires sophisticated monitoring capacity and trained personnel, but its use has shown increased survival.

The client must be placed on a ventilator and have a Swan-Ganz catheter inserted. Pentobarbital is the drug of choice, and the client is given a loading dose of 5 to 10 mg/kg by slow intravenous injection. While the drug is infused, the client's blood pressure (MAP) is closely monitored because pentobarbital is a cardiac depressant. If the loading dose is sufficient to reduce ICP, a maintenance dose of 100 to 200 mg/hr is administered until pressure is under control. Pentobarbital is tapered slowly. It is important to monitor the serum level of the drug daily; the dose should be reduced if the serum levels exceed 5 mg/100 ml.

Assessment of the pupils should continue while the client is being treated. Even though the client is in a deep coma, the pupils will dilate if the brain stem becomes compressed. If pupils become dilated, the physician should be notified. Arterial pressure must be monitored closely, and systemic arterial pressure should not be allowed to fall below 70 mm Hg. Temperature should also be monitored because barbiturates reduce metabolism and have a concurrent cooling effect on the body. If temperature falls below 91.4°F (33°C), the patient should be warmed.

MECHANICAL VENTILATION

Hyperventilation, induced by a ventilator or by manual ventilation, is an important adjunct to management. It induces hypocapnia, which reduces cerebral blood volume and ICP. This intervention may be lifesaving while a client is being prepared for other treatments. Manual hyperventilation is sometimes done during ICP elevations or when sudden clinical signs of deterioration appear.

Surgical Management

Various surgical techniques are used to treat clients with increased ICP. Optimally, the cause is located and removed. Other techniques include (1) surgical placement of a shunt to allow drainage if CSF is blocked and (2) decompressive surgery. The latter is done by removing some brain tissue (e.g., part of the temporal lobe) to give the remaining structures room to expand. If compliance is low at surgery, the bone flap removed to gain access to the brain is not replaced or the dura may not be closed. Subsequent surgery is then required to repair the defect.

Nursing Management

Whether or not hyperventilation is used, pay meticulous attention to maintaining respiratory function. Assess an intubated client often. Frequent arterial blood gas samples are drawn. Acid-base imbalances are corrected to ensure adequate oxygenation.

Maintain a patent airway by suctioning to prevent buildup of carbon dioxide and elevation of ICP. Adequately oxygenate intubated clients before each passage of a suction catheter. Because hyperinflation as well as the addition of positive end-expiratory pressure raises ICP, keep the passage of a suction catheter as brief as possible. Never exceed 15 seconds. The use of lidocaine via the endotracheal tube may reduce elevations in ICP. Do not suction via the nose because drainage may indicate CSF leak and it is important to be able to observe it. (See discussion of suctioning in Chapter 37.)

It is also important to prevent venous obstruction. Raise the head of the bed 30 degrees. Avoid turning the client's head sharply to either side, and keep the head in alignment with the rest of the body. Maintain a regular bowel program because excessive strain can cause a Valsalva maneuver, which can result in venous back-up and increased ICP.

Fluid administration for clients with increased ICP is controversial. Administer fluid exactly as prescribed. Currently the tendency is to use a slightly hypertonic solution (e.g., 5 per cent dextrose in half-normal saline). Such fluid remains in the vascular space and therefore contributes less to cerebral edema. Balanced salt solutions are generally used, but other solutions may be required if complications occur that render the client hemodynamically unstable.

It is important to avoid the use of fluid (e.g., dextrose 5 per cent in water) that moves rapidly into the brain to cause edema. Remember to document the fluid administered with medications and in keeping monitoring devices open (e.g., indwelling arterial catheter lines). A large amount of fluid can be administered by these routes. The types and amounts of such fluids must be taken into account.

The actual amount of fluid infused per hour is determined by various factors. Never infuse more than the prescribed amount. If fluid therapy falls behind, consult the physician. This is especially important for a client with low intracranial compliance. Also remember that mechanical ventilation causes a client to retain fluid.

Increased temperature in clients with increased ICP raises the metabolic rate and aggravates ICP further. Therefore, hyperthermia requires vigorous treatment with cooling measures and prescribed medication.

• SUMMARY

Directions. In the space provided, rewrite the above selection in your own words, focusing on the main ideas and major details.

• COMPREHENSION QUESTIONS

Directions. Below are 10 multiple-choice questions. Circle the letter of the best answer from the four choices.

1 An example of brain tissue is:

a hypocapnia

b dexamethasone

c hyperventilation

d part of the temporal lobe

2 Mannitol is a:

a fluid

b diuretic

c brain tissue

d edematous tissue

3 A controversial method for decreasing brain swelling is the use of:
a diuretics
b antacids
c steroids
d carbon dioxide

4 Treatment of seizures after head injury requires:
a anticonvulsants
b mannitol
c diuretics
d steroids

5 Increased temperature of clients with increased ICP raises:
a fluid retention
b venous obstruction
c salt balance
d the metabolic rate

6 A mainstay in the treatment of ICP is:
a sporadic ventilation
b continuous controlled hyperventilation
c building up carbon dioxide
d elevating ICP

7 Edema may be caused by:
a any amount of fluid
b dehydration
c fluid moving rapidly into the brain
d increasing body temperature

8 The passage of a suction catheter should not exceed:
a 30 seconds
b 15 minutes
c 5 minutes
d 15 seconds

9 Barbiturate-induced coma may be used to:
a protect the brain
b prevent seizures
c cure edema
d avoid hyperthermia

10 A patient in a therapeutic coma requires:
a some nursing care
b home supervision
c intense nursing care
d big intake of barbiturates

Comprehending? Yes ___ No ___

• CRITICAL THINKING/EVALUATION

Were you successful in applying active reading strategies to this selection? Explain.

References

Arnold, E., and Boggs, K. (Eds.) (1995). *Interpersonal Relationships: Professional Communication Skills for Nurses* (2nd ed). Philadelphia: W. B. Saunders Co.

Black, J., and Matassarin-Jacobs, E. (1996). *Luckmann and Sorensen's Medical-Surgical Nursing: A Psychophysiologic Approach* (4th ed). Philadelphia: W. B. Saunders Co.

Bolander, V. (Ed.) (1994). *Sorensen and Luckmann's Basic Nursing: A Psychophysiologic Approach* (3rd ed). Philadelphia: W. B. Saunders Co.

Ignatavicius, D., et al (Eds.) (1995). *Medical-Surgical Nursing: A Nursing Diagnosis Approach* (2nd ed). Philadelphia: W. B. Saunders Co.

Iyer, P. W., et al. (1995). *Nursing Process and Nursing Diagnosis* (3rd ed). Philadelphia: W. B. Saunders Co.

Lehne, R. (1994). *Pharmacology for Nursing Care* (2nd ed). Philadelphia: W. B. Saunders Co.

Lewis, N. (Ed.) (1961). *Roget's New Pocket Thesaurus in Dictionary Form.* New York: Washington Square Press.

Matteson, M., and McConnell, E. (1988). *Gerontological Nursing: Concepts and Practice.* Philadelphia: W. B. Saunders Co.

Mish, F. (Ed.) (1988). *Webster's Ninth New Collegiate Dictionary.* Massachusetts: Merriam-Webster, Inc.

O'Toole, M. (Ed.) (1992). *Miller-Keane Encyclopedia and Dictionary of Medicine, Nursing, and Allied Health* (5th ed). Philadelphia: W. B. Saunders Co.

Ulrich, S., et al. (1994). *Medical-Surgical Nursing Care Planning Guides* (3rd ed). Philadelphia: W. B. Saunders Co.

Varcarolis, E. (Ed.) (1994). *Foundations of Psychiatric Mental Health Nursing* (2nd ed). Philadelphia: W. B. Saunders Co.

Glossary

abbreviation(s) A shortened form of a written word or phrase used in place of the whole.
abuse Improper use or treatment.
acronym A word formed from the initial letters of a compound term.
adaptation Adjustment to environmental conditions.
adventitious Coming from another place or source.
affect The external expression of emotion attached to ideas or mental representations of objects.
afferent Toward a center or specific site of reference.
afterbirth The placental and fetal membranes expelled from the uterus after childbirth.
aggravates Worsens.
agoraphobia Fear of open and public spaces.
align To bring into line or alignment.
allegation(s) A statement by a party to a legal action of what he undertakes to prove.
alleviates Relieves.
Alzheimer's disease Irreversible senile dementia characterized by intellectual deterioration, disorganization of the personality, and functional disabilities in carrying out the tasks of daily living.
ambulatory care Care of patients who are not confined to bed.
analgesia Absence of sensibility to pain.
analogy Likeness.
anatomy The science dealing with the form and structure of living organisms.
angina Spasmodic choking or suffocative pain.
anonymity The quality or state of being anonymous.
anonymous Not named or identified.
anorexia Lack or loss of appetite for food.
anti-inflammatory Effective against a response provoked by physical, chemical and biologic agents.
antonyms Words of opposite meaning.
anxiety Painful or apprehensive uneasiness of mind over an impending or anticipated ill.
appendicitis Inflammation of the vermiform appendix.
applicable Relevant.
approximate To come close.
arbitrary Based on or determined by individual preference.
arthritis Inflammation of a joint.
aspirate To remove fluid.
assert To state or declare positively and often forcefully or aggressively.
assessment Appraisal.
assumption The supposition that something is true.
asthma Condition caused by spasmodic constriction of bronchi.
ataxia Failure of muscular coordination.
auscultation Listening for sounds produced within the body.
autonomy Self-directing freedom.
avoidance An act or practice of avoiding or withdrawing from something.

basophils Any structure, cells, or histologic elements staining readily with basic dyes.
benign Not malignant.
biomechanics The application of mechanical laws to living structures.
bulimia nervosa An eating disorder characterized by binge eating followed by purging behavior such as vomiting or laxative abuse.

cancer Malignant tumor.
caption(s) The explanatory comment or designation accompanying a pictorial illustration.
cardiovascular Pertaining to the heart and blood vessels.
care plan A nurse's systematic strategies for taking care of patients.
cervical Pertaining to the neck or the cervix uteri.
charting The keeping of a clinical record of the important facts about a patient and the progress of his or her illness.
chronic Persisting for a long time.
chronological order Of, relating to, or arranged in or according to the order of time.
clarify To make understandable.
clotting The formation of a jellylike substance over the ends or within the walls of a blood vessel, with resultant stoppage of the blood flow.
coagulation The creation of a clot.
cognitive Having to do with that operation of the mental process by which we become aware of

objects of thought and perception, including all aspects of perceiving, thinking, and remembering.
collaborate To work together.
collegiate Designed for or characteristic of college students.
complication A factor that makes difficulty.
components Parts.
concept Something conceived in the mind; thought, notion.
concise Marked by brevity of expression or statement; free from all elaboration and superfluous detail.
concrete To make actual or real.
congestive Pertaining to the atypical accumulation of blood.
consistency Firmness of constitution or character; persistency.
construct Compose.
controversy A discussion marked especially by the expression of opposing views; dispute.
conversely Reversed in order, relation, or action.
conversion Changeover.
coping The process of contending with life difficulties in an effort to overcome or work through them.
core Central and often foundational part.
corticosteroids Hormones produced by the adrenal cortex; also, their synthetic equivalents.
credence Something believed to be true.
cyrtometer An instrument that measures the curves of the body.

deficits Lack or impairment in a functional capacity.
delegate To appoint.
deposit To place, especially for safekeeping (or as a pledge).
detrimental Obviously harmful.
deviation Noticeable or marked departure from accepted norms of behavior.
diacritical mark An accent near or through an orthographic or phonetic character or combination of characters indicating a phonetic value different from that given the unmarked or otherwise marked element.
diaphoresis Perspiration.
dilemma A difficult or persistent problem.
diphtheria An acute childhood disease affecting throat membranes.
discs (disks) Circular or rounded flat plates.
disruption Something that stops the normal course of events.
diuretics Drugs that cause increased urination.
DNA Deoxyribonucleic acid.
document To support with written information.
dressings Materials used for protecting a wound.
dysfunction Impaired or abnormal functioning.

edema An abnormal accumulation of fluid in the intercellular spaces of the body.
elaborate To expand on something in detail.
electro-oculogram A graphic representation of the electrical activity associated with eye movements.
endocrine Pertaining to internal secretions; hormonal.
enhance(s) To add or contribute to.
enzyme Any protein that acts as a catalyst, increasing the rate at which a chemical reaction takes place.
epidermis The outermost and nonvascular layer of the skin.
episode An event that is distinctive and separate, although part of a larger series.
epistaxis Hemorrhage from the nose.
etymology The history of a linguistic form (as a word) shown by tracing its development since its earliest recorded occurrence in the language where it was found.
euphoria A feeling of well-being or elation.
exacerbate(ion) To make more violent, bitter, or severe.
excessive Exceeding the usual, proper, or normal.
excitation A changed condition resulting from stimulation.
exocrine Secreting externally via a duct.
exotic Strikingly or excitingly different or unusual.
expedient Faster and easier.
external Of, or relating to, or connected with the outside or an outer part.
extracurricular Lying outside one's regular duties or routines.
extraneous Unrelated.

feedback The return to a point of evaluative or corrective information about an action or process.
fibrinogenemia The absence of fibrinogen in blood.
flexibility A ready capability to adapt to new, different, or changing requirements.
footnote A note of reference, explanation, or comment usually placed below the text on a printed page.
former First mentioned in order of two things mentioned or understood.
friction The rubbing of one body against another.
fulcrum The support about which a lever turns.

gastrointestinal Pertaining to the stomach and intestines.
generativity Pertaining to reproduction.
gestures The use of motions of the limbs or body as a means of expression.
glossary A collection of textual glosses or specialized terms with their meanings.
gout A hereditary form of arthritis in which uric acid appears in excessive quantities in the blood and may be deposited in the joints and other tissues.
graphic Pertaining to a visual representation.
gravity The quality of having weight.
gynecology The branch of medicine dealing with diseases of the genital tract in women.

habitual Resorted to on a regular basis.
hallucinations Sensory impressions that have no basis in external stimulations.
haphazard Marked by lack of plan, order, or direction.
hematoma A localized collection of clotted blood in an organ.
hemoglobin An allosteric protein found in erythrocytes that transports molecular oxygen (O_2) in the blood.
hepatitis Inflammation of the liver.
hindrance Impediment.
holistic Pertaining to the whole human being (biological, psychological, and social).
hormones Chemical transmitters produced by cells.
hypertension Persistently high blood pressure.
hyperventilation Abnormal prolonged deep breathing.
hyponatremia Deficiency of sodium in the blood; salt depletion.
hypotension Lowered blood pressure.
hysterectomy Surgical removal of the uterus.

idiom The language peculiar to a people or to a district, community, or class.
immobility Incapable of being moved.
immune system The body's ability to recognize and dispose of substances it interprets as foreign and harmful to its well-being.
immunosuppressive Pertaining to the stopping of the forming of antibodies.
impairments Injury.
impending About to occur.
incision A cut or wound made by a sharp instrument.
incorporated To unite or work into something already existing so as to form an indistinguishable whole.
inference Deduction.
inflammatory Pertaining to a response elicited by injury or destruction of tissues.
ingrained Forming a part of the essence or innermost being.
inguinal hernia Hernia occurring in the groin, or inguina where the abdominal folds of flesh meet the thighs.
inherent Innate.
interaction Mutual or reciprocal reaction.
internal Situated near the inside of the body.
interventions Interference in the affairs of another to accomplish a goal.
intricate Having many complexly interrelating parts or elements.
irrigate To wash a body cavity or wound by a stream of water or fluid.

jargon Specialized vocabulary of a particular field or subject.

legend An explanatory list of the symbols on a map or chart.
lethargy An abnormal degree of fatigue.
leverage The action of a lever or the mechanical advantage gained by it.
life-style A way of living.
limitation Restraint.
locus A point.

major Greater in importance.
maladaptive Marked by poor or inadequate adaptation.
malnutrition Poor nourishment resulting from improper diet or from some defect in metabolism that prevents the body from using its food properly.
mandates Requires.
mandatory Containing a command.
manipulate To control for one's own purposes.
maximize To make the most of.
medulla The central or inner portion of an organ.
melanin A dark, sulfur-containing pigment normally found in the hair, skin, ciliary body, choroid of the eye, pigment layer of the retina, and nerve cells.
melena Darkening of the feces by blood pigments.
metabolic Having to do with the disposition of the nutrients absorbed into the blood following digestion.
midbrain Part of the brain stem.
minor Inferior in importance.
miscommunication Failure to communicate clearly.

mobility The ability to move in one's environment with ease and without restriction.
momentum A property of a moving body that determines the length of time required to bring it to rest when under the action of a constant force or movement.
monitoring To watch, observe, or check, especially for a special purpose.
moral Of or relating to principles of right and wrong in behavior.
motivated To have provided a reason or cause for action.
multidisciplinary Pertaining to many fields of study.
multitude A great number.
musculoskeletal Pertaining to the muscles and skeleton.
mutations Permanent, transmissible changes in the genetic material.
myalgia Muscular pain.
myocardial infarction Heart attack.
myth An unfounded or false notion.
myxedema The lack of thyroxine.
myxorrhea A flow of mucus.

naloxone A narcotic antagonist structurally related to oxymorphone used as an antidote to narcotic overdosing and as an antagonist for pentazocine overdose.
neologisms Made-up words with special meanings.
neuron Nerve cell.
nitroglycerin A chemical well known as an explosive, but also having medical uses.
nonbiologic Not pertaining to living organisms.

obesity Excessive accumulation of fat in the body; increase in weight beyond that considered desirable with regard to age, height, and bone structure.
objective Free from bias.
obstacle Something that impedes progress or achievement.
occipitoatlantal Junction between back of head and beginning of spine.
ombudsmen People who investigate complaints.
ostomy Formation of artificial opening.
outcomes Effects, results.
overwhelmed Upset.

pallor Paleness, as of skin.
palpitation A heartbeat that is unusually rapid, strong, or irregular enough to make a person aware of it.
pancreas A large, elongated, racemose gland located transversely behind the stomach, between the spleen and duodenum.
paralysis Loss or impairment of motor function in part caused by a lesion of the neural or muscular mechanism.
pathogen Any disease-producing agent or microorganism.
pelvic Pertaining to the pelvis, the lower portion of the trunk of the body.
percussion In medical diagnosis, striking a part of the body with short, sharp blows of the fingers in order to determine the size, position, and density of the underlying parts by the sound obtained.
permeability Pertaining to the ability to pass through.
pharmacology The study of drugs.
physiology The science that treats the functions of the living organism and its parts and of the physical and chemical factors and processes involved.
pivotal Key.
portable Capable of being carried or moved about.
postoperative After a surgical operation.
posture An attitude of the body.
precise Exactly or sharply defined or stated.
prefix An affix attached to the beginning of a word or an inflectional form.
pregnant Containing unborn young within the body.
prematurity Underdevelopment; the condition of a premature infant.
pressure The burden of physical or mental distress.
priority Taking precedence (as in importance).
procrastination To put off intentionally the doing of something that should be done.
pronunciation To present in printed characters the spoken counterpart of a written word.
proposals Suggestions.
psychobiology The branch of psychology that studies the relationship between physiologic processes and behavior.
psychosocial Pertaining to or involving both psychic and social aspects.
psychotherapy Any number of related techniques for treating mental illness by psychological methods.
pulmonary Pertaining to the lungs, or to the pulmonary artery.
pulse The beat of the heart as felt through the walls of the arteries.
purification To clear from material defilement or imperfection.

rapport Agreement and harmony.

receptive Able to receive and transmit stimuli.
refine To perfect or complete.
regardless Despite everything.
regimen Regulated activity designed to achieve certain ends.
reinforce To strengthen by additional assistance.
remission A diminution or abatement of symptoms of a disease.
repertoire A list or supply of capabilities.
resuscitate Restoring life or consciousness of one apparently dead, or whose respirations have ceased.
retirement Withdrawal from work.
revisions Alterations.
root The main part of the word.

sabotage An act or process tending to hamper or hurt.
sanitary Promoting or pertaining to health.
schema A mental code of experience that includes a particular organized way of perceiving cognitively.
schizophrenia A mental disorder.
scleroma Hardening of the skin.
scoliosis Lateral deviation in the normally vertical line of the spine.
secrete To produce and discharge a substance.
seizures Convulsions.
self-concept The way a person feels, thinks or views himself or herself.
self-directedness Motivated or guided by self.
sensory Pertaining to sensations or to any response of the senses (hearing, sight, touch, etc.) to incoming stimuli.
shrugging Gesturing with the shoulder.
socialism A system of society or group living in which there is no private property.
somatic Pertaining to or characteristic of the body.
spasmodic The nature of a spasm, a sudden involuntary contraction of a muscle or group of muscles.
specialized Designed or fitted for one particular purpose or occupation.
spinal cord That part of the central nervous system lodged in the spinal canal, extending from the foramen magnum to the upper part of the lumbar region.
spiritual Pertaining to the spirit.
stability The strength to stand or endure; firmness.
statistics A branch of mathematics dealing with the collection, analysis, interpretation, and presentation of masses of numerical data.
statute A law enacted by the legislative branch of the government.
sterile Free from living microorganisms.
streamlined Stripped of nonessentials.
stringent Rigorous.
suffix An affix occurring at the end of a word, base, or phrase.
summarize Covering the main points succinctly.
superego In psychoanalytic theory, a part of the psyche derived from both the id and the ego, which acts, largely unconsciously, as a monitor.
supplemented Something that completes or makes an addition.
support To provide with substantiation.
symptoms Indications of disease perceived by the patient.
syncope Fainting.
syndrome An assortment of symptoms resulting from a single cause, and constituting a distinct common health problem.
synonym One of two or more words or expressions of the same language that have the same or nearly the same meaning in some or all senses.
synthesis The production of a substance by the union of chemical elements, groups, or similar compounds.
systematic Methodical in procedure or plan.

tachycardia A heart rate that is too rapid.
thesaurus A book of words and their synonyms.
thrombus An aggregation of blood factors frequently causing vascular obstruction.
tonsillectomy Excision of tonsils.
transmit To send or convey from one person to another.
trauma A wound or injury, especially produced by extreme force.

unabridged Complete; being the most complete of its class.
unilateral Done or undertaken by one person or party.
upheld Supported.

validation State of being confirmed.
variety The quality or state of having different forms or types.
verify To establish the truth, accuracy, or reality of.
vertebrae The separate segments composing the spine.
visualize To form a mental image.
vital signs The signs of life, namely pulse, respiration, and temperature.

wheezing Breathing with a whistling sound.
word parts Prefixes, roots, and suffixes.

Answer Key

CHAPTER 1

Exercise 1–1
Answers will vary

Exercise 1–2
Answers will vary

Exercise 1–3
Answers will vary

Vocabulary Check
1 d
2 a
3 c
4 d
5 a
6 c
7 b
8 b
9 a
10 c

Critical Thinking Log
Answers will vary

CHAPTER 2

Five Prereading Strategies
1 Prereading Strategies
2 Using prereading strategies for active reading. The five prereading strategies are: read the title, introduction and summary, boldface headings, key words, and look at graphic aids.
3 Prereading Strategies
Key words
Questions to think about before readings
Five prereading strategies
Vocabulary
Summary
4 Answers will vary
5 Yes

Exercise 2–1
1 Several different types of care plans in use
2 Individually Constructed
Advantages
Disadvantages
Standardized
Advantages
Disadvantages
Computerized
Medical Diagnosis
Nursing Diagnosis
Individually Constructed
Advantages
Disadvantages
Summary
3 extraneous
inflammatory
trauma
regimen
analgesia
impending
document
credence
multidisciplinary
4 Yes: Table 6–1 Acute Pain; Figure 6–2 Computerized Care Plan
5 This selection is about the following care plans: individualized, standardized, or computerized.

Vocabulary Check
1 b
2 d
3 a
4 d
5 c
6 b
7 b
8 a
9 c
10 d

Critical Thinking Log
Answers will vary

CHAPTER 3

Exercise 3–1
Answers will vary

Exercise 3–2
Answers may vary but should contain the following ideas: When nurses communicate with other professionals, it is sometimes best to communicate in written form in order to create a permanent record and to lessen misunderstandings.

Exercise 3–3
Answers will vary

Exercise 3–4
Answers will vary

Exercise 3–5
1 Nursing journal
2 General nursing journal
3 Encyclopedia or general nursing textbook
4 General nursing text
5 Nursing journal
6 Encyclopedia

Exercise 3–6
Answers will vary

Vocabulary Check
1 c
2 d
3 c
4 a
5 d
6 b
7 a
8 c
9 a
10 d

Critical Thinking Log
Answers will vary

CHAPTER 4

Exercise 4–1

TABLE 4–1 Prefixes, Roots, Suffixes

	Definition	Example	Definition of Example	Your Example
Prefixes				
1 anti	Against	Anti-inflammatory	An agent that acts against inflammation	Answers will vary
2 *dys	Bad, difficult	Dysfunction	Functioning badly	Answers will vary
3 *endo	Within	Endocrine	Secreting from within	Answers will vary
4 ex	Out	Exhale	To breathe out	Answers will vary
5 fore	Before, in front of	Foresight	To know beforehand	Answers will vary
6 *hem hemato	Relating to the blood	Hemoglobin	A red matter in the blood	Answers will vary
7 *hydra hydro	Relating to water	Hydrocephalus	Water on the brain	Answers will vary
8 *hyper	Over, above, beyond	Hyperactive	Overactive	Answers will vary
9 *hypo	Under	Hypodermic	Injected under the skin	Answers will vary
10 *idio	Relating to the individual organ, distinct	Idiomuscular	Relating to an individual muscle	Answers will vary
11 inter	Between	Interstate	Between states	Answers will vary
12 mal	Poor, bad	Malpractice	Poor practice	Answers will vary
13 *micro	Small	Microscope	An instrument used to see small objects	Answers will vary

TABLE 4–1 Prefixes, Roots, Suffixes *(Continued)*

	Definition	Example	Definition of Example	Your Example
***Prefixes** (Continued)*				
14 *neuro	Nerve	Neurobiology	Biology of the nervous system	Answers will vary
15 non	Not	Nonviable	Not capable of developing into a living thing	Answers will vary
16 *ortho	Straight, normal	Orthodontia	The practice of straightening teeth	Answers will vary
17 retro	Backward	Retroactive	Back, toward the past	Answers will vary
18 semi	Half	Semicircle	Half circle	Answers will vary
19 sub	Under	Subconscious	Beneath conscious knowledge	Answers will vary
20 tele	Distant, far	Television	Broadcasting images over a distance	Answers will vary
21 Answers will vary	Answers will vary	Answers will vary	Answers will vary	Answers will vary
22 Answers will vary	Answers will vary	Answers will vary	Answers will vary	Answers will vary
23 Answers will vary	Answers will vary	Answers will vary	Answers will vary	Answers will vary
24 Answers will vary	Answers will vary	Answers will vary	Answers will vary	Answers will vary
25 Answers will vary	Answers will vary	Answers will vary	Answers will vary	Answers will vary
Roots				
1 *arteri arterio	Artery	Arteriosclerosis	Thickening of the walls of the arteries	Answers will vary
2 *arthro arthr	Joint	Arthritis	Disease involving pain and stiffening of the joint	Answers will vary
3 *cardi cardio	Heart	Cardiovascular	Pertaining to the heart and blood vessels	Answers will vary
4 dem, demo	People	Democracy	Government of the people	Answers will vary
5 *derm dermo	Skin	Dermatologist	Skin doctor	Answers will vary
6 fac, fact	Make, do	Factory	Place where things are made	Answers will vary
7 geo	Earth	Geology	Study of the earth	Answers will vary
8 *gyne	Woman	Gynecology	Branch of medicine, dealing with women's diseases	Answers will vary
9 later	Side	Unilateral	One-sided	Answers will vary
10 mit, miss	Send	Transmit	To send across	Answers will vary
11 *nephro nephr	Kidney	Nephritis	Inflammation of the kidney	Answers will vary
12 neur, neuro	Nerve	Neurology	Study of nerves	Answers will vary
13 *oste osteo	Bone	Osteoporosis	Disease of the bones	Answers will vary
14 *path	Disease	Pathology	Study of disease	Answers will vary
15 port	Carry	Transport	To carry across	Answers will vary
16 *psych	Mind	Psychology	Study of the mind	Answers will vary
17 *soma	Body	Somatic	Referring to the body	Answers will vary
18 spec spect	To look at	Spectator	One who watches	Answers will vary
19 ven veno	Vein	Venous	Pertaining to veins	Answers will vary

Table continued on following page

TABLE 4–1 Prefixes, Roots, Suffixes *(Continued)*

	Definition	Example	Definition of Example	Your Example
Roots *(Continued)*				
20 vers	Turn	Reversible	Able to be turned	Answers will vary
21 Answers will vary	Answers will vary	Answers will vary	Answers will vary	Answers will vary
22 Answers will vary	Answers will vary	Answers will vary	Answers will vary	Answers will vary
23 Answers will vary	Answers will vary	Answers will vary	Answers will vary	Answers will vary
24 Answers will vary	Answers will vary	Answers will vary	Answers will vary	Answers will vary
25 Answers will vary	Answers will vary	Answers will vary	Answers will vary	Answers will vary
Suffixes				
1 able, ible	Capable of	Reachable	Capable of being reached	Answers will vary
2 ation	Act of	Purification	The act of making pure	Answers will vary
3 *cide	Causing death	Pesticide	Capable of killing pests	Answers will vary
4 *cyte	Cell	Blastocyte	Undifferentiated embryonic cell	Answers will vary
5 *ectomy	Excision	Tonsillectomy	The removal of the tonsils	Answers will vary
6 er, or, ant	Person who	Actor	One who acts	Answers will vary
7 ful	Full of	Dreadful	Full of dread	Answers will vary
8 graph	Picture or record	Phonograph	Record player	Answers will vary
9 gram	Instrument that records	Cardiogram	Records heart function	Answers will vary
10 ism	Doctrine	Socialism	Doctrine of public ownership	Answers will vary
11 itis	Inflammation of	Appendicitis	Inflammation of the appendix	Answers will vary
12 *meter	Measure of	Centimeter	Measure of metric length	Answers will vary
13 ology	Study of	Biology	Study of living things	Answers will vary
14 *oplasty	Plastic surgery	Rhinoplasty	Plastic surgery of the nose	Answers will vary
15 *osis	Condition of	Psychosis	Pathological condition of the mind	Answers will vary
16 *ostomy	Opening	Colostomy	An artificial opening created in the large intestine	Answers will vary
17 *phobia	Fear	Agoraphobia	Fear of open space	Answers will vary
18 rupt	Break, burst	Interrupt	To break in	Answers will vary
19 scope	See	Telescope	Instrument for seeing far	Answers will vary
20 *tomy	Cutting	Hysterectomy	Removal of the uterus	Answers will vary
21 Answers will vary	Answers will vary	Answers will vary	Answers will vary	Answers will vary
22 Answers will vary	Answers will vary	Answers will vary	Answers will vary	Answers will vary
23 Answers will vary	Answers will vary	Answers will vary	Answers will vary	Answers will vary
24 Answers will vary	Answers will vary	Answers will vary	Answers will vary	Answers will vary
25 Answers will vary	Answers will vary	Answers will vary	Answers will vary	Answers will vary

Exercise 4–2
Answers will vary

Exercise 4–3
Answers will vary

Exercise 4–4

Postinjury Phase. Ideally, accidental injuries should be prevented, but in some instances this simply is not possible. Therefore nurses should attend to optimizing postinjury prevention efforts, to minimize the long-range effects of an injury. Many communities have emergency call systems, such as "Lifeline," that allow older people at risk of falling ready access to postfall assistance. The systems work by activating a central emergency call board (such as in an emergency room) when the client pushes a button. These buttons are generally small and may be worn on light clothing. Other alternatives include daily checking systems, in which neighbors, friends, or family phone the older person each day.

An example of a fall-related injury prevention protocol developed for a nursing home is shown on this page. It includes both preinjury and postinjury interventions to reduce injury.

Evaluation

Criteria for evaluation of nursing care for those with potential for injury are:

1. What is the incidence of injury in the target client population? How does it compare with national averages?
2. What is the incidence of functional impairment attributable to injury in the client population?
3. Are the patients assessed for potential for specific injuries: fall-related injury, other trauma, burns, poisoning?
4. Are steps taken to reduce the at-risk individual's likelihood of sustaining injury?
5. Is the client's lifestyle adversely affected by the injury prevention program?
6. What is the cost of the injury prevention program to the individual, family, and facility or agency?

NONCOMPLIANCE

Definition and Scope of Problem

Noncompliance is a term with many definitions and connotations. Even leading experts on nursing diagnosis offer quite different definitions. Carpenito defines noncompliance as "personal behavior that deviates from health-related advice given by health care professionals." Gordon defines it as "failure to participate in carrying out the plan of care *after indicating initial intention to comply*." The North American Nursing Diagnosis Association has developed yet another definition: "A person's informed decision not to adhere to a therapeutic recommendation."

Compliance is a concern of nurses because the goal of compliance is improved health status. Despite inconsistencies in definition, there is widespread agreement that achieving compliance is problematic in many different categories of patients. Research on compliance shows that noncompliance is found in patients of all ages, social classes, and ethnic groups; it is found in all types of health care delivery systems and in patients whose symptoms vary from nonexistent to life-threatening.

Noncompliance is most often seen in the community setting, where patients have greater control over their daily routines and are more likely to have competing demands on their time. In institutional settings there are fewer opportunities for noncompliance, because many self-care activities are either closely supervised or done for the patient.

The extent of noncompliance by the elderly is thought to be high by some observers, with medication noncompliance rates averaging about 50 per cent. However, variations in the definition of noncompliance used in studies and measurement difficulties make accurate estimates of the extent of this problem among the elderly difficult to obtain.

Most of the compliance literature focuses on younger adults. Sackett and Snow's review of 31 compliance studies shows that one third of the studies specifically exclude the elderly, and only 2 of 31 are specific to this population. Much of what we know about compliance in the elderly has been extrapolated from studies of age-heterogeneous groups with specific chronic diseases, such as diabetes and hypertension. The literature that considers the elderly as a discrete group calls attention to sensory deficits and memory impairment as two important contributors to noncompliance.

different kinds

high blood pressure

Vocabulary Check

1 d
2 a
3 c
4 d
5 b
6 a
7 c
8 d
9 a
10 c

Critical Thinking Log

Answers will vary

CHAPTER 5

Exercise 5–1

Answers are provided in the following paragraph in the text.

Exercise 5–2

Answers will vary but should be based on the direct definition given in each sentence.

Exercise 5–3

1 or psychogenic fugue
2 (depressive neurosis)
3 decode
4 —that is, psychotic symptoms . . .
5 (itching)

Exercise 5–4

1 general
2 manipulates
3 specific channel for transmitting and receiving messages
4 they cannot live without it
5 situation in which the interaction occurs.

Exercise 5–5

Students will write their own definitions based on the following ideas:

1 movements are slow, facial expressions are decreased, gaze is fixed
2 hepatitis, mononucleosis, multiple sclerosis, cancer
3 attitudes, beliefs, feelings, worries, convictions
4 posture, rhythm of movement, gestures accompanying a verbal message
5 dialogue that is descriptive, problem focused and supportive of the client's strength.

Exercise 5–6

1. **Serum sickness** is a complex of symptoms that occurs after the administration of foreign serum or certain drugs. It is caused by a collection of immune complexes in the walls of vessels in the skin, joints, and the glomeruli of the kidney. The most common causes of serum sickness today are penicillin and related drugs and some horse serum antitoxins. (Ignatavicius, p. 537)
2. **Impulsiveness** is an action that is abrupt, unplanned, and directed toward immediate gratification. Thinking things over or considering the effects of the action on others does not occur. These clients have a history of unpredictable and hasty decisions. Frustration is poorly tolerated and often precipitates an impulsive response. A client's impulsive behavior has been described as erratic, self-serving, and thoughtless. In certain situations, the antisocial client's impulsive behavior is able to generate fear and aggression in others. (Varcarolis, p. 383)
3. Bandler and Grindler (1975) offer a different approach to the study of communication in their conceptual model, defined as **neurolinguistic programming** (NLP). This conceptual model focuses on the way a person takes in and internally processes verbal information. According to these theorists, people make sensory-based interpretations about the realities they observe. (Arnold and Boggs, p. 18)
4. Nurses learn about themselves through self-reflection and the feedback of others. **Self-reflection** is a mental process by which we are able to consciously examine the meaning of our motives and actions. It is a mental

faculty available only to humans. (Arnold and Boggs, p. 70)

5. The roles people assume represent an effort to influence the judgments of others about their self-concept. As a result, they emphasize certain parts of the self-concept and suppress those aspects they consider less desirable. Jung (1965) calls this public expression of self the **"persona."** The persona represents all the surface masks a person wears to bridge the gap between the inner self and society's expectations of the self. (Arnold and Boggs, p. 131)

Exercise 5–7

Word	*Definition*	*Context*	*Glossary*	*Dictionary*	*Medical Dictionary*
1. systemic	referring to whole body		√	√	√
2. prevalence	widespread	√		√	
3. immune	protection	√	√	√	√
4. synovial membrane	a layer in a joint		√		√
5. adjacent	next to	√		√	
6. articular cartilage	joint cartilage		√		√
7. pannus	inflammation from rheumatoid arthritis	√	√		√
8. adhesions	fibrous band of tissue		√		√
9. proximal	nearest to a certain point				√
10. distal	farthest from a point	√			√
11. boutonnière	buttonhole	√		√	
12. remissions	lessening or stopping of symptoms		√		√
13. exacerbations	worsening of symptoms	√			√
14. splinting	to immobilize an injury	√			√
15. judicious	careful	√		√	

Vocabulary Check

1 a

2 c

3 b

4 d

5 a

6 d

7 a

8 b

9 d

10 a

Critical Thinking Log

Answers will vary

CHAPTER 6

1 Two

2 \in-sizh-n\

3 Noun

4 Fifteenth century

5 Three
First definition

Exercise 6–1

1 Carcinogen

2 Cardiac

3 Hematoma

4 Hemophilia

5 Menopause

6 Nematodes

7 Perioperative

8 Peripheral

9 Peritonitis

10 Sinusitis

Exercise 6–2

1 ___8___ Scoliosis

2 ___7___ Cyst

3 ___1___ Myotomy

4 ___9___ Pathogen

5 ___2___ Glomerulitis

6 ___10___ Scoliosis

7 ___5___ Myxorrhea

8 3 Bulimia
9 6 Afterbirth
10 4 Distillation

Exercise 6–3
1 Aorta
2 Chorea
3 Diuretic
4 Hypogastric
5 Phosphate
6 Spina bifida
7 Technologist
8 Convolution
9 Dysgraphia
10 Mercury

Exercise 6–4
1 2
2 4
3 2
4 1c
5 1a
6 2
7 1a
8 1
9 3
10 1

Exercise 6–5
1 f
2 t
3 f
4 t
5 t

Thesaurus Entry
Noun

Exercise 6–6
The nurse drew out her notebook from the desk in the
jot down
station. She wanted to note some of the happenings she
observed *attendant*
noticed during her shift. In particular the nurse wanted
distasteful
to object to some of the objectionable occurrences on the
impartial
floor. However, she wanted to be objective, so the
end *protest*
objective of her observation would not be to object against
impressions
the other nurse, but to get him to change his notions on
care for
what it is to nurse a patient.

Vocabulary Check
1 b
2 d
3 a
4 b
5 d
6 a
7 a
8 c
9 a
10 a

Critical Thinking Log
Answers will vary

CHAPTER 7

Exercise 7–1
Answers will vary

Vocabulary Check
1 d
2 a
3 c
4 b
5 b
6 d
7 d
8 c
9 b
10 a

CHAPTER 8

Exercise 8–1
1 Gestures
2 Examination
3 Systems
4 Texture
5 Description

Exercise 8–2

1 a Too narrow
b Correct
c Not mentioned
d Too broad

2 a Too broad
b Not mentioned
c Correct
d Too narrow

3 a Too broad
b Not mentioned
c Correct
d Too narrow

4 a Correct
b Too narrow
c Too broad
d Not mentioned

5 a Correct
b Too narrow
c Not mentioned
d Too broad

Exercise 8–3

1 Assessing clients through the classification process

2 Validation of data interpretation

3 Factors which interface with nurse's ability to collect data

4 Language barriers between nurse and client

5 Reasons for nurses to carry their own malpractice insurance

Exercise 8–4

Answers will vary

Exercise 8–5

Types of data collected by nurse during assessment

Topic: Various types of angina pectoris
Main idea: There are several types of angina pectoris

Topic: Reasons for mental illness
Main idea: Increasing care is needed for patient with Alzheimer's disease as it progresses.

Topic: Religious institutions and the elderly
Main idea: Churches and other religious institutions serve the elderly in many ways.

Topic: Hospitalization and patient's identity crisis
Main idea: Nurse considers the patient's autonomy and allows the client to make decisions.

Topic: How antisocial clients affect the nurse
Main idea: Clients with antisocial personality disorders evoke strong emotions in nurses.

Exercise 8–6

Topic: Nurse's responsibility to report peer negligence
Unstated main idea: A nurse must report peer negligence through appropriate channels to protect the patient.

Topic: Silence in communication
Unstated main idea: Silence can also be used to emphasize an important point in a verbal communication—a brief silence following an important verbal message.

Topic Allergic and nonallergic asthma
Unstated main idea: Asthma is triggered by allergenic and nonallergenic factors.

Topic: Communication with ill children
Unstated main idea: In later childhood, the ability to verbally communicate with the nurse improves.

Topic: Symptoms of depression
Unstated main idea: There are many indicators of depression.

Exercise 8–7

Topic: Ethical theories
Main idea paragraph 1: Ethical theories describe approaches for resolving dilemmas commonly faced by nurses.

Main idea paragraph 2: There are two major ethical theories used to help nurses resolve health care dilemmas: deontology and utilitarianism.

Main idea paragraph 3: One of the flaws with this approach is that most situations have extenuating circumstances.

Main idea paragraph 4: The utilitarian approach states that actions are right or wrong on the basis of the consequences of the actions. Utilitarians focus on the results of actions rather than on their motivations. This view is quite different from the deontological position, which would maintain that the nurse must tell the truth without exception.

Main idea of the entire passage: There are two ethical theories that nurses use to resolve dilemmas: deontology and utilitarianism; however, both these theories have limitations.

Vocabulary Check

1 d
2 b
3 b
4 a
5 b
6 c
7 c
8 a
9 a
10 b

Critical Thinking Log

Answers will vary

CHAPTER 9

Exercise 9–1

4 types of MS—main idea

Benign—20% have this kind
mild attacks
minimal disability

Exacerbation-remission—25% of cases
increasingly frequent attacks
mild or moderate course

Chronic relapsing or progressive—most frequent
no remissions
progressive deterioration over several years

Chronic progressive or combined—similar to chronic relapsing
initial presentation more insidious
becomes progressive

Exercise 9–2

Answers will vary but should conform to the examples given in the chapter.

Exercise 9–3

• COLLABORATIVE MANAGEMENT

Assessment

HISTORY

Careful attention to the history of a client with a possible infectious disease helps the nurse determine risk factors for infection. The age of a client, history of cigarette smoking or alcohol use, current illness or disease (such as diabetes), past and current medication use, familial predisposition, and poor nutritional status may place the client at increased risk for a number of infectious diseases.

The nurse must assess the drug and sexual habits of the patient.

The nurse also determines whether the client has been exposed to infectious agents. A history of recent exposure to someone with similar clinical symptoms or to contaminated food or water, as well as the time of exposure, assists in identifying a possible source for infection. Nurses may find this information helpful for determining the incubation period for the disease and thus for providing a clue to its cause.

Contact with animals, including pets, may facilitate exposure to infection. The nurse asks the client about recent contact with animals at home, at work, or in the course of leisure activities, such as hunting. The nurse also asks the client about recent contact with insects.

The nurse obtains a travel history from the client. Travel to areas both within and outside the client's home country may expose a susceptible client to infectious organisms not encountered in the local community.

A thorough sexual history may reveal sexual behavior associated with increased risk of sexually transmitted diseases. The nurse should obtain a history of intravenous drug use and a transfusion history to assess the client's risk for hepatitis B, hepatitis C, and human immunodeficiency virus (HIV) infections.

Vocabulary Check

1 b
2 c
3 a
4 d
5 b
6 d
7 a
8 b
9 c
10 c

Critical Thinking Log

Answers will vary

CHAPTER 10

Example 10–1

First, 1973—current 1982 every—continued

Example 10–2

depends—affect, connections

Example 10–3

differs from

Example 10–4
also

Exercise 10–1
1 Simple listing
2 Comparison-contrast
3 Cause-effect
4 Cause-effect
5 Chronological (time order)

Exercise 10–2

1 Organizational pattern	Simple listing
Topic	Three layers of skin
Main idea	Skin is the largest body organ and has three layers.
Major details	Epidermis
	Dermis
	Subcutaneous tissue
2 Organizational pattern	Simple listing
Topic	
Main idea	Reasons for bathing
	People bathe for reasons other than hygiene.
Major details	Relax
	Time alone
	Stimulant
3 Organizational pattern	Simple listing
Topic	Statutory law
Main idea	Nurses can influence statutory law, which is created by state legislatures or U.S. Congress.
4 Organizational pattern	Compare and contrast
Topic	Similarities and differences between nursing diagnosis and medical diagnosis
Main idea	Nursing dignoses are not medical diagnoses although there are similarities between the two.
Major details	

Similarities	**Differences**
Obtaining person's history	Focus
	Specific goals and objective
	Medical diagnosis to learn source of symptoms
Performing physical exam	Nursing diagnosis to describe combination of signs and symptoms
Organizing data base	
Analyzing data obtained	
Use of:	
Physical skills	
Intellectual skills	
Assessment skills	
Observational skills	

Purpose of diagnosis: to identify problem and plan solution

5 Organizational pattern	Chronological (time order)
Topic	Development of infant posture and locomotion
Main idea	The infant gradually progresses in skill of locomotion and walks alone at about 12 to 14 months.

Major details
Birth: legs tucked up
2–3 months: legs extended
5–6 months: sits with support
6½–7½ months: sits without support
8–9 months: creeps
9–11 months: pulls up on furniture
11–12 months: stands alone, walks with help
12–14 months: walks alone

Exercise 10–3
1 c
2 c
3 b
4 a
5 d
6 b
7 d
8 a
9 c
10 d

Vocabulary Check
1 c
2 b
3 a
4 b
5 c
6 d
7 b
8 d
9 a
10 c

Critical Thinking Log
Answers will vary

CHAPTER 11

Exercise 11–1
1 *Medical-Surgical Nursing—A Psychophysiologic Approach,* Third Edition.
2 Joan Luckmann and Karen Creason Sorensen
3 W.B. Saunders Company
4 No

Exercise 11–2
1 The addition of special features is designed to assist the nurse in the clinical setting to allow a clear transition from the book to the bedside.
2 1 Pain
  2 Perioperative care
  3 Shock
  4 Chronic conditions

Exercise 11–3
1 Seven
2 Cardiovascular disorders
3 Unit 6
4 1809

Exercise 11–4
1 Temporary teeth that are shed in childhood.
2 Answers will vary.

Exercise 11–5
1 *Neurological and Neurosurgical Nursing,* Second Edition.
2 *The New England Journal of Nursing*

Exercise 11–6
1 Reference values for therapeutic drug monitoring
2 Four

Exercise 11–7
1 909
2 2–244

Exercise 11–8
Answers will vary.

Exercise 11–9
Answers will vary.

Exercise 11–10
1 The psychosocial health assessment
2 ____________
3 ____________
4 C
5 Answers will vary
6 Answers will vary
7 Answers will vary
8 Answers will vary
9 Answers will vary

Exercise 11–11
Answers will vary

Vocabulary Check
1 b
2 a
3 c
4 b
5 b
6 c
7 b
8 c
9 a
10 b

Critical Thinking Log
Answers will vary

CHAPTER 12

Exercise 12–1
1 There are two views of an older woman using a walker.
2 In the left picture, she seems to have problems using the walker.
3 This is a person being fitted to use a walker.
4 The equipment suggests that with a proper fitting walker, a person can have better body alignment.
5 Answers will vary

Exercise 12–2
1 Pathophysiologic condition that requires cautious use or complete avoidance of certain antihypertensive drugs.
2 Pathophysiologic conditions, drugs to be avoided or use with caution, reasons for concern.
3 These drugs can injure the fetus.
4 Thiazides, furosemide.
5 The purpose is to show which drugs prescribed for high blood pressure should not be given to patients suffering from other medical conditions and why.

Exercise 12–3
1 Adult dosages for antidepressants.

2 7.

3 Nardil.

4 20 mg/day.

5 Selective serotonin reuptake blockers.

Exercise 12–4

1 Some major complications of immobility

2 Pressure sores
Pneumonia
Urinary tract

3 Depression
Insomnia
Sensory deprivation

Exercise 12–5

1 Diagram of the nursing process.

2 Assessment, diagnosis, planning, implementation, and evaluation.

3 The nursing process is cyclical.

4 Implementation.

5 Assessment.

Exercise 12–6
Answers will vary

Vocabulary Check

1 d
2 d
3 b
4 d
5 b
6 a
7 b
8 c
9 c
10 a

Critical Thinking Log
Answers will vary

CHAPTER 13

Exercise 13–1
Answers will vary

Exercise 13–2
Answers will vary

Exercise 13–3

—Free radicals are "highly reactive cellular components derived from atoms or molecules in which an electron pair has been transiently separated into two electrons that exhibit independence of motion."

—Lipofuscin is a pigmented material rich in lipids and proteins that accumulates in many organs with aging.

—Lipofuscin appears to have some relationship to free radicals and the process of aging because the substance is associated with oxidation of unsaturated lipids.

Exercise 13–4
Answers will vary

Exercise 13–5
Answers will vary

Exercise 13–6
Answers will vary

Exercise 13–7

1 %
2 ?
3 ′
4 ″
5 →
6 ←
7 @
8 5
9 ×
10 $

Exercise 13–8

Two major types of skin glands
  Sebaceous glands
    Originate in dermis
    Secrete sebum
  Sweat glands
    Eccrine
      Promote body cooling
    Apocrine
      Responsible for body odor
Sebaceous glands' function diminishes with age
  In men decrease is minimal
  More so in women after menopause
Sweat glands change with age
  Decrease in size
  Decrease in number
  Decrease in function
    Older people have difficulty sweating
    Impairs older people's ability to maintain body temperature

Exercise 13–9
Answers will vary

Exercise 13–10
Answers will vary

Exercise 13–11
Answers will vary

Exercise 13–12
Answers will vary

Exercise 13–13
Answers will vary

Vocabulary Check
1 a
2 d
3 c
4 b
5 d
6 b
7 c
8 d
9 a
10 d

Critical Thinking Log
Answers will vary

CHAPTER 14

Exercise 14–1
Answers will vary

Exercise 14–2
Answers will vary

Map

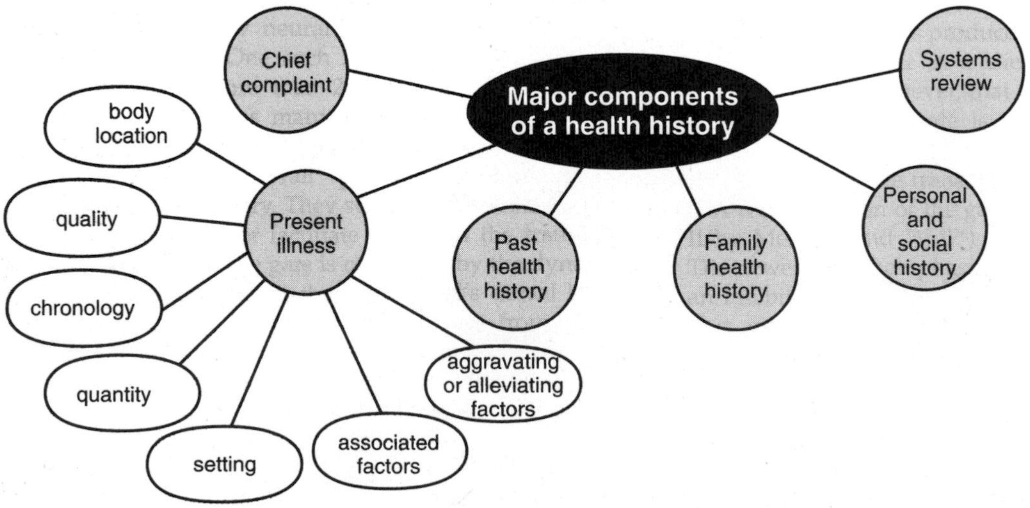

Major components of a health history
Chief complaint
Present illness
body location
quality
chronology
quantity
setting
associated factors
aggravating or alleviating factors
Past health history
Family health history
Personal and social history
Systems review

Exercise 14–3
Sample Answers

Outline
Major Components of a Health History
A. Chief Complaint
B. Present Illness
  1. body location
  2. quality
  3. quantity
  4. chronology
  5. setting
  6. aggravating or alleviating factors
  7. associated factors
C. Past Health History
D. Family Health History
E. Personal and Social History
F. Systems Review

List
Chief Complaint
Present Illness
  body location
  quality
  quantity
  chronology
  setting
  aggravating or alleviating factors
  associated factors
Past Health History
Family Health History
Personal and Social History
Systems Review

Vocabulary Check
1 d
2 a
3 b
4 c
5 c
6 a
7 d
8 c
9 a
10 b

Critical Thinking Log
Answers will vary

CHAPTER 15

Exercise 15–1
1 d
2 c
3 a
4 c
5 d

Exercise 15–2
1 b
2 b
3 b
4 c
5 a

Exercise 15–3
1 d
2 c
3 b
4 a
5 c

Exercise 15–4
1 b
2 b
3 b
4 c
5 a

Exercise 15–5
Part I
1 third
2 the legal system
3 governor
4 state
5 American Nurses Association
Part II
1 e
2 d
3 a
4 c
5 b
Part III
1 b
2 d
3 c
4 b
5 c
6 a
7 d
8 b
9 a
10 a
Part IV
1 F
2 T
3 T
4 F
5 T

Exercise 15–6
Answers will vary

Exercise 15–7
Answers will vary

Exercise 15–8
Answers will vary

Vocabulary Check
1 d
2 d
3 a
4 d
5 c
6 b
7 b
8 b
9 b
10 a

Critical Thinking Log
Answers will vary

READING SELECTION 1

Preview Question
Answers will vary

Vocabulary
Answers will vary

Summary
Answers will vary

Comprehension Questions
1 c
2 a
3 d
4 b
5 d
6 a
7 c
8 a
9 d
10 b

Critical Thinking/Evaluation
Answers will vary

READING SELECTION 2

Preview Question
Answers will vary

Vocabulary
Answers will vary

Summary
Answers will vary

Comprehension Questions
1 d
2 a
3 b
4 d
5 c
6 b
7 d
8 d
9 a
10 d

Critical Thinking/Evaluation
Answers will vary

READING SELECTION 3

Preview Question
Stage 1—vascular stage
Stage 2—cellular exudate stage
Stage 3—tissue repair and replacement stage

Vocabulary
Answers will vary

Summary
Answers will vary

Comprehension Questions
1 a
2 b
3 d
4 d
5 a
6 d
7 c
8 a
9 b
10 a

READING SELECTION 4

Preview Question
Head and neck
Vertebral spine
Upper and lower extremities

Vocabulary
Answers will vary

Summary
Answers will vary

Comprehension Questions
1 b
2 d
3 b

4 b
5 a
6 c
7 d
8 b
9 a
10 d

Critical Thinking/Evaluation
Answers will vary

READING SELECTION 5

Preview Question
The head

Vocabulary
Answers will vary

Summary
Answers will vary

Comprehension Questions
1 b
2 c
3 d
4 a
5 d
6 c
7 a
8 d
9 b
10 c

READING SELECTION 6

Preview Question
Answers will vary

Vocabulary
Answers will vary

Summary
Answers will vary

Comprehension Questions
1 a
2 b
3 d
4 c
5 b
6 b
7 d
8 c
9 d
10 a

Critical Thinking/Evaluation
Answers will vary

READING SELECTION 7

Preview Question
(a) Anatomy and physiology of the external, middle, and inner ear
(b) Answers will vary

Vocabulary
Answers will vary

Summary
Answers will vary

Comprehension Questions
1 a
2 d
3 b
4 c
5 a
6 d
7 b
8 c
9 a
10 d

READING SELECTION 8

Preview Question
How the blood flows through the heart

Vocabulary
Answers will vary

Summary
Answers will vary

Comprehension Questions
1 c
2 d
3 a
4 b
5 a
6 d
7 b
8 b
9 a
10 c

READING SELECTION 9

Preview Question
The scalp, skull or brain

Vocabulary
Answers will vary

Summary
Answers will vary

Comprehension Questions
1 b
2 c
3 c
4 d
5 a
6 d
7 b
8 c
9 c
10 d

Critical Thinking/Evaluation
Answers will vary

READING SELECTION 10

Preview Question
(a) No
(b) They are pathologic.

Vocabulary
Answers will vary

Summary
Answers will vary

Comprehension Questions
1 b
2 b
3 a
4 c
5 d
6 a
7 b
8 a
9 c
10 b

Critical Thinking/Evaluation
Answers will vary

READING SELECTION 11

Preview Question
It allows the surgeon to directly visualize the heart during the operation.

Vocabulary
Answers will vary

Summary
Answers will vary

Comprehension Questions
1 d
2 b
3 c
4 b
5 a
6 d
7 b
8 a
9 d
10 a

Critical Thinking/Evaluation
Answers will vary

READING SELECTION 12

Preview Question
Elderly women with osteoporosis

Vocabulary
Answers will vary

Summary
Answers will vary

Comprehension Questions

1 b
2 c
3 d
4 b
5 c
6 b
7 d
8 a
9 c
10 b

Critical Thinking/Evaluation
Answers will vary

READING SELECTION 13

Preview Question
Respiratory depression
Circulating depression
Nausea and vomiting
Paresthesia
Physical dependence
Tolerance

Vocabulary
Answers will vary

Summary
Answers will vary

Comprehension Questions

1 b
2 a
3 c
4 a
5 c
6 b
7 a
8 d
9 a
10 c

Critical Thinking/Evaluation
Answers will vary

READING SELECTION 14

Preview Question
It explains many aspects of pain and how pain may be controlled by thoughts, emotion and action.

Vocabulary
Answers will vary

Summary
Answers will vary

Comprehension Questions

1 d
2 a
3 b
4 c
5 a
6 b
7 d
8 d
9 b
10 c

Critical Thinking/Evaluation
Answers will vary

READING SELECTION 15

Preview Question
Two examples of what happens when intracranial volume is increased by coughing, vomiting, suctioning, straining, etc.

Vocabulary
Answers will vary

Summary
Answers will vary

Comprehension Questions

1 d
2 b
3 c
4 a
5 d
6 b
7 c
8 d
9 a
10 c

Critical Thinking/Evaluation
Answers will vary

Index

Note: Page numbers in *italics* refer to illustrations; page numbers followed by t refer to tables.